Sexuality and Illness

This evidence-based guide educates and informs health professionals about promoting sexual well-being in the context of challenges from physical and mental health.

Sexuality is an important aspect of quality of life for many people but can be affected by a wide variety of health conditions, such as cardiovascular disease, mental illness, menopause, diseases of aging, neurological diseases and spinal cord injuries, combat injuries, and cancer. Building readers' confidence in initiating and encouraging open communication on this often-neglected topic, *Sexuality and Illness* includes case studies that illustrate how to talk about sexuality and support patients with concerns about it. Making recommendations for practice and further reading, it takes into account gender, sexual, race, and ethnic diversity.

This accessible text demystifies a topic that is sometimes difficult to discuss. It is essential reading for healthcare practitioners interested in providing comprehensive and person-centered care.

Anne Katz practices as a sexuality counsellor in Winnipeg, Manitoba, Canada. She is the author of 13 books on sexuality in cancer and cancer survivorship. She is internationally known as an engaging speaker and educator and the host of "Sexually Speaking with Dr. Anne Katz" podcast.

Sexuality and Illness

A Guidebook for Health Professionals

Anne Katz

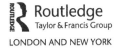

Routledge
Taylor & Francis Group

LONDON AND NEW YORK

First published 2022
by Routledge
2 Park Square, Milton Park, Abingdon, Oxon OX14 4RN

and by Routledge
605 Third Avenue, New York, NY 10158

Routledge is an imprint of the Taylor & Francis Group, an informa business

British Library Cataloguing-in-Publication Data
A catalogue record for this book is available from the British Library

Library of Congress Cataloging-in-Publication Data
A catalog record has been requested for this book

ISBN: 978-0-367-70336-3 (hbk)
ISBN: 978-0-367-70335-6 (pbk)
ISBN: 978-1-003-14574-5 (ebk)

DOI: 10.4324/9781003145745

Typeset in Times New Roman
by Deanta Global Publishing Services, Chennai, India

For my best man

Contents

Boxes

1   Introduction

Sexuality is defined by the World Health Organization as that "experienced and expressed in thoughts, fantasies, desires, beliefs, attitudes, values, behaviors, practices, roles and relationships." On the other hand, sexual health is

> a state of physical, mental and social well-being in relation to sexuality. It requires a positive and respectful approach to sexuality and sexual relationships, as well as the possibility of having pleasurable and safe sexual experiences, free of coercion, discrimination and violence
>
> (WHO, 2006) (https://www.who.int/teams/sexual-and-rep roductive-health-and-research/key-areas-of-work/sexual-healt h/defining-sexual-health).

We are all sexual beings, from infancy to death; but how that is expressed differs by age, gender, relationship status, social norms, and health status. The latter is the context for this book. It is well established that illness impacts on physical and emotional sexual function in multiple ways. Despite the evolving research in this area, this generally remains a neglected topic in health care.

Sexual health is a very important aspect of quality of life in healthy adults as well as those experiencing health problems (Flynn et al., 2016). Sexual dysfunction in both men and women carries with it burdens that are poorly researched, articulated, and largely ignored (Balon, 2017). These include interpersonal conflict and distress, quality of life, emotional functioning, and financial costs. In men, sexual dysfunction is associated with both psychological and physical health (Tan, Tong, & Ho, 2012). In turn, physical and mental illnesses are risk factors for sexual dysfunction (McCabe et al., 2016). This bi-directional relationship should spur health care providers to consider sexual dysfunction in their clinical assessment of individuals presenting for care (Brotto et al., 2016).

Why should you read this book?

If sexuality is an important part of quality of life and if it is both a factor contributing to and a negative response to disease, as well as acute and chronic ill health, then should health care providers of all types consider this when treating patients? I hope that your response would be a resounding 'yes'!

This book is divided into three sections. The first section provides an overview of human sexuality, from the past to our present understanding of how sex 'works.' Four models of the human sexual response cycle are presented with an additional two models that conceptualize

DOI: 10.4324/9781003145745-1

sexual dysfunction. Chapter 3 addresses communication about sexuality and sexual functioning by health care providers. Five models are presented to facilitate the conversation with patients/clients as well as providing guidance on how to take a sexual history. Chapter 4 discusses sexual development from a lifespan perspective, from adolescence to old age, including sexual aging.

The second section provides the latest evidence on the role that many different diseases/conditions impact on sexuality. These include medical and mental conditions as well as the impact of trauma and disability. Cancer treatment in both men and women is known to have a significant impact on sexuality and sexual function and this is described in two separate chapters. Chapter 11 discusses cancer in adolescence and young adulthood, a time when sexual identity and relationships are established and where developmental milestones are impacted during treatment. The section ends with a chapter on infertility and the sexual challenges of treatments to enable conception.

The third section of the book focuses on interventions for sexual dysfunction for men and women in two separate chapters. This is important as many health care providers have limited knowledge of what can be done when a patient/client discloses that they are having sexual problems.

All chapters include resources that can be suggested to patients/clients but that also serve to further increase knowledge and confidence for the health care provider.

References

Balon, R. (2017). Burden of sexual dysfunction. *Journal of Sex and Marital Therapy, 43*(1), 49–55. doi: 10.1080/0092623x.2015.1113597

Brotto, L., Atallah, S., Johnson-Agbakwu, C., Rosenbaum, T., Abdo, C., Byers, E.S., … Wylie, K. (2016). Psychological and interpersonal dimensions of sexual function and dysfunction. *Journal of Sexual Medicine, 13*(4), 538–571. doi: 10.1016/j.jsxm.2016.01.019

Flynn, K.E., Lin, L., Bruner, D.W., Cyranowski, J.M., Hahn, E.A., Jeffery, D.D., … Weinfurt, K.P. (2016). Sexual satisfaction and the importance of sexual health to quality of life throughout the life course of U.S. adults. *Journal of Sexual Medicine, 13*(11), 1642–1650. doi: 10.1016/j.jsxm.2016.08.011

McCabe, M.P., Sharlip, I.D., Lewis, R., Atalla, E., Balon, R., Fisher, A.D., … Segraves, R.T. (2016). Risk factors for sexual dysfunction among women and men: A consensus statement from the fourth international consultation on sexual medicine 2015. *Journal of Sexual Medicine, 13*(2), 153–167. doi: 10.1016/j.jsxm.2015.12.015

Tan, H.M., Tong, S.F., & Ho, C.C.K. (2012). Men's health: Sexual dysfunction, physical, and psychological health: Is there a link? *Journal of Sexual Medicine, 9*(3), 663–671. doi: 10.1111/j.1743-6109.2011.02582.x

2 Our understanding of human sexuality in the 21st century

This chapter will explore how we view sexuality and sexual functioning. From the work of Masters and Johnson in the 1960s to the present day conceptualization of sexuality, our thinking about sexuality has changed from a linear, male-oriented perspective to a more bio-psycho-social approach from researchers such as Dr Rosemary Basson. Four models of the human sexual response cycle are presented with an additional two models that conceptualize sexual dysfunction. All of these models present insight into the 'how' of the human sexual response. As with all conceptual models, they have limitations and should be seen as resources to support our understanding rather than being the definitive explanation of any particular circumstance. A 'one size fits all' approach should be used with caution.

The past: Masters and Johnson and Kaplan

For centuries, sexuality and sex remained unexplained, mysterious, and often misunderstood. At times it was celebrated and accepted as part of life while for many years, sexuality was condemned, vilified, controlled by religion, and by the norms and values of society. In the middle of the 20th century, Alfred Kinsey, a focus of some notoriety, was perhaps the first sex researcher; he conducted qualitative interviews with students in one of his courses in which they provided him with detailed sexual histories. From these interviews he published, along with colleagues, the landmark book, *Sexual Behavior in the Human Male* in 1948 and a second book, *Sexual Behavior in the Human Female* in 1953 (Brown & Fee, 2003). Both books were academic; however, they garnered a great deal of public interest, not to mention criticism from religious leaders. The backlash against the second book in particular is believed to have led to his early death from stress contributing to cardiac disease and ultimately, pneumonia.

A few years later, a scientific approach to understanding sexual functioning, albeit from a strictly heterosexual perspective, was initiated by William Masters and Virginia Johnson. An entertaining if not completely accurate depiction of their work was presented on the Showtime series, *Masters of Sex*. This TV series gave audiences a glimpse of their research from which much of our understanding of sexual functioning persisted until the early years of the 21st century. Masters and Johnson described a four-phase model of the human sexual response. The first phase, excitement refers to vascular engorgement of the genitals and breasts. The second phase, plateau, is described as advanced arousal in which further engorgement occurs as well as raised heart rate and respiration. The third phase is that of orgasm with intense contractions of the pelvic floor muscles and whole-body pleasurable sensations. Finally, in the fourth phase, resolution occurs, and blood leaves the genitals and the body returns to its pre-arousal state. This model was assumed to be the same for both

DOI: 10.4324/9781003145745-2

men and women and the phases were presented as linear. This model has been accepted for decades, and is still found in text books, and the four phases used as the basis for clinical enquiry into sexual problems, even though it leaves out an important aspect of sexuality, the mental processes that are involved in wanting sex as well as experiencing sexual satisfaction.

A student of theirs, Helen Singer Kaplan, added an important component to her model of the human sexual response, that of desire (Kaplan, 1979). Her three-part model encompassed desire, excitement, and orgasm. While inclusion of desire was a significant contribution to our understanding of the human sexual response, her model was generally understood to be linear. While she never intended it to be interpreted that way, instead suggesting that any of the three phases could occur independently of the others. This has led to the common (mis) understanding that desire is a precursor to arousal; newer models suggest otherwise as presented in the next section.

Zilbergeld and Ellison (1980) proposed a five-and-a-half-part model with distinct stages – interest, arousal, physiologic readiness (erection in men and vaginal lubrication in women), orgasm, and satisfaction. The phase of orgasm was divided into two – physiological (muscle contractions) and subjective (pleasurable sensations) – hence the 'five-and-a-half part.'

A bio-psycho-social approach in the 21st century

A more comprehensive approach that includes not only physical or emotional experience but also contextual factors is the circular model described by Basson (2015). This model focuses on the experience of desire or libido as part of the female sexual response cycle and suggests that women do not follow the linear experience of spontaneous desire as the norm but rather that reactive desire occurs in an overlapping fashion with arousal. The key to understanding this model is that rather than experiencing spontaneous desire, it is often only felt when the woman is physically and/or psychologically aroused. Further, Basson suggests that women have multiple reasons to engage sexually that are psychosocial in nature and include factors such as avoiding conflict with a partner, wanting emotional intimacy with the partner, and/or as an expression of love. According to the model, if the result of sexual activity is perceived as rewarding to the woman, this increases her motivation for another encounter, whether she experiences an orgasm or not (Chivers, 2017).

Given that both the Masters and Johnson and Kaplan's models are seen as more reflective of male sexual functioning, can Basson's circular model of responsive desire be applied to men? Connaughton and colleagues (Connaughton, McCabe, & Karantzas, 2016) found that men with sexual problems were more likely to endorse responsive rather than spontaneous desire and they tended to focus on relational and contextual factors. This may be indicative of their need to find non-sexual motivation to engage in sexual activity. Similar findings were described by other researchers (Giraldi, Kristensen, & Sand, 2015) who report that men endorse the Masters and Johnson or Kaplan model when they are not experiencing sexual difficulties but when they have erectile dysfunction or are not satisfied with their sex life, they then endorse the Basson circular model. Other researchers have found that there is a great deal of variability in the male sexual response with adherence to one particular model not supported (Busby, Leonhardt, Leavitt, & Hanna-Walker, 2019). Also contradicting the common perception that men are like machines, always ready for sex with unlimited libido, is the more recent understanding that for men, cognitive and emotional factors are important drivers of libido (Nimbi, Tripodi, Rossi, & Simonelli, 2018).

Models of sexual dysfunction

There are also models that depict the concept of sexual dysfunction, predominately in the area of oncology. Bober and Varela (2012) presented an integrative bio-psycho-social model that includes biological factors such as neurologic side effects of treatment, physical changes such as scars or amputations, and hormonal changes. Psychological impacts include emotional and cognitive changes as a result of the diagnosis of a potentially life-threatening disease as well as the experience of anxiety and depression, changes in relationships as well as self- and sexual image alteration. The model also includes socio-cultural issues such as religious beliefs and social norms related to sexuality. These factors are important to address when responding to a complaint of altered sexual functioning in the clinical setting.

Katz and Dizon (2016) describe a bio-psycho-social model for men with cancer that moves away from the mainly biomedical understanding to include the impact of treatment and physical changes on a man's sexuality. Societal norms are acknowledged to influence how he sees his sexual performance and the sentinel role of the partner and communication is highlighted. These factors ultimately influence the satisfaction of the man and his partner and should be addressed when assessing sexual problems in men during and after cancer treatment.

Conclusion

Models are important to our understanding of how things work, and this includes the complex nature of the human sexual response. While credit must be given to those who first described the physiological details of sexual functioning, our current understanding incudes a more comprehensive description that goes beyond sexual organs. Models of sexual dysfunction can also help to explain factors that are important to understand from a clinical perspective and going beyond the purely biomedical is important because people live not just in their bodies but also as part of relationships and the larger society.

References

Basson, R. (2015). Human sexual response. *Handbook of Clinical Neurology*, *130*, 11–18. doi: 10.1016/b978-0-444-63247-0.00002-x

Bober, S.L., & Varela, V.S. (2012). Sexuality in adult cancer survivors: Challenges and intervention. *Journal of Clinical Oncology*, *30*(30), 3712–3719. doi: 10.1200/jco.2012.41.7915

Brown, T.M., & Fee, E. (2003). Alfred C. Kinsey: A pioneer of sex research. *American Journal of Public Health*, *93*(6), 896–897. doi: 10.2105/ajph.93.6.896

Busby, D.M., Leonhardt, N.D., Leavitt, C.E., & Hanna-Walker, V. (2019). Challenging the standard model of sexual response: Evidence of a variable male sexual response cycle. *Journal of Sex Research*, *57*, 1–12. doi: 10.1080/00224499.2019.1705960

Chivers, M.B.L. (2017). Controversies of women's sexual arousal and desire. *European Psycholgist*, *22*(1), 5–26. doi: 10.1027/1016-9040/a000274

Connaughton, C., McCabe, M., & Karantzas, G. (2016). Conceptualization of the sexual response models in men: Are there differences between sexually functional and dysfunctional men? *Journal of Sexual Medicine*, *13*(3), 453–463. doi: 10.1016/j.jsxm.2015.12.032

Giraldi, A., Kristensen, E., & Sand, M. (2015). Endorsement of models describing sexual response of men and women with a sexual partner: An online survey in a population sample of Danish adults ages 20–65 years. *Journal of Sexual Medicine*, *12*(1), 116–128. doi: 10.1111/jsm.12720

Kaplan, H.S. (1979). *Disorders of sexual desire*. New York: Simon & Schuster.

Katz, A., & Dizon, D.S. (2016). Sexuality after cancer: A model for male survivors. *Journal of Sexual Medicine*, *13*(1), 70–78. doi: 10.1016/j.jsxm.2015.11.006

Nimbi, F.M., Tripodi, F., Rossi, R., & Simonelli, C. (2018). Expanding the analysis of psychosocial factors of sexual desire in men. *Journal of Sexual Medicine*, *15*(2), 230–244. doi: 10.1016/j.jsxm.2017.11.227

Zilbergeld, B., & Ellison, C. (1980). Desire discrepancies and arousal problems in sex therapy. In S. Leiblum & L. Pervin (Eds.), *Principles and practice of sex therapy* (pp. 65–101). New York: Guilford Press.

3 Communicating about sexuality with patients

Two of the most common reasons that health care providers report for avoiding a discussion about sexual side effects of illness and the treatment thereof are embarrassment and not wanting to be seen as invading a patient's privacy. This chapter will provide the reader with models that facilitate a discussion about sexuality. The most common models include the PLISSIT model, the Ex-PLISSIT model, the 5 As model, the BETTER model, and the CARD model. This chapter will also provide guidance on how to conduct a sexual history as well as addressing ways in which the clinician can become more comfortable talking to patients about this important aspect of quality of life and a common side effect of many illnesses and their treatments.

How do clinicians communicate with patients?

Communication between health care provider and patient has a direct effect on patient satisfaction (McFarland, Johnson Shen, & Holcombe, 2017). The communication style of the health care provider is a factor; the closer the communication style of the health care provider to that of the patient, the greater the patient's satisfaction is likely to be (Trant et al., 2019). This is important in talking about sexuality, as the biomedical language used by the health care provider may result in dissatisfaction with care, not to mention lack of understanding; health care providers may use biomedical language to hide their embarrassment when talking about sex or sexuality. This contradicts the notion of patient-centered communication. The principles of patient-centered communication include careful listening to the patient, knowing their medical history, explaining things in a way that the patient understands, and providing easy to understand answers to the patient's questions (Platonova, Qu, & Warren-Findlow, 2019). However, a large study using data from a national survey of US adults found that only 42–46% of those surveyed reported that health care providers spent enough time with them, answered their questions, or helped them with feelings of uncertainty related to their health (Spooner, Salemi, Salihu, & Zoorob, 2016). Clinicians often assume that asking about a patient's sexual functioning will take a lot of time, but many patients just want validation that their concerns are real and a referral for help is available.

Talking about sexuality and sexual functioning is a neglected aspect of patient care. Health care providers may experience the same embarrassment talking about this as their patients do; however, there is evidence that women, particularly those under the age of 40, see sexual health as an important part of their well-being and want to talk about this (Fairchild, Haefner, & Berger, 2016). Personal history, religious and cultural backgrounds, and the lack of knowledge about the specifics of sexuality and sexual dysfunction are barriers to open and honest conversations in the clinical setting. When asked, clinicians cite multiple reasons for not

DOI: 10.4324/9781003145745-3

asking about sexuality in patient encounters. These include time constraints, fear of offending the patient, discomfort in talking to a much younger patient or someone of a similar age as their parents or grandparents or to someone of a different gender/sex, lack of training or knowledge, and lack of financial compensation (Althof, Rosen, Perelman, & Rubio-Aurioles, 2013). The perception that there are limited treatments available to treat sexual problems is an additional barrier (Kingsberg, Faught, Pinkerton, Parish, Gudeman, Krop, & Simon, 2019).

Recent studies suggest that discussions about the impact of cancer and other diseases on sexuality are not common. In a systematic review of 29 studies from ten countries, 29% of which were from the United States, 88% of the health care providers said that they had a discussion about the sexual side effects of cancer while only 50% of the patients recalled such a conversation. This was heavily influenced by the sex of the patient; 60% of the men reported that the health care provider had talked about this compared to just 28% of the women. Older age of the health care provider and male sex of the patient were more likely to result in a discussion; the latter is perhaps influenced by the proportion of male patients seen by male urologists. Twenty-one percent of the health care providers said they had assessed sexual functioning in their patients but only 10% of the patients reported this (Reese et al., 2017). Women may also not see their sexual problems as a medical issue and may assume that it is part of aging and not something that can be mitigated (Kingsberg et al., 2019).

In a study of older women in the United States, less than 25% reported a discussion on sexual functioning with a physician; this was more likely to occur if the woman had a chronic disease (Bergeron et al., 2017). Barriers exist in the palliative care setting as well, despite health care providers caring for end of life patients being prepared to talk about other sensitive topics (Leung, Goldfarb, & Dizon, 2016). Adolescents, those in both sexual minority and sexual majority populations, report that physicians need to discuss sexuality more frequently with them and, importantly, need to ask parents to leave the room so that an open discussion can be held (Fuzzell, Fedesco, Alexander, Fortenberry, & Shields, 2016). Another area where communication is less than optimal is in fertility care, where individuals dealing with fertility specialists report gaps (Klitzman, 2018). The impact of different diseases on sexuality will be discussed in the following chapters.

Taking a sexual history

Key to discovering and understanding an individual's or couple's sexual problem(s) is to take a sexual history. This cannot be replaced by a questionnaire and is used as an important addition to any information gained from a screening tool mentioned above. It is important to indicate to the patient that you are going to take a sexual history, and this may be done with an opening statement such as "It is important to know about your sexual and relationship histories. I ask all my patients about this because these are an important part of overall health. Do you have any questions or concerns about this?"

There are a number of principles on which the history should be based. Taking a sexual history should be done in a culturally respectful manner, taking into account the patient's background and lifestyle as well as the context of their relationship status. It is crucial to avoid assumptions sexual orientation, gender identity, sexual activity, or relationship status (Rubin et al., 2018).

The clinician taking the history should be knowledgeable and comfortable with the topic. The history should use a patient-centered approach, with direct questions while at the same time allowing the patient to tell their story, in their own words, and at a pace that is comfortable for them. Reassuring the patient of the confidential nature of the enquiry and using a non-judgmental tone and attitude will allow the patient to open up about something that is private and sensitive (Althof et al., 2013).

A simple way of starting the sexual history is to ask these four questions:

* What concerns do you have about your sexuality or sexual functioning at this time?
* What changes have you noticed over time or since you were last here?
* How satisfied are you with your sexuality or sexual functioning now?
* Has your sexuality or sexual function been affected by your _____ (insert disease) or treatments for this?

The Centers for Disease Control and Prevention (CDC) have created a 5 P Plus guide to the sexual history that addresses the following: partners, practices, past history of sexually transmitted infections (STI), protection from sexually transmitted infections, and pregnancy plans. Detailed instructions for using this model can be found at https://www.cdc.gov/std/t reatment/sexualhistory.pdf. The Plus refers to the addition of questions about a history of trauma or violence, any concerns or problems, and distress or satisfaction related to sexual activity (Rubin et al., 2018).

If the patient reports a concern about any aspects of sexuality, it is necessary to conduct a more specific history that includes body image, relationship functioning, and questions about changes to desire, arousal, orgasm, satisfaction, pain, and any anxiety associated with any of these topics.

There is a paucity of literature on the topic of communication with male patients about sexuality despite the importance of asking about erectile dysfunction that is a warning sign of cardiovascular disease (Zhao et al., 2019). One study showed positive outcomes when patients were asked to complete an investigator-developed questionnaire that was then used as a prompt for further discussion (Hartmann & Burkart, 2007). More than two-thirds of the participants in the study expressed relief that their sexual problem(s) were identified, and they were willing to discuss this.

However, sexual history taking is not ubiquitous in primary care. In one study of adults aged 50–80, physician-initiated discussion took place 50% of the time during the periodic health exam (Ports, Barnack-Tavlaris, Syme, Perera, & Lafata, 2014). Another study found that primary care providers seldom initiated a complete sexual history based on the 5P model described above (Palaiodimos et al., 2020). In 65% of the patient visits, no sexual history was taken; a partial sexual history was taken in 34% of the visits; and all five components of the 5P model were included in just 1% of the visits. Women were more likely to be asked about their sexual history, and older patients were less likely to be asked about this.

Models for assessment of sexual problems

The most common models for assessing sexual problems include the PLISSIT model (Annon, 1974), the Ex-PLISSIT model (Taylor & Davis, 2007), the 5 As model (Bober, Carter, & Falk, 2013), the BETTER model (Mick, Hughes, & Cohen, 2003; Mick, 2007), and the CARD model (Wang, Pierdomenico, Brandt, & Lefkowitz, 2015). These models are simple to use and predicated on engaging the patient in a description of what they are experiencing. These are distinct from sexual health assessment or questionnaires that assess specific aspects of sexual functioning.

PLISSIT

This model is derived from the psychology literature and has been used widely. The model is divided into four phases: permission, limited information, specific suggestion, and intensive therapy. The first phase, permission, refers to giving the patient permission to express their concerns or describe their symptoms. Having a prepared statement that opens the discussion is an example of giving permission. Most patients will be satisfied with a response that is described as limited information. This normalizes and validates the patient's experience and provides a basic level of information to address the patient's concern. The third phase, specific suggestion, is information or a recommendation that is more detailed. Finally, the fourth phase, intensive therapy, refers to care that is outside the expertise of the health care provider. A referral to a specialist such as a sex therapist, gynecologist, endocrinologist, or urologist may be necessary to address the symptoms or experience of the patient. An example of how to use the PLISSIT model is provided in Box 3.1.

Box 3.1 Using the PLISSIT model in the maternity unit

P: Permission

"After having a baby, many women want to know when they can resume sexual activity. What information do you need?"

LI: Limited information

"The usual advice is to avoid sexual intercourse until after your 6-week follow-up, but it might be good to try before that appointment so that you can report any concerns to your OB-GYN."

SS: Specific suggestions

"Breastfeeding tends to lower your estrogen levels, so you may notice some vaginal dryness. Using a lubricant for sex will make things more comfortable for you. I have a list of lubricants that you can buy at any drugstore."

IT: Intensive therapy

"Because you tore during delivery, it is a good idea to see a pelvic floor physiotherapist about 6 weeks from now. I will send a referral and their office will call with an appointment date and time."

Ex-PLISSIT

This model expands on the PLISSIT model by including reflection and review at each of the phases of the PLISSIT model. Reflection provides the practitioner with a way to recognize their own biases, beliefs, and attitudes. Reviewing with the patient on what they have understood allows the practitioner to correct misunderstandings and/or provide additional information to the patient. The model also instructs practitioners to include the permission stage for all the other stages, suggesting that patient consent is needed before providing limited or specific information. Finally, this model allows for referral to a specialist at any time, rather than regarding this as a 'last option.'

5 As

This model is well known to most practitioners as it is widely used for counseling about tobacco cessation. However, the authors suggest a slight modification in the order of the steps. The first A refers to "ask"; much like the PLISSIT model, it refers to an opening statement inviting the patient to disclose their symptom(s) or experience. The second A in this context is 'assess.' This comes third in the original model after 'advice.' There is a risk that in the context of sexuality assessment, providing advice first will ignore a deeper description by the patient. So 'assess' follows 'ask' and this is where the patient can more fully describe what they are experiencing. 'Advise' follows this assessment and allows for providing the patient with specific information that addresses their concern(s). The fourth A, 'assist,' refers to providing resources to the patient, including referral to a specialist. Finally, the last A, 'arrange,' refers to the practitioner arranging follow-up to allow the patient to provide feedback; it is useful to learn about the resolution of the problem(s) and the need for additional help. An example of how to use the 5 As model is provided in Box 3.2.

Box 3.2 Using the 5 As model in the cardiology unit

Ask: "What questions do you have about resuming sexual activity after your heart attack?"

Assess: "Were you taking Viagra or any other medication to help you achieve erections before this?"

Advice: "You should not use Viagra or other similar medications if you are taking nitrates for chest pain."

Assist: "We have a pamphlet that talks about resuming sexual activity safely. I will include it with your other discharge information."

Arrange: "I will make a note to check in with you when you are back here for your appointment with the cardiologist. And here's my contact information if you have questions at any time."

BETTER

This model, developed for use in the oncology setting, is similar to the other models presented. It encourages practitioners to bring up the topic (B) with an introductory statement. This is followed by explaining (E) that sexual functioning is important to quality of life. The nurse can then tell (T) the patient that resources will be found to address their problem(s) and if the timing is not right (second T), they can ask for help at any time. The nurse is encouraged to educate (E) the patient about the sexual side effects of the treatment, and finally, the nurse should record (R) the discussion in the patient's chart. An example of how to use the BETTER model is presented in Box 3.3.

Box 3.3 Using the BETTER model in oncology

B: Bring up the topic
"Women treated for breast cancer often have questions about sex during and after treatment. What questions do you have?"

E: Explain that sexuality is important for quality of life
"While you may not feel like it now, you will want to have sex again one day! And it's important for your relationship and general well-being."

T: Tell the patient that resources will be found to answer her questions
"We have some pamphlets that have useful advice for you, but I can also try and answer any questions you may have at this time."

T: While the timing may not be right, there is always help available if she needs it
"You've received a lot of information today and you may be feeling overwhelmed. If you don't have any questions now, you can call me or any of the other nurses at any time and we will try to help."

E: Educate about the sexual side effects of treatment
"Women with breast cancer often experience challenges with their body image, even after reconstruction of their breast. We have a sexuality counselor on staff who works with women to address this concern."

R: Record the discussion in the patient's chart
"Patient informed about changes to sexuality and offered help from the sexuality counselor when needed."

CARD

This model is similar to the others described and has four distinct phases. The first phase (C) is an opening statement such as, "Cancer treatment can affect your sexual health, which is important to many women and couple's quality of life." The next phase is to ask (A) if the patient has any concerns or questions; specific symptoms can be mentioned to the patient to prompt a response. The patient is then asked if they would be interested in further resources or a referral (R) and finally the discussion is documented (D) in the patient's chart.

Measuring alterations in sexual functioning

Some practitioners may be interested in using an instrument to measure sexual functioning in the clinical setting. There are many measures available but some of them are dated and do not address sexual minorities, single people, or other sociodemographic variables. Measures designed for research are often long and patients may balk at completing a questionnaire with 50–100 items. In addition, some questionnaires have not been validated and have been used in a single study only and their utility in clinical practice is not established. Hatzichristou and colleagues (Hatzichristou et al., 2016) have published a detailed list of measures that is useful. They comment that questionnaires should be used as an adjunct to taking a good sexual history and not in place of a face-to-face discussion with the patient.

These are the most common sexuality questionnaires:

1. The International Index of Erectile Function (IIEF)

   The IIEF is a 15-item patient-reported questionnaire (IIEF-15) that has a shortened version, the IIEF-5, previously known as the Sexual Health Inventory for Men (SHIM). Both of these measures have been used widely in both research and clinical practice despite concerns about validity and reliability (Neijenhuijs, Holtmaat, et al., 2019). A major concern is that the cut-off scores for both are not clearly established but it is recommended that 25 for the IIEF-15 and 21 for the IIEF-5 be used clinically to diagnose erectile dysfunction. A significant criticism of these measures is that they do not include any measure of distress or desire, two domains that are regarded as important in the experience of sexual dysfunction (Bravi et al., 2020). The measures are also not useful for men who are not currently sexually active (Forbes, Baillie, & Schniering, 2014).

2. The Female Sexual Function Index (FSFI)

   This self-report measure is available in both long (19 item; FSFI-19) and short form (6 item; FSFI-6). Developed more than 20 years ago (Rosen et al., 2000), the long form assesses sexual functioning over 6 domains (desire, arousal, lubrication, orgasm, satisfaction, and pain) but lacks the inclusion of a measure of distress and is not useful for women who are not sexually active (Meston, Freihart, Handy, Kilimnik, & Rosen, 2020). Despite these limitations, both measures are regarded as adequate screening tools (Neijenhuijs, Hooghiemstra, et al., 2019).

3. Measures of Distress

   There are a number of questionnaires that assess sexual distress (Santos-Iglesias, Mohamed, & Walker, 2018). Questionnaires specific to women include the Female Sexual Distress Scale (FSDS) with 12 items and a revised version, the FSDS-R, with 13 items. One measure for men only is the Sexual Distress Scale (SDS) that also has been revised (SDS-R); these measures have 12 and 13 items respectively. The Multidimensional Sexuality Questionnaire (MSQ) can be used for both men and women. There are other scales that can be used to measure distress in specific populations experiencing sexual problems such as men or women with cancer as well as others that include a sub-scale for distress.

4. Patient-reported Outcomes Measurement Information System (PROMIS)

   Twenty-four PROMIS measures are available that measure multiple aspects of sexual functioning and satisfaction including desire, arousal, orgasm, and bother (akin to distress) in the general population as well as for those experiencing chronic illnesses such as cancer. Measures are available in both long and short form and in multiple languages. They are available for download without cost and have been shown to be psychometrically sound. The website HealthMeasures (https://www.healthmeasures.net/index.php) also provides scoring and interpretation of the measures, and clinicians and researchers can use selective domains within the various PROMIS measures to customize for specific sexual populations and/or symptoms (Weinfurt et al., 2015).

Conclusion

This chapter has provided information on the importance of communication about sexuality with patients as well as how to take a sexual history. For those clinicians who want to use a more structured approach, a variety of models and measures have been presented to guide discussions and/or collect data. No one approach is better than the other, and in practice, formal measures are not used often as they may not capture the nuances of facial expression and body language present in face-to-face discussions where questions can be asked and answered.

References

Althof, S.E., Rosen, R.C., Perelman, M.A., & Rubio-Aurioles, E. (2013). Standard operating procedures for taking a sexual history. *Journal of Sexual Medicine, 10*(1), 26–35. doi: 10.1111/j.1743-6109.2012.02823.x

Annon, J. (1974). *The behavioral treatment of sexual problems*. Honolulu, HI: Enabling Systems.

Bergeron, C.D., Goltz, H.H., Szucs, L.E., Reyes, J.V., Wilson, K.L., Ory, M.G., & Smith, M.L. (2017). Exploring sexual behaviors and health communication among older women. *Health Care for Women International, 38*(12), 1356–1372. doi: 10.1080/07399332.2017.1329308

Bober, S., Carter, J., & Falk, S. (2013). Addressing female sexual function after cancer by internists and primary care providers. *Journal of Sexual Medicine, 10*(Suppl. 1), 112–119. doi: 10.1111/jsm.12027

Bravi, C.A., Tin, A., Montorsi, F., Mulhall, J.P., Eastham, J.A., & Vickers, A.J. (2020). Erectile function and sexual satisfaction: The importance of asking about sexual desire. *Journal of Sexual Medicine, 17*(2), 349–352. doi: 10.1016/j.jsxm.2019.09.024

Fairchild, P.S., Haefner, J.K., & Berger, M.B. (2016). Talk about sex: Sexual history-taking preferences among urogynecology patients and general gynecology controls. *Female Pelvic Medicine and Reconstructive Surgery, 22*(5), 297–302. doi: 10.1097/spv.0000000000000291

Forbes, M., Baillie, A., & Schniering, C. (2014). Critical flaws in the female sexual function index and the international index of erectile function. *Journal of Sex Research, 51*(5), 485–491. doi: 10.1080/00224499.2013.876607

Fuzzell, L., Fedesco, H.N., Alexander, S.C., Fortenberry, J.D., & Shields, C.G. (2016). "I just think that doctors need to ask more questions": Sexual minority and majority adolescents' experiences talking about sexuality with healthcare providers. *Patient Education and Counseling, 99*(9), 1467–1472. doi: 10.1016/j.pec.2016.06.004

Hartmann, U., & Burkart, M. (2007). Erectile dysfunctions in patient–physician communication: Optimized strategies for addressing sexual issues and the benefit of using a patient questionnaire. *Journal of Sexual Medicine, 4*(1), 38–46. doi: 10.1111/j.1743-6109.2006.00385.x

Hatzichristou, D., Kirana, P.S., Banner, L., Althof, S.E., Lonnee-Hoffmann, R.A., Dennerstein, L., & Rosen, R.C. (2016). Diagnosing sexual dysfunction in men and women: Sexual history taking and the role of symptom scales and questionnaires. *Journal of Sexual Medicine, 13*(8), 1166–1182. doi: 10.1016/j.jsxm.2016.05.017

Kingsberg, S.A., Schaffir, J., Faught, B.M., Pinkerton, J.V., Parish, S.J., Iglesia, C.B., … Simon, J.A. (2019). Female sexual health: Barriers to optimal outcomes and a roadmap for improved patient-clinician communications. *Journal of Women's Health (Larchmt), 28*(4), 432–443. doi: 10.1089/jwh.2018.7352

Kingsberg, S.S., Faught, J., Pinkerton, B., Parish, J., Gudeman, S., & Krop, J. (2019). Female sexual health: Barriers to optimal outcomes and a roadmap for improved patient–clinician communications. *Journal of Women's Health, 28*(4), 432–443. doi: 10.1089/jwh.2018.7352

Klitzman, R. (2018). Impediments to communication and relationships between infertility care providers and patients. *BMC Women's Health, 18*(1), 84. doi: 10.1186/s12905-018-0572-6

Leung, M.W., Goldfarb, S., & Dizon, D.S. (2016). Communication about sexuality in advanced illness aligns with a palliative care approach to patient-centered care. *Current Oncology Reports, 18*(2), 11. doi: 10.1007/s11912-015-0497-2

McFarland, D.C., Johnson Shen, M., & Holcombe, R.F. (2017). Predictors of satisfaction with doctor and nurse communication: A national study. *Health Communication, 32*(10), 1217–1224. doi: 10.1080/10410236.2016.1215001

Meston, C.M., Freihart, B.K., Handy, A.B., Kilimnik, C.D., & Rosen, R.C. (2020). Scoring and interpretation of the FSFI: What can be learned from 20 years of use? *Journal of Sexual Medicine, 17*(1), 17–25. doi: 10.1016/j.jsxm.2019.10.007

Mick, J.M. (2007). Sexuality assessment: 10 strategies for improvement. *Clinical Journal of Oncology Nursing*, *11*(5), 671–675. doi: 10.1188/07.cjon.671-675

Mick, J., Hughes, M., & Cohen, M. (2003). Sexuality and cancer: How oncology nurses can address it better. *Oncology Nursing Forum*, *30*, 152–153.

Neijenhuijs, K.I., Holtmaat, K., Aaronson, N.K., Holzner, B., Terwee, C.B., Cuijpers, P., & Verdonck-de Leeuw, I.M. (2019). The international index of erectile function (IIEF)–A systematic review of measurement properties. *Journal of Sexual Medicine*, *16*(7), 1078–1091. doi: 10.1016/j.jsxm.2019.04.010

Neijenhuijs, K.I., Hooghiemstra, N., Holtmaat, K., Aaronson, N.K., Groenvold, M., Holzner, B., … Verdonck-de Leeuw, I.M. (2019). The female sexual function index (FSFI)–A systematic review of measurement properties. *Journal of Sexual Medicine*, *16*(5), 640–660. doi: 10.1016/j.jsxm.2019.03.001

Palaiodimos, L., Herman, H.S., Wood, E., Karamanis, D., Martinez-Rodriguez, C., Sanchez-Lopez, A., … Leider, J. (2020). Practices and barriers in sexual history taking: A cross-sectional study in a public adult primary care clinic. *Journal of Sexual Medicine*, *17*(8), 1509–1519. doi: 10.1016/j.jsxm.2020.05.004

Platonova, E.A., Qu, H., & Warren-Findlow, J. (2019). Patient-centered communication: Dissecting provider communication. *International Journal of Health Care Quality Assurance*, *32*(2), 534–546. doi: 10.1108/ijhcqa-02-2018-0027

Ports, K.A., Barnack-Tavlaris, J.L., Syme, M.L., Perera, R.A., & Lafata, J.E. (2014). Sexual health discussions with older adult patients during periodic health exams. *Journal of Sexual Medicine*, *11*(4), 901–908. doi: 10.1111/jsm.12448

Reese, J.B., Sorice, K., Beach, M.C., Porter, L.S., Tulsky, J.A., Daly, M.B., & Lepore, S.J. (2017). Patient-provider communication about sexual concerns in cancer: A systematic review. *Journal of Cancer Survivorship*, *11*(2), 175–188. doi: 10.1007/s11764-016-0577-9

Rosen, R., Brown, C., Heiman, J., Leiblum, S., Meston, C., Shabsigh, R., … D'Agostino, R. (2000). The female sexual function index (FSFI): A multidimensional self-report instrument for the assessment of female sexual function. *Journal of Sex and Marital Therapy*, *26*(2), 191–208. doi: 10.1080/009262300278597

Rubin, E.S., Rullo, J., Tsai, P., Criniti, S., Elders, J., Thielen, J.M., & Parish, S.J. (2018). Best practices in North American pre-clinical medical education in sexual history taking: Consensus from the summits in medical education in sexual health. *Journal of Sexual Medicine*, *15*(10), 1414–1425. doi: 10.1016/j.jsxm.2018.08.008

Santos-Iglesias, P., Mohamed, B., & Walker, L.M. (2018). A systematic review of sexual distress measures. *Journal of Sexual Medicine*, *15*(5), 625–644. doi: 10.1016/j.jsxm.2018.02.020

Spooner, K.K., Salemi, J.L., Salihu, H.M., & Zoorob, R.J. (2016). Disparities in perceived patient-provider communication quality in the United States: Trends and correlates. *Patient Education and Counseling*, *99*(5), 844–854. doi: 10.1016/j.pec.2015.12.007

Taylor, B., & Davis, S. (2007). The extended PLISSIT model for addressing the sexual wellbeing of individuals with an acquired disability or chronic illness. *Sexuality and Disability*, *25*(3), 135–139. doi: 10.1007/s11195-007-9044-x

Trant, A.A., Szekely, B., Mougalian, S.S., DiGiovanna, M.P., Sanft, T., Hofstatter, E., … Pusztai, L. (2019). The impact of communication style on patient satisfaction. *Breast Cancer Research and Treatment*, *176*(2), 349–356. doi: 10.1007/s10549-019-05232-w

Wang, L.Y., Pierdomenico, A., Brandt, R., & Lefkowitz, A. (2015). Female sexual health training for oncology providers: New applications. *Sexual Medicine*, *3*(3), 189–197. doi: 10.1002/sm2.66

Weinfurt, K.P., Lin, L., Bruner, D.W., Cyranowski, J.M., Dombeck, C.B., Hahn, E.A., … Flynn, K.E. (2015). Development and initial validation of the PROMIS® sexual function and satisfaction measures version 2.0. *Journal of Sexual Medicine*, *12*(9), 1961–1974. doi: 10.1111/jsm.12966

Zhao, B., Hong, Z., Wei, Y., Yu, D., Xu, J., & Zhang, W. (2019). Erectile dysfunction predicts cardiovascular events as an independent risk factor: A systematic review and meta-analysis. *Journal of Sexual Medicine*, *16*(7), 1005–1017. doi: 10.1016/j.jsxm.2019.04.004

4 Sexuality across the lifespan from adolescence to old age

This chapter presents an overview of sexual development and behaviors across the lifespan. Numerous models that have been developed to explain sexual development are presented because there is no single widely accepted definitive model or description. Misconceptions about sexuality from adolescence to old age abound; these include assumptions about promiscuity in younger individuals and asexuality in older adults. We are sexual beings from infancy until death and each stage of life presents key developmental tasks that should be met for general health and well-being. Biology and society affect our sexual development and how we understand who we are as sexual beings. Societal influences are highly relevant and 'teach' individuals what is acceptable in terms of sexual behavior, sexual roles, and sexual relationships.

Theories of sexual development

One of the first models of sexual identity is that of Freud's five-stage theory that begins with a focus on oral sensations (the infant breastfeeding, putting objects into the mouth) and developing over time to a focus on phallic pleasure (Brandon-Friedman, 2019). Many of Freud's ideas have been criticized including the notion of female orgasm being immature (clitoral) as opposed to mature orgasm (vaginal). Erickson's eight-stage model has greater relevance. The fifth and sixth stages reflect sexual development in adolescence and young adulthood. Identity versus role confusion, the fifth stage, describes the developmental tasks of adolescence when identity separate from family is supposed to occur; this stage encompasses self-discovery, social bonds with peers, and sexual experimentation. The sixth stage, intimacy versus isolation, occurs in young adulthood when lasting relationships are formed and sexuality becomes integrated into these relationships (Brandon-Friedman, 2019). Sexual development in sexual minority individuals was described by Cass (1979) based largely on white males. The six stages of this model include identity confusion, identity comparison, identity tolerance, identity acceptance, identity pride, and identity synthesis. This model has been criticized as being applicable only to men, being linear, and not addressing racial and ethnic factors that influence sexual identity in addition to changes in society since the model was first published. Sexual fluidity also is not considered (Kenneady & Oswalt, 2014).

Cacciatore and colleagues (2019) propose an 11-part model of sexuality beginning in infancy.

1. Infants discover their own bodies and toddlers are curious about adult bodies (birth to 4 years)
2. Toddlers and young children begin to express affection for friends (3–8 years)

DOI: 10.4324/9781003145745-4

3. Toddlers and children 3–8 years 'fall in love' with a parent
4. Children between 6 and 12 years move their affection to an 'idol,' often a teacher
5. Between the ages of 8 and 15, feelings of love toward a friend or someone familiar
6. Up to age 15, adolescents begin to talk about love with peers and parents
7. Young adolescents start professing their love for a peer by sending messages to them (10–16 years)
8. In early- to middle adolescence (11–16), holding hands is common in burgeoning relationships
9. At the same age, kissing and hugging become part of relationships
10. Between 13 and 16, physical touching and exploring of the other persons' body is common
11. Between 14 and 16 is often when adolescents begin to have sexual intercourse

This model has been used to plan age- and stage-appropriate sexuality education and stands in stark contrast to the abstinence-only programs that have not been shown to prevent sexual activity, unintended pregnancy, or sexually transmitted infections (STIs).

Sexual development in adolescence

Much of the research on adolescent sexuality focuses on the adverse effects of sexual activity. In contrast, the National Commission on Adolescent Sexual Health (Haffner, 1995) states that:
Sexual health encompasses sexual development and reproductive health, as well as such characteristics as the ability to develop and maintain meaningful interpersonal relationships; appreciate one's own body; interact with both genders in respectful and appropriate ways; and express affection, love, and intimacy in ways consistent with one's own values.

> Further, "responsible adolescent intimate relationships should be consensual, non-exploitive, honest, pleasurable, and protected against unintended pregnancies and sexually transmitted diseases, if any type of intercourse occurs" (Haffner, 1995).

Fortenberry (2014) suggests that adolescents learn about sexuality through formal and informal channels. Formal education occurs in school-based sex education programs that generally focus on prevention of STIs and pregnancy prevention. Informal learning comes from parents, siblings, same- and older aged friends, religious institutions, and importantly, the media. But adolescents also learn from their own sexual experiences. Key to sexual development is the awareness of the adolescent of the sexual desire of others and this is influenced by neural and hormonal systems. Fortenberry states that this combination of maturation, learning, and experience results in mostly positive changes; however, sexual problems in this age group are not well understood or addressed. Shame, guilt, absence of pleasure, and pain are not uncommon in this age group and not well articulated in the literature. The occurrence of sexual dysfunction is not unheard of among late adolescents and young adults but does not appear to curtail sexual activity although they do report a negative impact on sexual satisfaction (Moreau, Kågesten, & Blum, 2016).

Another conceptual model of adolescent sexuality (Vasilenko, Kreager, & Lefkowitz, 2015) depicts adolescent sexual activity as putting the individual at risk for poor physical health such as contracting STIs. The self-perception of their sexual activity also affects future mental and social outcomes. Sexual behaviors are influenced by demographic (gender, ethnicity), situational (substance use, condom use), and cultural factors (media, values). The authors suggest that later initiation of sexual activity leads to more positive outcomes.

A more positive perspective on sexuality in this age group highlights the importance of masturbation and self-discovery for the development of healthy sexuality in adulthood. However, the authors also point out that physical readiness for sexual behavior is not the same as emotional or cognitive readiness (Cacciatore et al., 2019).

Sexual development in young adulthood

According to Erikson, young adulthood is when intimate relationships are formed. When someone recognizes that they cannot change to please the person they are with and that they do not expect the other person to change, this is a hallmark of moving from adolescence to early or young adulthood. The intimacy here is not strictly sexual but rather reflects the ability to connect emotionally with another in a committed relationship. Forming an intimate relationship is the opposite of what Erikson called 'isolation' that may be exemplified by self-absorption and a reluctance to reciprocate love. DeLamater and Friedrich (2002) state that developing the skills to talk effectively with a sexual partner as well as being able to decide about pregnancy and protection against STIs are hallmarks of sexual maturity in young adulthood. It is important to recognize that sexual development includes not only physical and mental/emotional maturity but also that societal influences play an important role (Gilleard & Higgs, 2016) and perhaps never more so than in early adulthood where identity is partially or wholly cemented. What is clear is that young adulthood is a time when sexual orientation can change over time and in response to changing circumstances (Kaestle, 2019).

In recent years, the acceptance of a range of sexual identities has been increasingly accepted. This encompasses both opposite- and same-sex identity as well as those who regard themselves as asexual. Some young adults define themselves as sexually fluid, defined as flexibility in sexual responsiveness across the lifespan and impacted by social and cultural factors as well as by specific relationships (Kaestle, 2019). While it is often regarded as something that is more common in women rather than men, one study found no statistical difference between women reporting fluidity (64%) and men (52%) (Katz-Wise, 2015).

Asexuality, defined as the lack of sexual attraction, is a somewhat controversial sexual identity that has historically been seen as related to sexual trauma, psychopathology, or personality disorder (Brotto & Yule, 2017). There are questions about whether this is a unique form of sexual orientation, mental illness, paraphilia, or sexual dysfunction. In a review of the topic, Brotto and Yule (2017) suggest that there is some evidence that asexuality is indeed a sexual orientation; some individuals identifying within this spectrum as experiencing sexual attraction some of the time (called Gray As) while others, called demisexuals, experience attraction after developing a strong romantic attraction to someone.

Young adulthood is also the stage when individuals embark on childbearing and rearing. Pregnancy itself changes one's sexuality and sexual self-image. Raising children presents unique challenges to sexuality, with lack of privacy and fatigue causing a loss of sexual connection for many couples. This dissipates as children grow and eventually leave home, but it can take a concerted effort to re-engage sexually with a partner. The inability to conceive, infertility, is a source of sexual problems as you will see in Chapter 12.

Sexual development in middle adulthood

The mid-40s are a time of transition from young- to middle adulthood. This is Erikson's 7th stage characterized by generativity versus stagnation or self-absorption. Generativity refers to caring about the generation that comes after us and can be operationalized as having children and guiding them or developing mentoring relationships in work or professional settings. Altruism and generosity are key components of this stage and contrast stagnation. Sexual changes occur during middle adulthood with peri-menopausal symptoms appearing for women and erectile decline starting for men. It is during mid-life that many men and women develop health conditions that become chronic such as diabetes, cardiovascular disease, and cancer. These all affect sexual functioning as do their treatments (Polland, Davis, Zeymo, & Venkatesan, 2018). A large community-based study found that one-third of the women experienced loss of sexual desire beginning in the fourth decade and continuing into the sixth decade (Zheng, Islam, Bell, Skiba, & Davis, 2020). It is important to note that sexual problems affect overall satisfaction with sexual life (Quinn-Nilas, Milhausen, McKay, & Holzapfel, 2018) and one partner's sexual problems affect the sexual functioning of the other partner (Jiann, Su, & Tsai, 2013). Couples should therefore be treated together when addressing sexual problems in one partner (Jannini & Nappi, 2018).

Menopause

Menopause is a major milestone for women in terms of general health as well as sexual functioning. Mid-life changes in ovarian hormones are hallmarks of the menopausal transition that occurs 4–6 years before the cessation of menses (Bacon, 2017). Abnormal menstrual bleeding, vasomotor symptoms and vulvo-vaginal dryness (now termed the genito-urinary syndrome of menopause [GSM]) impact negatively on a woman's sexual functioning during this transition and cause significant distress (Simon et al., 2018). Women report loss of libido, pain with intercourse (El Khoudary et al., 2019) as well as body image changes (Moral et al., 2018). Women regard sex as an important part of life and wish to continue their sexual relationship despite these symptoms (Thornton, Chervenak, & Neal-Perry, 2015). However, health care providers often neglect to talk about the sexual aspects of menopause (Simon et al., 2018), focusing instead of the other symptoms and missing an opportunity to provide information and interventions that help with the sexual problems that exist.

Andropause

In recent years, attention has been drawn to what some call andropause, a condition in men equated with menopause in women. It is also called the male menopause, partial androgen deficiency of the aging male or late onset hypogonadism (Pines, 2011). This is characterized as declining levels of testosterone that are alleged to impact negatively on sexual desire and erections (Corona, Isidori, Aversa, Burnett, & Maggi, 2016). This is a controversial issue suggesting that this condition is under-reported and under-treated (Harrison, 2011) while others suggest that this is a medicalized issue heavily influenced by pharmaceutical companies (Marshall, 2012). However, Tharakan and colleagues (Tharakan, Miah, Jayasena, & Minhas, 2019) suggest that the link between declines in testosterone and sexual function is inconclusive and testosterone supplementation is not without side effects and risk. These medications are heavily promoted in both direct-to-consumer and medical advertising. Studies have shown that testosterone supplementation does not have a benefit for sexual function, both in treating erectile problems and in improving libido (Huo et al., 2016). Seeing declining hormone levels as the only cause of sexual problems is reductionist, as many other factors including biological, psychological, relational, and cultural play an influential role (Nimbi, Tripodi, Rossi, Navarro-Cremades, & Simonelli, 2020). The role that obesity and other physiological factors play is also important to consider as well as medications (Basaria, 2013).

Sexual development in old age

Erikson described the developmental stage of old age as the balance between integrity and despair. With age comes wisdom and this is a significant strength in terms of facing adversity in an aging body. One of the challenges in discussing anything related to aging is the definition of what old, elderly, or senior means in today's society. In the 1980s, 40 was regarded as 'over the hill'; today's 40-year olds are having babies and see themselves as young. Retirement age used to be 55 but now people in their 70s are working as consultants, using their expertise and experience to guide others. And both men and women are sexually active well after the age of 70 as described in a large national study (Herbenick et al., 2010). In this study, 28.2% of men in their 70s had intercourse in the previous month and 42.9% in the past year. Women of the same age had slightly fewer encounters; 11.9% in the past month and 21.6% in the past year.

Sexual activity decreases with age, predominately because of ill health in both sexes and absence of a partner for women. However, agism plays a large role in our society and if an older person believes that sex is something only for young people, they may give up engaging in an activity that remains enjoyable and important for emotional connection as well as for general well-being (Bauer, Haesler, & Fetherstonhaugh, 2016). Older adults may focus more on touching and sensual activities rather than sexual intercourse (Gore-Gorszewska, 2020). Positive factors that help to maintain sexual activity of all kinds include increased time and opportunity (Heath, 2019). Positive mental health contributes to continued sexual engagement (Kleinstäuber, 2017) and depression is associated with less sexual activity (Jackson et al., 2019). While some elderly couples state that their sexual life has changed due to illness of the partner, others say that this opens the relationship to other non-penetrative opportunities (Roney & Kazer, 2015). Multiple barriers exist for older individuals and couples receiving help for sexual problems. Communication with health care providers is one barrier with fewer than 20% of women in one study reporting a conversation about sexuality with a health care provider (March, 2018). Other barriers include health care providers' lack of knowledge as well as stigma and discrimination (Ezhova et al., 2020). Health care providers who have training in sexuality are more likely to address the issue with older patients and offer interventions, both medical and psychosocial than providers who are not trained (Levkovich, Gewirtz-Meydan, & Ayalon, 2020).

Conclusion

The development of the sexual self begins in early childhood and continues through old age. Each stage of life has developmental milestones for sexuality, and they build on each other. From the exploration of what it means to live in a male or female body to the sexual discoveries of adolescence, there are no deadlines in the experience, and individuals will achieve these milestones in their own time as well as in part, according to the norms of the culture and society they live in.

References

Bacon, J.L. (2017). The menopausal transition. *Obstetrics and Gynecology Clinics of North America*, *44*(2), 285–296. doi: 10.1016/j.ogc.2017.02.008

Basaria, S. (2013). Reproductive aging in men. *Endocrinology and Metabolism Clinics of North America, 42*(2), 255–270. doi: 10.1016/j.ecl.2013.02.012

Bauer, M., Haesler, E., & Fetherstonhaugh, D. (2016). Let's talk about sex: Older people's views on the recognition of sexuality and sexual health in the health-care setting. *Health Expectations, 19*(6), 1237–1250. doi: 10.1111/hex.12418

Brandon-Friedman, R.A. (2019). Youth sexual development: A primer for social workers. *Social Work, 64*(4), 356–364. doi: 10.1093/sw/swz027

Brotto, L.A., & Yule, M. (2017). Asexuality: Sexual orientation, paraphilia, sexual dysfunction, or none of the above? *Archives of Sexual Behavior, 46*(3), 619–627. doi: 10.1007/s10508-016-0802-7

Cacciatore, R., Korteniemi-Poikela, E., & Kaltiala, R. (2019). The steps of sexuality—A developmental, emotion-focused, child-centered model of sexual development and sexuality education from birth to adulthood. *International Journal of Sexual Health, 31*(3), 319–338. doi: 10.1080/19317611.2019.1645783

Cass, V.C. (1979). Homosexual identity formation. *Journal of Homosexuality, 4*(3), 219–235. doi: 10.1300/J082v04n03_01

Corona, G., Isidori, A.M., Aversa, A., Burnett, A.L., & Maggi, M. (2016). Endocrinologic control of men's sexual desire and arousal/erection. *Journal of Sexual Medicine, 13*(3), 317–337. doi: 10.1016/j.jsxm.2016.01.007

DeLamater, J., & Friedrich, W.N. (2002). Human sexual development. *Journal of Sex Research, 39*(1), 10–14. doi: 10.1080/00224490209552113

El Khoudary, S.R., Greendale, G., Crawford, S.L., Avis, N.E., Brooks, M.M., Thurston, R.C., … Matthews, K. (2019). The menopause transition and women's health at midlife: A progress report from the study of women's health across the Nation (swan). *Menopause, 26*(10), 1213–1227. doi: 10.1097/gme.0000000000001424

Ezhova, I., Savidge, L., Bonnett, C., Cassidy, J., Okwuokei, A., & Dickinson, T. (2020). Barriers to older adults seeking sexual health advice and treatment: A scoping review. *International Journal of Nursing Studies, 107*, 103566, doi: 10.1016/j.ijnurstu.2020.103566

Fortenberry, J.D. (2014). Sexual learning, sexual experience, and healthy adolescent sex. *New Directions for Child and Adolescent Development, 144*(144), 71–86. doi: 10.1002/cad.20061

Gilleard, C., & Higgs, P. (2016). Connecting life span development with the sociology of the life course: A new direction. *Sociology, 50*(2), 301–315. doi: 10.1177/0038038515577906

Gore-Gorszewska, G. (2020). "What do you mean by sex?" A qualitative analysis of traditional versus evolved meanings of sexual activity among older women and men. *Journal of Sex Research*, 1–15. doi: 10.1080/00224499.2020.1798333

Haffner, D. (1995). Facing facts: Sexual health for America's adolescents. Retrieved from https://eric.ed.gov/?id=ED391779

Harrison, J. (2011). 'Talking about my generation': A state-of-the-art review of health information for men in the andropause. *Health Information and Libraries Journal, 28*(3), 161–170. doi: 10.1111/j.1471-1842.2011.00950.x

Heath, H. (2019). Sexuality and sexual intimacy in later life. *Nursing Older People, 31*(1), 40–48. doi: 10.7748/nop.2019.e1102

Herbenick, D., Reece, M., Schick, V., Sanders, S.A., Dodge, B., & Fortenberry, J.D. (2010). Sexual behavior in the United States: Results from a national probability sample of men and women ages 14–94. *Journal of Sexual Medicine*, 7 Suppl. 5, 255–265. doi: 10.1111/j.1743-6109.2010.02012.x

Huo, S., McGarvey, S., Hill, E., Tügertimur, B., Hogenmiller, A., … Fugh-Berman, A. (2016). Treatment of men for "low testosterone": A systematic review. *PLOS ONE, 11*(9), e0162480. doi: 10.1371/journal.pone.0162480

Jackson, S.E., Firth, J., Veronese, N., Stubbs, B., Koyanagi, A., Yang, L., & Smith, L. (2019). Decline in sexuality and wellbeing in older adults: A population-based study. *Journal of Affective Disorders, 245*, 912–917. doi: 10.1016/j.jad.2018.11.091

Jannini, E.A., & Nappi, R.E. (2018). Couplepause: A new paradigm in treating sexual dysfunction during menopause and andropause. *Sexual Medicine Reviews, 6*(3), 384–395. doi: 10.1016/j.sxmr.2017.11.002

Jiann, B.P., Su, C.C., & Tsai, J.Y. (2013). Is female sexual function related to the Male Partners' erectile function? *Journal of Sexual Medicine, 10*(2), 420–429. doi: 10.1111/j.1743-6109.2012.03007.x

Kaestle, C.E. (2019). Sexual orientation trajectories based on sexual attractions, partners, and identity: A longitudinal investigation from adolescence through young adulthood using a U.S. representative sample. *Journal of Sex Research, 56*(7), 811–826. doi: 10.1080/00224499.2019.1577351

Katz-Wise, S.L. (2015). Sexual fluidity in young adult women and men: Associations with sexual orientation and sexual identity development. *Psychology and Sexuality, 6*(2), 189–208. doi: 10.1080/19419899.2013.876445

Kenneady, D.A., & Oswalt, S.B. (2014). Is Cass's model of homosexual identity formation relevant to today's society? *American Journal of Sexuality Education, 9*(2), 229–246. doi: 10.1080/15546128.2014.900465

Kleinstäuber, M. (2017). Factors associated with sexual health and well being in older adulthood. *Current Opinion in Psychiatry, 30*(5), 358–368. doi: 10.1097/yco.0000000000000354

Levkovich, I., Gewirtz-Meydan, A., & Ayalon, L. (2020). Communicating with older adults about sexual issues: How are these issues handled by physicians with and without training in human sexuality? *Health and Social Care in the Community*, 1–10. doi: 10.1111/hsc.13172

March, A.L. (2018). Sexuality and intimacy in the older adult woman. *Nursing Clinics of North America, 53*(2), 279–287. doi: 10.1016/j.cnur.2018.01.005

Marshall, B.L. (2012). Medicalization and the refashioning of age-related limits on sexuality. *Journal of Sex Research, 49*(4), 337–343. doi: 10.1080/00224499.2011.644597

Moral, E., Delgado, J.L., Carmona, F., Caballero, B., Guillán, C., González, P.M., … Nieto Magro, C. (2018). The impact of genitourinary syndrome of menopause on well-being, functioning, and quality of life in postmenopausal women. *Menopause, 25*(12), 1418–1423. doi: 10.1097/gme.0000000000001148

Moreau, C., Kågesten, A.E., & Blum, R.W. (2016). Sexual dysfunction among youth: An overlooked sexual health concern. *BMC Public Health, 16*(1), 1170. doi: 10.1186/s12889-016-3835-x

Nimbi, F.M., Tripodi, F., Rossi, R., Navarro-Cremades, F., & Simonelli, C. (2020). Male sexual desire: An overview of biological, psychological, sexual, relational, and cultural factors influencing desire. *Sexual Medicine Reviews*. doi: 10.1016/j.sxmr.2018.12.002

Pines, A. (2011). Male menopause: Is it a real clinical syndrome? *Climacteric, 14*(1), 15–17. doi: 10.3109/13697137.2010.507442

Polland, A., Davis, M., Zeymo, A., & Venkatesan, K. (2018). Comparison of correlated comorbidities in male and female sexual dysfunction: Findings from the third national survey of sexual attitudes and lifestyles (Natsal-3). *Journal of Sexual Medicine, 15*(5), 678–686. doi: 10.1016/j.jsxm.2018.02.023

Quinn-Nilas, C., Milhausen, R.R., McKay, A., & Holzapfel, S. (2018). Prevalence and predictors of sexual problems among midlife Canadian adults: Results from a national survey. *Journal of Sexual Medicine, 15*(6), 873–879. doi: 10.1016/j.jsxm.2018.03.086

Roney, L., & Kazer, M.W. (2015). Geriatric sexual experiences: The seniors tell all. *Applied Nursing Research, 28*(3), 254–256. doi: 10.1016/j.apnr.2015.04.005

Simon, J.A., Davis, S.R., Althof, S.E., Chedraui, P., Clayton, A.H., Kingsberg, S.A., … Wolfman, W. (2018). Sexual well-being after menopause: An International Menopause Society White Paper. *Climacteric, 21*(5), 415–427. doi: 10.1080/13697137.2018.1482647

Tharakan, T., Miah, S., Jayasena, C., & Minhas, S. (2019). Investigating the basis of sexual dysfunction during late-onset hypogonadism. *F1000 Research, 8*. doi: 10.12688/f1000research.16561.1

Thornton, K., Chervenak, J., & Neal-Perry, G. (2015). Menopause and sexuality. *Endocrinology and Metabolism Clinics of North America, 44*(3), 649–661. doi: 10.1016/j.ecl.2015.05.009

Vasilenko, S.A., Kreager, D.A., & Lefkowitz, E.S. (2015). Gender, contraceptive attitudes, and condom use in adolescent romantic relationships: A dyadic approach. *Journal of Research on Adolescence, 25*(1), 51–62. doi: 10.1111/jora.12091

Zheng, J., Islam, R.M., Bell, R.J., Skiba, M.A., & Davis, S.R. (2020). Prevalence of low sexual desire with associated distress across the adult life span: An Australian cross-sectional study. *Journal of Sexual Medicine, 17*(10), 1885–1895. doi: 10.1016/j.jsxm.2020.07.007

5 How medical conditions affect sexuality and sexual functioning

Sexual functioning is dependent on healthy vascular, neurologic, and hormonal functioning. There is strong evidence that diseases affecting these processes adversely affect all aspects of the human sexual response cycle. For example, diabetes is a condition that profoundly affects both nerves and blood vessels, resulting in problems with sexual arousal. It is well established that erectile problems in an otherwise healthy man predicts cardiovascular disease and recognition of this association can prevent a significant cardiac event. This chapter will address these conditions as well as others such as stroke, renal disease, sexually transmitted infections including HIV/AIDS, obesity, inflammatory diseases, neurologic conditions such as multiple sclerosis and Parkinson's, and pain.

Cardiovascular disease

The link between cardiovascular disease and sexual dysfunction in men is well established. Sexual functioning, particularly arousal, is dependent on vascular and neural factors primarily but hormonal and psychological factors also play a role. The factors that have a major impact on cardiovascular health are also involved in arousal difficulties. These include hypertension, insulin resistance, dyslipidemia, obesity, smoking, sedentary lifestyle, and depression. The metabolic syndrome is highly correlated with both cardiovascular disease and erectile dysfunction (Svatikova & Kopecky, 2020). The role of inflammation is also important; hypertension is associated with endothelial and smooth muscle cells damage resulting in arterial stiffness, reducing blood flow to the penis (Calmasini, Klee, Webb, & Priviero, 2019).

Sexual problems in men with cardiovascular disease are well described with older age, anxiety and depression, hypertension, diabetes, and being treated with beta-blockers being highly associated with sexual dysfunction. Women have the same associations but they are assessed less often for cardiovascular disease (Rundblad et al., 2017). The risk of cardiovascular disease in men with erectile dysfunction (ED), especially severe dysfunction, is significant. In a meta-analysis of studies, the risk of cardiovascular disease was increased by 43%, coronary heart disease by 59%, stroke by 34%, and all-cause mortality by 33% (Zhao et al., 2019).

The penis is said to be the canary in the coal mine for cardiovascular disease. Erectile problems predate a cardiac event by 2–5 years (Hackett et al., 2016) and thus investigation of the onset of ED in an otherwise healthy man in his 40s is vital to both diagnose silent cardiovascular disease and encourage lifestyle changes to mitigate the outcomes of cardiac disease. Currently there is no evidence of the same risk for future cardiac events for women (Miner, Esposito, Guay, Montorsi, & Goldstein, 2012). Vascular ED is usually slow in onset with decreased rigidity and maintenance of an erection as well as a decrease in early morning

DOI: 10.4324/9781003145745-5

erections and nocturnal erections (Martin Miner et al., 2019). The occurrence of ED in these men may provide a teachable moment that should not be overlooked; simply writing a prescription for medication to treat the ED misses a vital opportunity to diagnose and treat heart disease. However, medications used to treat many co-morbidities also cause sexual dysfunction; diuretics, beta-blockers, and anti-depressants are all associated with impaired sexual function (Polland, Davis, Zeymo, & Venkatesan, 2018). Most of the research in this area has been focused on men so it is unclear if similar side effects exist for women (Santana et al., 2019).

Interventions to reduce the risk of cardiovascular disease in overweight individuals include encouragement to lose 10% or more of body weight and to get 20–30 minutes of physical exercise five times a week. High-protein, low-carbohydrate and low-fat diets have shown some efficacy in lowering both cardiovascular and erectile dysfunction risks. Smoking cessation is important as is avoiding excessive alcohol intake (Hackett et al., 2016).

Response of couples to alterations in sexual response

Sexuality is often affected when one or both partners in a couple have a chronic illness. The sexual side effects of cardiovascular disease and its treatments have been described above; in addition to the physical signs and symptoms, anxiety about the health of the affected partner will affect the sexual relationship. It has been shown that satisfaction with the couple relationship suffers when one of them has cardiac disease (Günzler, Kriston, Harms, & Berner, 2009). Quarrels increase and less communication occurs as well as fewer displays of tenderness. Sexual satisfaction is also decreased in many couples (Byrne, Murphy, D'Eath, Doherty, & Jaarsma, 2017); however, the reasons for this are not clear.

In the event that one of the partners has experienced a myocardial infarction (MI), anxiety and lack of information affect the sexual relationship. Men report more negative impacts on sexual functioning than women one year after the incident while women report little change but often their pre-morbid sexual function was worse than men (Thylén & Brännström, 2015). The partner of the person who has had a MI has a significant influence on the sexual relationship and if they are worried that sexual activity is harmful, sexual activity will cease or decrease (López-Medina, Gil-García, Sánchez-Criado, & Pancorbo-Hidalgo, 2016). The American Heart Association (Steinke et al., 2013) states that sexual activity can resume one week after an uncomplicated MI but couples are often reluctant to engage in sexual activity. It is not uncommon for the couple to misinterpret physical sensations during sexual activity where heart rate and respiration increase; in reality, sexual intercourse is considered low risk in terms of cardiac effort (Stein, Sardinha, & Araújo, 2016).

Communication with health care providers

As with many other illnesses, information from health care providers about sexual functioning is less than optimal. Multiple studies report that communication is often lacking or insufficient (Rundblad et al., 2017) with few being offered counseling about sexuality and relationships. In a study of registered nurses working in cardiac in-patient units, 75% stated that they are not knowledgeable enough to discuss this with patients and that sexuality is not a priority for patients while in hospital (Kolbe, Kugler, Schnepp, & Jaarsma, 2016). In another study, patients reported that they were comfortable talking about sexuality but the cardiac nurses providing education said that the patients were not comfortable (D'Eath et al., 2018). The interpretation of patient comfort or discomfort can result in no discussion about sexuality and a knowledge gap for patients and their partners, resulting in long-term consequences.

Recommendations for the care of individuals with cardiac disease

The importance of counseling about sexual function, anxiety, depression, and fear is highlighted in recommendations from the American Heart Association. Counseling should include a review of medications and potential side effects on sexual functioning, the role of exercise in health promotion, avoidance of any stress related to sexual activity by choosing a familiar setting for sexual activity, not engaging in anal sex, and reporting of any cardiac symptoms experienced while engaging in sexual activity (Steinke et al., 2013).

PDE5-I medications (sildenafil, tadalafil, vardenafil, etc.) are safe to use in men experiencing ED if they have stable cardiovascular disease; this class of medication should not be used in men who are taking nitrates to control chest pain due to the risk of hypotension (Levine et al., 2012). Men with more complicated or unstable disease should seek the recommendation from their cardiologist about sexual activity and the use of erectile aids.

Box 5.1 Case study

Case study

Bob is 54-years old and like many men his age, has only sought medical care when injured. This summer he and his wife Marg celebrated their 25th wedding anniversary with a trip to Mexico. They had a great time but on two occasions, he was not able to achieve an erection. Marg told him not to worry about it; he had been drinking quite a lot and she suggested this was the reason. But Bob was concerned and went to the medical clinic at a nearby drugstore. He was seen by a physician assistant who insisted on taking his blood pressure. Bob was annoyed; he needed to get back to work and what did this have to do with his penis?

The PA looked a little worried and asked Bob to wait for 5 minutes and then he would measure his blood pressure again. Bob was having none of this; he stormed out of the clinic, shouting at the receptionist that this was the dumbest place he had ever been to and the PA was the stupidest person he had ever met. He didn't tell Marg about any of this and for the next couple of weeks, he didn't make any attempt to have sex. When Marg asked him if everything was okay, he said he was stressed about work and that was the end of that.

But he was worried and he half joking asked one of his work friends, Noel, if he ever had problems 'getting it up.' Noel laughed, patted him on the back, and said he would bring Bob a 'little blue helper' the next day. Bob was a little embarrassed when Noel handed him the pills; there were two in the package and he dropped it into his lunch bag. That weekend he took one after lunch and was pleased with the result; he and Marg had sex for the first time in weeks and it was great. His erection was firmer than it had been in ages and Marg even commented on that. But what was he going to do about getting more of them? Once again Noel had the answer; he had a buddy who was a pharmacist who kept him supplied. He would connect Bob with this guy, no problem.

Months went by. Bob continued using the 'little blue helpers' and had no problem getting more from the pharmacist. He knew this was likely not what he should be doing, but Noel seemed to have no problem with this, so he continued getting pills. One day he was out in the yard, taking down the lights from the big tree in their front yard, when he felt a tightness in his chest. He stopped for a moment, took a deep breath, and then felt himself falling off the ladder and onto the grass.

Stroke

The physical and psychological impacts of stroke on the individual and their partner are significant, with global sexual changes occurring in both men and women (Tamam, Tamam, Akil, Yasan, & Tamam, 2008). Depending on the extent of neurological damage, the early stages of recovery, the individual may need a great deal of assistance with activities of daily living including personal hygiene, eating, and drinking as well as mobility. Those who have experienced this report alterations to body image, increased reliance on the partner, and post-stroke fatigue that impacts on libido; these contribute to a lack of self-worth and major challenges to their relationship (Thompson & Ryan, 2009). Irritability and anger are also reported that lead to guilt about the burden placed on the partner and over time, the partner is seen increasingly as a friend and not a romantic or sexual partner. Women who have experienced a stroke report a general lack of caring about personal hygiene and attractiveness that erodes their self-confidence (Lever & Pryor, 2017). In this study, women reported feeling vulnerable during attempts at sexual activity.

Some individuals who have had a stroke report that the emotional connection with their partner was enhanced, particularly if there was good communication between them (Nilsson, Fugl-Meyer, von Koch, & Ytterberg, 2017). Others reported a decrease in satisfaction with life in general, sex itself, and the partnered relationship and the partners also reported less satisfaction (Fugl-Meyer, Nilsson, von Koch, & Ytterberg, 2019). There are no increased risks from sexual activity for those who have suffered a stroke but finding sexual positions that are comfortable and allow for physical touch may be challenging due to physical deficits (Steinke et al., 2013). It is often assumed that stroke only happens to older adults but it can and does occur in younger individuals when the potential effect on the sexual relationship may lead to relationship stress and breakdown.

Communication with health care providers

Communication with health care providers about anticipated changes is inconsistent with multiple barriers cited. These include time constraints, lack of knowledge, agism, and a perception that this is not a priority for patients. This perception is an obstacle to patients receiving the information and help that they need (Richards, Dean, Burgess, & Caird, 2016). The topic of sexuality may not be considered important in rehabilitation programs, and staff have been seen laughing about the topic in conversation. In addition, lack of policy requiring attention to be paid to this and lack of education for staff in addition to the personal level of comfort talking about sexuality prevent discussion about this with patients and their partner (Vikan et al., 2019). When asked, couples suggested that information about sexuality and changes to sexual functioning should be addressed in the sub-acute and chronic phases of the illness (McGrath, Lever, McCluskey, & Power, 2019); they identified high priority topics that they would like included in patient education. These include:

- Being told about resuming sexual activity
- Myths about sexuality after stroke
- Communicating with health care providers
- Expressing emotional closeness with new and established partners
- Changes to emotions, body image and physical function
- Managing guilt and anger in relationships
- Changes to self-confidence and self-concept
- Fear of rejection by partner(s)
- Fatigue
- Sexual pleasure

Diabetes

It is well established that diabetes mellitus (DM) affects sexual function in both women (Pontiroli, Cortelazzi, & Morabito, 2013) and men (Bebb, Millar, & Brock, 2018); this is especially noticeable in individuals with Type 2 diabetes where 68% of women experience sexual problems and 82% of men have erectile problems (Bąk et al., 2017). Those with Type 1 diabetes are also affected with 35% of women and 50% of men reporting problems. Men report erectile dysfunction, but women experience more global effects including decreased libido, arousal, orgasm and, sexual satisfaction. Diabetes is also associated with hypogonadism in men which results in loss of libido (Kizilay, Gali, & Serefoglu, 2017). Depression is associated with sexual dysfunction in both men and women with Type 2 DM (Corona, Giorda, Cucinotta, Guida, & Nada, 2014) and Type 1 DM (Tagliabue et al., 2011) as are diabetes-associated complications (Rutte et al., 2015). In younger women, diabetes is also associated with urinary tract infections and dyspareunia (Cichocka, Jagusiewicz, & Gumprecht, 2020).

The impact of DM on young adults is especially important; this is a life stage where romantic and sexual partnerships are established, and sexual dysfunction can have a significant impact on establishing these relationships. The need to disclose their illness to a potential partner may be an obstacle for some (Monaghan, Helgeson, & Wiebe, 2015) but others report that this is not a concern (Pinhas-Hamiel et al., 2017). Young adults with Type 1 DM report that they are concerned about both hypo- and hyperglycemia during sexual activity and if they use an insulin pump, there are additional concerns about the presence of the pump, how to manage it during sex, and physical discomfort associated with its placement on the body (Santos, Pascoal, & Barros, 2020).

Sexual minority men and women report higher rates of diabetes than their heterosexual counterparts in some studies (Caceres et al., 2017). Men who have sex with men report a host of psycho-sexual problems (Jowett, Peel, & Shaw, 2012) related to having diabetes. These include the negative outcome of erectile dysfunction during casual sex which may be interpreted as lack of attraction to a partner. The presence of an insulin pump may be seen as a sign of HIV infection because DM is a side effect of anti-retroviral medication. The presence of a candida infection in the ano-perineal area, common in diabetes, could be aversive to a sexual partner and the need to have food or beverage nearby during sex in case of hypogly-cemia is also problematic. There is a paucity of literature on the sexual experiences of sexual minority women with diabetes beyond studies about increased risk due to obesity, tobacco-and alcohol use.

Management of diabetes-associated sexual problems

Tight glycemic control is important in preventing the onset of sexual dysfunction in both men and women (Kizilay et al., 2017). First line treatment for men with erectile dysfunc-tion is the use of PDE-5i but lack of effectiveness and cost present barriers (Corona, Giorda, Cucinotta, Guida, & Nada, 2016). Men with hypogonadism can be treated with supplemental testosterone but consideration should be given to the side effects of this therapy and the evi-dence of this being helpful in reducing body mass, blood glucose levels, or sexual function is mixed (Bebb et al., 2018). Treatment of depression with SSRIs and SNRIs is problem-atic due to the known sexual side effects of these classes of drugs but bupropion has been shown to have fewer side effects. In one study, 58% of individuals with DM and depression showed improvements in sexual function when treated with bupropion (Sayuk, Gott, Nix, & Lustman, 2011).

For women experiencing sexual problems, management should focus on the specific symptom with moisturizers and lubricants for vulvo-vaginal dryness or estrogen supplemen-tation. Testosterone is not FDA approved for women.

Counseling and lifestyle changes such as eating a healthy diet, physical exercise, and maintaining a healthy diet are all beneficial for dealing with sexual dysfunction with men and women living with both Type 1 and Type 2 diabetes.

Renal disease

Sexual dysfunction is common in men and women with chronic kidney disease and is associ-ated with other risk factors such as age, diabetes (Navaneethan et al., 2010), and depression (Theofilou, 2012). Sexual complaints include loss of libido, arousal problems (erectile dys-function in men and vulvo-vaginal dryness in women), problems with achieving orgasm, as well as decreased or absent ejaculation (Holley & Schmidt, 2010). Kidney transplantation improves survival and quality of life for those with renal disease but sexual problems persist after transplant in 50% of recipients (van Ek et al., 2017). Depression is common among those who receive a kidney transplant (Luo et al., 2020).

Communication with health care providers

Despite the high prevalence of sexual problems in this population, communication about this is rare. Nurses who have extended contact with these patients due to the chronic nature of the disease and the need for dialysis have multiple opportunities to discuss this but rarely do (Ho & Fernández, 2006; Yodchai, Hutchinson, & Oumtanee, 2018). Reasons for the lack of communication are similar to those given for not addressing this in other populations; these include the age of the patient, culture and ethnicity, and language (van Ek et al., 2018). Physicians are no less reluctant; just 11% of nephrologists reported treating sexual problems in their patients on dialysis (Green et al., 2012). Nephrologists in another study stated that they waited for the patient to raise the topic (van Ek et al., 2015); 96% said that they discussed sexual dysfunction in less than half of their patients. Ninety one percent of renal surgeons said a discussion was the responsibility of the nephrologist and 63% of nephrologists felt that it was the responsibility of the patient's primary care provider (Green et al., 2012).

Sexually transmitted infections

Despite the obvious association between sexual activity and sexually transmitted infections (STIs), there is little research in this area. Most of the available evidence focuses on the human immunodeficiency virus (HIV) and the human papilloma virus (HPV). There is limited literature that focuses on psychological effects of being diagnosed with genital herpes, or dyspareunia associated with pelvic inflammatory disease secondary to gonorrhea and chlamydia in women. Chronic pelvic pain syndrome in men secondary to prostatitis is mentioned as well as some controversy related to other sexual problems such as ejaculatory and erectile problems (Sadeghi-Nejad, Wasserman, Weidner, Richardson, & Goldmeier, 2010). A more recent review found that people diagnosed with an STI experience significant sexual dysfunction in addition to avoidance of sex (Haapa, Suominen, Paavilainen, & Kylmä, 2018).

a) Human immunodeficiency virus

HIV in women impacts on menopausal symptoms that may be worse in HIV-infected women (Cejtin, 2012) with vulvo-vaginal atrophy experienced by up to 96% along with vasomotor symptoms. Dyspareunia is common (Tariq, Delpech, & Anderson, 2016) and overall, women living with HIV are less likely to be sexually active (Narasimhan, Payne, Caldas, Beard, & Kennedy, 2016). The reasons for this include fatigue, decreased desire as well as feeling unattractive usually as a result of the physical changes due to lipodystrophy and/or lipoatrophy, common side effects of highly active anti-retroviral therapy (HAART) (Carlsson-Lalloo, Rusner, Mellgren, & Berg, 2016). Lipodystrophy refers to abnormal fat deposition in the abdominal area (visceral adipose tissue), the breasts, as well as causing a 'buffalo hump'; widely distributed lipomas are also common. On the other hand, lipoatrophy refers to fat loss on the face and/or limbs (Lake et al., 2017). The easily recognizable physical changes are known to cause stigma and embarrassment that impact on sexual desire. Sexual problems may be underestimated in women living with HIV due to lack of assessment. In one study, 60% of physicians working in HIV clinics did not ask about this (Bell et al., 2006).

Sexual problems are common in men living with HIV infection. Depression and anxiety are recognized as contributing to libido and erectile function, but the disease also causes hypogonadism that adds to the man's distress and sexual performance. Much like women, the changes in appearance from lipoatrophy and lipodystrophy are signs of HIV infection that alert potential sexual partners to their disease status (Sadeghi-Nejad et al., 2010). Erectile dysfunction is very common in HIV-infected men with a relative risk of 2.32 (95% CI; 1.52–3.55; P < 001) in a recent meta-analysis (Luo et al., 2017). Earlier onset of erectile dysfunction has been found in HIV-infected men compared with men who are not infected (Zona et al., 2012). This could be related to the accelerated aging process associated with HIV infection as men in their 30s have reported ED. Highly active anti-retroviral therapy, particularly the protease inhibitors, are known to cause erectile dysfunction (Luo et al., 2017). There is also evidence that the use of oral agents for erectile dysfunction, often purchased from sources without a prescription, is associated with high-risk activities in men who have sex with men, leading to acquisition of STIs (Rosen et al., 2006). The use of these medications is also linked to the use of recreational drugs that in turn is associated with high-risk sexual activities (Sadeghi-Nejad et al., 2010).

b) Human papilloma virus

The prevalence of HPV infection among US men is 42.5% (Han, Beltran, Song, Klaric, & Choi, 2017), but despite this, there is little knowledge about how HPV infection impacts on male sexuality. Low-risk HPV (types 6 and 11) is known to cause genital warts. Penile, anal, and oral cancer are associated with types 16 and 18 (Palefsky, 2010) and are transmissible to women where they cause cervical cancer. It seems logical that penile lesions would have sexual concerns but there is no research supporting this but that does not mean that it does not occur.

HPV infection is associated with sexual dysfunction in women, beginning with decreased libido after diagnosis (Alay et al., 2020) and a multitude of alterations in sexual functioning including problems with arousal and lubrication, orgasm, and sexual satisfaction (Mercan et al., 2019). Women report being concerned about the response of their partner as well as the risk of infecting the partner. They are also worried about their attractiveness to their sexual partner, and their own sexual response (Nagele et al., 2016). Women with lesions on the vulva were more likely to be concerned than women with 'hidden' lesions such as those on the cervix. Women also report being worried that they would be perceived as being dirty or promiscuous (McCaffery, Waller, Nazroo, & Wardle, 2006).

Box 5.2 Assessment of a woman with HPV-related fear

You are asked to see a 36-year old woman who has been diagnosed with Stage 2 cervical cancer. The clinic nurse reports that the patient is very tearful and told her that she is scared that her husband is going to leave her. Using the PLISSIT model (Annon, 1974), here is an example of how you could have a conversation with her.

Permission: *Stacey the nurse at the clinic told me that you were very upset today when you learned of your diagnosis. How can I help you? I hope that I can answer any questions that you may have.*

Limited Information: *HPV-infection is very common; about 80% of adults have been exposed to the virus. Your partner is most likely to have been exposed as well.*

Specific Suggestion: *Have you thought about how you are going to tell your husband about this? He may be more supportive than you realize, and he is likely going to be really worried about you. Many women fear that this will have a negative effect on their relationship. Cervical cancer has nothing to do with anything you have done – this is not your fault. You can still have sex with your partner but depending on what treatment you have, you may have to avoid sex for a while. Your oncologist can give you more information about this.*

Intensive Therapy: *We have social workers on staff who can support you and your husband as you go through this. There is also a sexual medicine doctor who we refer to if you need to see a specialist.*

Obesity

It is well established that obesity has a negative impact on sexuality (Katz, 2017), especially for older women (Kwon & Schafer, 2017). Obesity is associated with a wide range of co-morbidities including diabetes, hypertension, and cardiovascular disease. There are psychosocial associations as well including poor body image as well as depression and anxiety. While there is limited evidence in clinical trials of the association between overweight/obesity and sexual dysfunction, studies have shown that increased body mass is associated with low sexual self-esteem in women in particular (Krychman, 2015). Being overweight or obese is associated with lower levels of sexual activity and an increase in sexual dysfunction in women as well as with greater sexual distress (Faubion et al., 2020). Women with polycystic ovarian syndrome (PCOS) are frequently overweight or obese and this has negative consequences on body image and sexual functioning (Kogure et al., 2019). Related to this are feelings of being sexually unattractive and decreased sexual satisfaction (Stapinska-Syniec, Grabowska, Szpotanska-Sikorska, & Pietrzak, 2018) as well as dyspareunia (Loh et al., 2020).

Nackers and colleagues (Nackers et al., 2015) showed in their large study of mid-life women that sexual desire and frequency of intercourse declined in women when they experienced greater than expected weight gain. However, not all overweight or obese women experience sexual problems related to their body mass; societal messages about sexual attractiveness may play a significant role in the development of sexual problems and the emergence of the body positive movement may play a role in greater self-acceptance and better sexual self-esteem for some women.

Sexual minority women tend to have higher body mass and are more likely to be overweight or obese than their heterosexual counterparts; in contrast, sexual minority men are less likely to be either overweight or obese (Azagba, Shan, & Latham, 2019). Sexual minority women may experience less influence of societal norms about body weight than heterosexual women (Bergeron & Senn, 1998); however, they may experience messages from within their community about how they should look (Kelly, 2007) and they may experience stigma associated with their weight depending on the norms within their community (Panza, Olson, Goldstein, Selby, & Lillis, 2020). Sexual minority women have a 44% higher risk of developing metabolic syndrome (Kinsky, Stall, Hawk, & Markovic, 2016) but the association of this related to sexual functioning is not clearly described in this population. Other risk factors for cardiovascular disease are also prevalent with smoking, heavy alcohol use in addition to obesity among sexual minority women (Caceres, Makarem, Hickey, & Hughes, 2019).

Obesity is also associated with pelvic floor dysfunction in women (Bilgic, Gokyildiz, Kizilkaya Beji, Yalcin, & Gungor Ugurlucan, 2019) with increased urinary frequency resulting in sexual dysfunction. The reasons for the dysfunction are multi-factorial and include the response of the sexual partner, fear of leakage during sexual activity, poor body image, and feeling unattractive.

Erectile dysfunction is associated with severe obesity in men (Ho et al., 2019) and the role of hypogonadism is seen as bi-directional with obesity linked to hypogonadism and hypogonadism resulting in overweight/obesity (Corona, Vignozzi, Sforza, Mannucci, & Maggi, 2015). The role of the metabolic syndrome that includes obesity, in the development of erectile dysfunction has been described earlier in this chapter. While sexual minority men experience less obesity than heterosexual men (Newlin Lew, Dorsen, & Long, 2018) perception about weight and the ideal body impact on body image and body dissatisfaction

(Tran et al., 2020). In a study of perceived weight in sexual minority men, 75% of obese participants saw themselves as being of normal weight, or perhaps merely overweight (Goedel, Krebs, Greene, & Duncan, 2017). Sexual minority men (Griffiths et al., 2018) experience weight stigma within their community that may also impact on sexual function.

Obesity in adolescents, an ever-growing problem in this age group, is known to cause problems with dating and romantic relationships (Becnel et al., 2017). Adolescent women who are overweight are less likely to date and engage in sexual activity, but when they do, they tend to participate in higher-risk sexual activity resulting in unplanned pregnancies and STIs. After bariatric surgery, 25% of young women reported a pregnancy and 18.7% were diagnosed with an STI, suggesting that these adolescents need more information and guidance about safer sex after surgery (Zeller et al., 2019).

Communication with health care providers

Talking about overweight or obesity is not easy but it can be framed within a conversation about healthy lifestyles (Kable et al., 2015). While female physicians are more likely to talk to patients about this (Dutton et al., 2014), patients are twice as likely to try to lose weight when instructed to do so by their physician of any gender (Pool et al., 2014). It is important to avoid the perception of judgment when having a discussion about weight (Gudzune, Beach, Roter, & Cooper, 2013). While barriers exist for weight loss, the impact on sexuality and sexual function may act as a strong motivator if the link is made clearly and compassionately by the health care provider.

Weight loss

For individuals who are experiencing sexual difficulties associated with weight, even a modest (5–10%) decrease in body weight will show improvement for both men and women over time (Ryan & Yockey, 2017). These improvements are thought to occur through multiple systems including endocrine effects (sex hormones), amelioration of cardiovascular disease, diabetes, and the metabolic syndrome as well as psychological factors such as improved body image, improvements in self-esteem, and depression (Rowland, McNabney, & Mann, 2017). While lifestyle changes (diet and physical activity) can contribute to weight loss, for those who are obese or morbidly obese and those with complications of diabetes or cardiovascular disease, a surgical approach to weight loss may be necessary.

Bariatric surgery has shown significant improvements in sexual functioning in women including improvements in body image (Conason, McClure Brenchley, Pratt, & Geliebter, 2017) as well as global improvements in desire, arousal, lubrication, orgasm, satisfaction, and sexual pain (Cherick et al., 2019; Gao et al., 2020). In men, bariatric surgery is associated with improved testosterone levels and erectile function (Glina, de Freitas Barboza, Nunes, Glina, & Bernardo, 2017; Lee et al., 2019). Long-term improvements persist in both women and men; however, treatment for depression mitigates this (Steffen et al., 2019).

Inflammatory conditions

Inflammatory bowel diseases (Crohn's and ulcerative colitis) are often diagnosed in adolescence or early adulthood at a time when body image is important in the development of romantic relationships. The treatment of these conditions along with the side effects of the disease process has a negative impact on sexual functioning and feelings of attractiveness (Marín et al., 2013). Sexual desire and satisfaction have been shown to worsen after diagnosis and the effects of corticosteroids on women and biologic agents on men contribute to sexual dysfunction. Depression and anxiety also have a significant impact on sexual desire and satisfaction (Eluri et al., 2018). As with many other chronic diseases, this is a topic that is rarely discussed by gastroenterologists (Leenhardt et al., 2019).

Individuals with arthritis experience a range of symptoms that impact on sexual function and satisfaction. These not only cause suffering for the individual but also affect relationships negatively. In a systematic review of studies on this topic (Restoux et al., 2020), challenges to sexual function were reported in a number of qualitative studies. These include erectile difficulty, decreased frequency of sexual activity, alterations in self-image and changes in romantic relationships. Sexual functioning is also impacted by pain, fatigue, fluctuations in the disease, embarrassment, and frustration. Sexual dysfunction may occur early in the disease process and has a significant impact on established and new relationships (Östlund, Björk, Valtersson, & Sverker, 2015).

Much of the research has focused on women who have a three-fold higher prevalence of sexual dysfunction than women without this condition (Puchner et al., 2019). Sexual dysfunction is due in part to the effects of pain and inflammation of the hips (Lavernia & Villa, 2016), shoulders, and knees that may preclude sexual intercourse due to pain and inflexibility. In one study, difficulty with sexual intercourse was associated with joint stiffness in 28% and pain in 18.5% (Dorner et al., 2018). However, other domains of sexual functioning are impacted including desire, arousal and lubrication, orgasm, and sexual satisfaction (Zhang et al., 2018). Depression may also play a role (Lin et al., 2017), much as it does in other chronic diseases.

Men with arthritis are twice more likely to experience sexual problems than their counterparts who do not have this condition (Zhao, Li, et al., 2018). Hand and finger pain may be a hindrance to men and impacts on their ability to use the man on top (missionary) position for intercourse (Östlund et al., 2015). Medications for arthritis, such as rituximab, may also play a role in sexual problems; however, this is often not shown in patient education material about the medication.

Relationship strain may occur due to the increased needs of the person with arthritis for help with daily activities. This can lead to the person with the condition being seen and treated as a patient by their partner rather than a sexual partner. Counseling for the couple as well as help with daily activities can be useful to mitigate the change in roles inherent in caring for someone who lives with mobility changes and pain. There are some strategies that can be helpful for sexual activity. These include adequate pain control as well as timing of medication to optimize comfort, using pillows, and adapting positions for sexual intercourse.

Communication with health care providers

Both men and women report that if a rheumatologist does not raise the topic of sexuality, they may not know if the sexual side effects they experience are related to the disease itself and whether this is something they can ask about (Helland, Dagfinrud, Haugen, Kjeken, & Zangi, 2017). Surgeons who perform joint replacement surgery almost never talk about this with their patients, especially with older patients (more than 60 years of age); however, older surgeons are more likely to discuss sexuality with their patients (Harmsen et al., 2017).

Neurologic disease

Both multiple sclerosis and Parkinson's disease, two common neurological conditions, are known to cause sexual dysfunction and relationship stress that itself impacts on sexuality for both the individual with the condition and their partner. In addition, the treatments for these conditions themselves cause sexual problems.

Multiple sclerosis

Sexual problems are common in both men and women with multiple sclerosis (MS), with 77% of men and 68% of women reporting some degree of sexual dysfunction (Petersen, Kristensen, Giraldi, & Giraldi, 2020). Associations between sexual dysfunction and MS include the age of the person with MS, poor quality of life, fatigue, incontinence, poor cognition, and worse physical function or disability (Polat Dunya, Tulek, Uchiyama, Haslam, & Panicker, 2020). Women have an almost two-fold increased risk of developing sexual problems (Zhao, Wang, et al., 2018) and problems increase with disease progression (Kisic-Tepavcevic et al., 2015); those with progressive MS experience worse sexual symptoms (Polat Dunya et al., 2020). However, the prevalence of sexual dysfunction in those with relapsing-remitting disease is also common with 41.8% of women experiencing loss of libido and 40.7% of men experiencing erectile dysfunction (Marck et al., 2016). While increased sexual dysfunction is seen in this population as they age, it has been reported in 70% of younger individuals with disease onset before the age of 42 (Calabrò et al., 2018). Women experience depression when sexual problems exist (Hösl et al., 2018) but the medications used to treat depression are themselves associated with sexual dysfunction (Marck et al., 2016). Fatigue is an important factor and as fatigue increases, so too does sexual dysfunction (Bartnik et al., 2017).

Relationships are also stressed by the illness in one of the couple with a 46% increased risk of relationship breakdown (Thormann et al., 2017). Relationships are negatively impacted by role changes due to physical disability, fatigue, depression, and decreased coping with the effects of the disease (Polat Dunya et al., 2020). Depression is related to relationship and sexual dissatisfaction as well as poor communication, particularly regarding sexual changes (Valvano et al., 2018). But some couples do thrive, and this appears to be related to the acceptance of the illness as well as the person with MS having a positive view of themselves (Wright & Kiropoulos, 2017). Similar attributes have been shown in the experience of spousal/partner care givers who accept the illness of a loved one and continue with their care-giving responsibilities due to the love and commitment that they feel. Despite this, challenges are part of the course of the disease with role changes and the need to undergo multiple losses (Appleton, Robertson, Mitchell, & Lesley, 2018).

Interventions to address sexual problems

Interventions to treat sexual problems in this population are limited. Counseling and supportive services are needed to address sexual dysfunction (Pöttgen et al., 2018) but these problems are often under-diagnosed (Delaney & Donovan, 2017). For men with erectile dysfunction, oral agents such as sildenafil, tadalafil, or vardenafil may be helpful but if the patient doesn't mention sexual problems, they will often go unaddressed; more individuals report bladder and bowel changes than sexual issues to their health care providers (Wang et al., 2018). There are, however, interventions that have shown promise in the mitigation of sexual dysfunction in women (Esteve-Ríos, Garcia-Sanjuan, Oliver-Roig, & Cabañero-Martínez, 2020); these include pelvic floor exercises, counseling, yoga, vibrators, and mindfulness-based psychoeducation. Using the PLISSIT model as a framework for counseling and referral was shown to be helpful in a single study (Khakbazan et al., 2016).

Individuals with MS want to know what sexual changes may occur with the disease so that they can anticipate and cope with the changes as well as prepare to find different ways of expressing their sexuality (Egerod, Wulff, & Petersen, 2018). A survey of Dutch urologists found that most do not screen for sexual dysfunction in women with MS (Scheepe, Alamyar, Pastoor, Hintzen, & Blok, 2017). Health care providers treating individuals with MS state that lack of time and knowledge are barriers to a conversation about sexuality in addition to the presence of family or friends at appointments (Tudor et al., 2018).

Parkinson's disease

Much like other chronic neurological diseases that affect motor function, Parkinson's disease (PD) can have a profound effect on sexuality and sexual function. Many individuals with PD experience some sort of sexual problem; this may be associated with medications such as beta-blockers and dopamine agonists used to mitigate the symptoms of the disease (Nasimbera et al., 2018) but co-morbidities commonly seen in older men may be part of the etiology (Ferrucci et al., 2016). Men with PD may experience a range of sexual problems including premature ejaculation that is particularly distressing and problems with orgasms for women are also reported as being most distressing (Jitkritsadakul, Jagota, & Bhidayasiri, 2015). Men may have higher libido than women with PD (Bronner et al., 2014) but decreased sexual interest is a common complaint of women across the lifespan and especially in women after menopause. Men and women with PD also experience depression; women commonly experience anxiety as well (Kotková & Weiss, 2013); both of these are commonly associated with decreased sexual function. A systematic review and meta-analysis suggest that men with PD are more likely to experience sexual dysfunction than women (Zhao et al., 2019) but single studies suggest high rates of sexual dysfunction in women (Varanda et al., 2016). Hypersexuality linked to impulse control is common in individuals treated with dopamine agonists as well as monoamine oxidase inhibitors type B (Reyes, Kurako, & Galvez-Jimenez, 2014). While sexual function may decline, the partner relationship may not and couples do report an increase in closeness (Buhmann et al., 2017).

Communication about sexual problems is limited with more men being counseled by neurologists than women (van Hees et al., 2017). Many of the same reasons for not having a discussion with patients have been reported (de Rooy et al., 2019) including not enough time and the patient not initiating the conversation.

Pain

Pain, acute or chronic, can cause alterations in sexual desire and frequency of sexual activity. Chronic pain is associated with fatigue, depression and anxiety, stress, and body image concerns; this is related to sexual problems in almost half of men and women (Finn, Morrison, & McGuire, 2018). There are certain conditions that by virtue of their anatomic location are the cause of significant impact on sexual functioning. Genito-pelvic pain affects both women and men and is the cause of a great deal of distress. Chronic widespread pain such as seen in individuals with fibromyalgia has some overlap with pelvic pain in women (Burri, Ogata, & Williams, 2017). Women with fibromyalgia report a global effect on sexuality with loss of libido, dyspareunia, decreased arousal, and pelvic floor dysfunction (Granero-Molina et al., 2018). In addition, body image is altered, and they fear the breakdown of their primary relationship. Because of the vague nature of the pain they suffer, they feel stigmatized and when consulting health care providers, their complaints are often trivialized and the impact on sexuality is ignored. Male partners are also affected (Romero-Alcalá et al., 2019); men have to face a new reality in their coupled sex life, and they report that they fear causing pain to their partner. In response, some men find that their desire decreases but they look for other ways to be physically connected.

Genito-pelvic pain in women

Genito-pelvic pain is often called vulvodynia which refers to vulvar pain of greater than three months duration without a clear cause. It can be localized or generalized, provoked or spontaneous, primary or secondary. The pain is usually described as burning, searing, and sharp (Pukall, 2016). The etiology of this pain may be related to inflammation, the use of oral contraceptives, recurrent yeast infections or pelvic floor dysfunction (S. Bergeron, N. O. Rosen, & C. R. Pukall 2020)(p. 182). It may also be the result of sexual trauma in childhood. Interpersonal factors are also involved; the relationship with the partner and their communication play a role as does the partner's response to the pain the woman experiences with genital touch or penetration. Central to the woman's experience of pain is anxiety that occurs before sexual activity as a consequence of this activity, and in the maintenance of the condition (p. 186). A great deal of distress is associated with this leading to avoidance of sexual as well as other touch, hypervigilance, and catastrophizing. Depression is not uncommon in women who live with this and may further influence both the woman's and her partner's response. It has been shown that on those days when the woman is feeling anxious or depressed, sexual activity results in pain and lower sexual function as well as greater sexual distress (Pâquet et al., 2018). Interstitial cystitis, a painful condition affecting the bladder and lower urinary tract, is also associated with sexual pain and dysfunction in women (Kim, Kim, & Yoon, 2019).

There is a lot of shame and guilt associated with this and some women have sex despite the pain that then leads to dissociation or a mind–body split (Shallcross, Dickson, Nunns, Mackenzie, & Kiemle, 2018). Some women report feeling invalidated by health care providers who told them their pain was psychosomatic and that nothing could be done for them (Braksmajer, 2018). Some women experience vulvar pain with arousal and this can be confusing; something that is pleasurable results in pain that is further compounded by friction and tissue trauma if sexual touch continues (Rosenbaum, Barnard, & Wilhite, 2015). Relationship distress may occur and as the woman continues to engage in sexual activity for her partner rather than for her own pleasure. Commonly these couples do not talk about what is happening and this increases the distress.

Assessment of sexual pain should include a comprehensive history of the pain and the cotton-swab test that is the standard assessment for provoked vestibulodynia. A complete medical and medication history should be taken and a physical examination as well as assessment of the pelvic floor is essential. Assessment of psychological functioning should also be done to identify anxiety and/or depression that may be amenable to treatment. Treatment options include pelvic floor physiotherapy, counseling, and as a last resort, vestibulectomy (Goldstein et al., 2016). Counseling for both the woman and the couple is essential to address the relationship and communication aspects of the condition. Women who experience sexual pain are more likely to judge themselves harshly and are not self-compassionate (sensitive to their own suffering) or may be unable to regulate their emotions to enable modification of their experience (Vasconcelos, Oliveira, & Nobre, 2020). Self-compassion may be protective of the couple and not just the woman experiencing sexual pain (Santerre-Baillargeon et al., 2018). It has also been suggested that empathy has a role to play; the empathetic responses to the partner's disclosure may decrease distress and increase sexual satisfaction in couples affected by female sexual pain (Bois et al., 2016).

Both cognitive behavioral therapy (CBT) and mindfulness-based cognitive therapy (MBCT) have been shown to be useful and it is important to individualize the counseling method for each woman (Brotto, Bergeron, Zdaniuk, & Basson, 2020). Compassion is a key aspect of mindfulness and this may in part play a role in the success of mindfulness-based therapy. It has also been shown that when women focus on their own sexual goals rather than on the partner's goals, pain is reduced. This self-focus may be hard for women to accept especially if they have been having sex to maintain the relationship or because they feel they have to (Corsini-Munt, Bergeron, & Rosen, 2020). The application of a cotton ball soaked in 4% aqueous lidocaine to the vulvar vestibule has been shown to reduce pain with penetration and reduction in sexual distress in survivors of breast cancer (Goetsch & Caughey, 2015) and this may be useful for women who experience pain with penetration.

Genito-pelvic pain in men

There has been less of a focus on pain in men although it is well known that chronic prostatitis and interstitial cystitis both cause genito-pelvic pain. Genito-pelvic pain in men is now termed urological chronic pelvic pain syndrome (UCPPS) with patterns of symptoms such as pelvic floor involvement similar to that of genito-pelvic pain in women (Bergeron, Pukall, Corsini-Munt, 2020, p. 187). Men who engage in anal intercourse may experience anodyspareunia, similar to the pain experienced by women with dyspareunia (p. 188). Men may also experience pain with orgasm (called dysorgasmia) (Clavell-Hernández, Martin, & Wang, 2018); this is not uncommon in men after surgery for prostate cancer and pain is reported in the penis, rectum, or abdomen.

Men who experience genito-pelvic pain report decreased desire, arousal, and orgasm and there is often some anticipation of failure before engaging in sex. The pain may also cause premature ejaculation as a way of 'getting it over quickly' especially in men who still engage in sex despite the pain (Pereira, Margarida Oliveira, & Nobre, 2016). Negative sexual thoughts are thought to mediate the relationship between sexual pain and sexual dysfunction (Pereira, Oliveira, & Nobre, 2018). Men with UCPPS also experience depression and their partners may experience their own sexual problems as well as depression (Smith, Pukall, Tripp, & Nickel, 2007). Psychological interventions are needed in a multi-disciplinary approach to management of male sexual pain.

Treatment of UCPPS may include analgesics or anti-biotics if an infectious cause is identified and if the pain does not resolve, referral for specialist care is advised including pain specialists, pelvic floor physiotherapy, and/or sex therapy (Rees, Abrahams, Doble, Cooper, & Group, 2015). Pelvic floor physiotherapy including soft tissue manipulation and myofascial release has been shown to help reduce baseline pelvic muscle tone that is an important element in genito-pelvic pain (Cohen, Gonzalez, & Goldstein, 2016). A Cochrane review (Franco et al., 2018) suggests that acupuncture may reduce pain but not the sexual dysfunction seen with this syndrome, and extracorporeal shock wave therapy may improve sexual dysfunction and pain but long-term studies are warranted.

Box 5.3 Case study

Martin and his partner Seth have been together for 10 years and were married a year ago in the presence of family and friends. Sex has always been important to them both but recently Seth began experiencing severe pain with orgasm. He tried to ignore this initially, but the pain did not go away and it was only when he had been avoiding sex with Martin for more than two weeks that he knew he had to do something about it. But he wasn't sure where to go for help. He was not 'out' to his primary care provider and didn't feel comfortable discussing this with him. Seth went to a community clinic that specialized in the care of gay and bisexual men, but Martin wasn't sure he wanted to go there either. He was scared that if someone he knew saw him there, they would think that he had HIV. This was a mess!

He looked up his symptoms on Google and from what he read, he thought he might have a urinary tract infection although he didn't have some of the symptoms that he read about. He wasn't going to the bathroom more than usual and his pain was mostly related to sex, or rather to orgasm. He finally went to a walk-in clinic close to his gym. He thought that if he saw someone he knew, he would tell them that he had hurt himself while working out. The wait was less than 20 minutes and he was taken into an examination room by a young guy who he thought he had seen at the gym. This made him nervous and he was about to leave when there was a knock on the door and a young woman appeared and introduced herself as the doctor on duty. Once again, he thought about running out of the clinic but then he reminded himself that Seth was going to ask him about why he was avoiding sex soon and he needed to find out what was wrong sooner rather than later.

Dr Bain took a thorough history and asked lots of questions. She thought it wasn't a urinary infection but just to be sure, she asked him to give a specimen of urine that would be sent for analysis. She sat quietly for a few minutes and then asked him if he had ever had a digital rectal examination. Martin felt himself go red in the face and he managed to stammer that no, he hadn't and why did she want to know that?

She explained that the pain he described might be due to infection of his prostate and again, Martin found himself completely embarrassed. Before he was even aware of it, he was lying on the examination bed and she was feeling around 'down there.' He nearly jumped off the table when she touched his prostate, even though she really was very gentle. It was over quite quickly, and soon he found himself leaving the clinic with a prescription in his hand. He has prostatitis and the doctor had told him that he would need to take the pills for a couple of months and that should clear things up. All he was left to wonder was how he was going to tell Seth what he had been hiding from him for weeks.

Conclusion

Chronic conditions affect all aspects of quality of life, including sexuality and sexual function. This chapter has highlighted the ways in which this occurs in the most common conditions in both men and women. There are limited interventions for the sexual problems that individuals and their partner face due to a paucity of research in this area. This doesn't mean that interventions won't work, just that research is needed.

References

Alay, I., Kaya, C., Karaca, I., Yildiz, S., Baghaki, S., Cengiz, H., ... Yasar, L. (2020). The effect of being diagnosed with human papillomavirus infection on women's sexual lives. *Journal of Medical Virology, 92*(8), 1290–1297. doi: 10.1002/jmv.25623

Annon, J. (1974). *The behavioral treatment of sexual problems*. Honolulu, HI: Enabling Systems.

Appleton, D., Robertson, N., Mitchell, L., & Lesley, R. (2018). Our disease: A qualitative meta-synthesis of the experiences of spousal/partner caregivers of people with multiple sclerosis. *Scandinavian Journal of Caring Sciences, 32*(4), 1262–1278. doi: 10.1111/scs.12601

Azagba, S., Shan, L., & Latham, K. (2019). Overweight and obesity among sexual minority adults in the United States. *International Journal of Environmental Research and Public Health, 16*(10). doi: 10.3390/ijerph16101828

Bąk, E., Marcisz, C., Krzemińska, S., Dobrzyn-Matusiak, D., Foltyn, A., & Drosdzol-Cop, A. (2017). Relationships of sexual dysfunction with depression and acceptance of illness in women and men with type 2 diabetes mellitus. *International Journal of Environmental Research and Public Health, 14*(9). doi: 10.3390/ijerph14091073

Bartnik, P., Wielgoś, A., Kacperczyk, J., Pisarz, K., Szymusik, I., Podlecka-Piętowska, A., ... Wielgoś, M. (2017). Sexual dysfunction in female patients with relapsing-remitting multiple sclerosis. *Brain and Behavior, 7*(6), e00699. doi: 10.1002/brb3.699

Bebb, R., Millar, A., & Brock, G. (2018). Sexual dysfunction and hypogonadism in men with diabetes. *Canadian Journal of Diabetes, 42*, Suppl. 1, S228–S233. doi: 10.1016/j.jcjd.2017.10.035

Becnel, J.N., Zeller, M.H., Noll, J.G., Sarwer, D.B., Reiter-Purtill, J., Michalsky, M., ... Biro, F.M. (2017). Romantic, sexual, and sexual risk behaviours of adolescent females with severe obesity. *Pediatric Obesity, 12*(5), 388–397. doi: 10.1111/ijpo.12155

Bell, C., Richardson, D., Wall, M., & Goldmeier, D. (2006). HIV-associated female sexual dysfunction – Clinical experience and literature review. *International Journal of STD and AIDS, 17*(10), 706–709. doi: 10.1258/095646206780071063

Bergeron, S., Rosen, N.O., & Pukall, C.R. (2020). Genital pain in women and men. In Y.M. Binik & K.S.K. Hall (Eds.), *Principles and practice of sex therapy* (6th ed., pp. 180–201). New York: The Guilford Press.

Bergeron, S.M., & Senn, C.Y. (1998). Body image and sociocultural norms. *Psychology of Women Quarterly, 22*(3), 385–401. doi: 10.1111/j.1471-6402.1998.tb00164.x

Bilgic, D., Gokyildiz, S., Kizilkaya Beji, N., Yalcin, O., & Gungor Ugurlucan, F. (2019). Quality of life and sexual function in obese women with pelvic floor dysfunction. *Women's Health, 59*(1), 101–113. doi: 10.1080/03630242.2018.1492497

Bois, K., Bergeron, S., Rosen, N., Mayrand, M.H., Brassard, A., & Sadikaj, G. (2016). Intimacy, sexual satisfaction, and sexual distress in vulvodynia couples: An observational study. *Health Psychology, 35*(6), 531–540. doi: 10.1037/hea0000289

Braksmajer, A. (2018). Struggles for medical legitimacy among women experiencing sexual pain: A qualitative study. *Women's Health, 58*(4), 419–433. doi: 10.1080/03630242.2017.1306606

Bronner, G., Cohen, O.S., Yahalom, G., Kozlova, E., Orlev, Y., Molshatzki, N., ... Hassin-Baer, S. (2014). Correlates of quality of sexual life in male and female patients with Parkinson disease and their partners. *Parkinsonism and Related Disorders, 20*(10), 1085–1088. doi: 10.1016/j.parkreldis.2014.07.003

Brotto, L.A., Bergeron, S., Zdaniuk, B., & Basson, R. (2020). Mindfulness and cognitive behavior therapy for provoked vestibulodynia: Mediators of treatment outcome and long-term effects. *Journal of Consulting and Clinical Psychology, 88*(1), 48–64. doi: 10.1037/ccp0000473

Buhmann, C., Dogac, S., Vettorazzi, E., Hidding, U., Gerloff, C., & Jürgens, T.P. (2017). The impact of Parkinson disease on patients' sexuality and relationship. *Journal of Neural Transmission (Vienna), 124*(8), 983–996. doi: 10.1007/s00702-016-1649-8

Burri, A., Ogata, S., & Williams, F. (2017). Female sexual pain: Epidemiology and genetic overlap with chronic widespread pain. *European Journal of Pain, 21*(8), 1408–1416. doi: 10.1002/ejp.1042

Byrne, M., Murphy, P., D'Eath, M., Doherty, S., & Jaarsma, T. (2017). Association between sexual problems and relationship satisfaction among people with cardiovascular disease. *Journal of Sexual Medicine, 14*(5), 666–674. doi: 10.1016/j.jsxm.2017.03.252

Caceres, B.A., Brody, A., Luscombe, R.E., Primiano, J.E., Marusca, P., Sitts, E.M., & Chyun, D. (2017). A systematic review of cardiovascular disease in sexual minorities. *American Journal of Public Health, 107*(4), e13–e21. doi: 10.2105/ajph.2016.303630

Caceres, B.A., Makarem, N., Hickey, K.T., & Hughes, T.L. (2019). Cardiovascular disease disparities in sexual minority adults: An examination of the behavioral risk factor surveillance system (2014–2016). *American Journal of Health Promotion, 33*(4), 576–585. doi: 10.1177/0890117118810246

Calabrò, R.S., Russo, M., Dattola, V., De Luca, R., Leo, A., Grisolaghi, J., … Quattrini, F. (2018). Sexual function in young individuals with multiple sclerosis: Does disability matter? *Journal of Neuroscience Nursing, 50*(3), 161–166. doi: 10.1097/jnn.0000000000000367

Calmasini, F.B., Klee, N., Webb, R.C., & Priviero, F. (2019). Impact of immune system activation and vascular impairment on male and female sexual dysfunction. *Sexual Medicine Reviews, 7*(4), 604–613. doi: 10.1016/j.sxmr.2019.05.005

Carlsson-Lalloo, E., Rusner, M., Mellgren, Å., & Berg, M. (2016). Sexuality and reproduction in HIV-positive women: A meta-synthesis. *AIDS Patient Care and STDs, 30*(2), 56–69. doi: 10.1089/apc.2015.0260

Cejtin, H.E. (2012). Care of the human immunodeficiency virus-infected menopausal woman. *American Journal of Obstetrics and Gynecology, 207*(2), 87–93. doi: 10.1016/j.ajog.2011.12.031

Cherick, F., Te, V., Anty, R., Turchi, L., Benoit, M., Schiavo, L., & Iannelli, A. (2019). Bariatric surgery significantly improves the quality of sexual life and self-esteem in morbidly obese women. *Obesity Surgery, 29*(5), 1576–1582. doi: 10.1007/s11695-019-03733-7

Cichocka, E., Jagusiewicz, M., & Gumprecht, J. (2020). Sexual dysfunction in young women with Type 1 diabetes. *International Journal of Environmental Research and Public Health, 17*(12), 4468.

Clavell-Hernández, J., Martin, C., & Wang, R. (2018). Orgasmic dysfunction following radical prostatectomy: Review of current literature. *Sexual Medicine Reviews, 6*(1), 124–134. doi: 10.1016/j.sxmr.2017.09.003

Cohen, D., Gonzalez, J., & Goldstein, I. (2016). The role of pelvic floor muscles in male sexual dysfunction and pelvic pain. *Sexual Medicine Reviews, 4*(1), 53–62. doi: 10.1016/j.sxmr.2015.10.001

Conason, A., McClure Brenchley, K.J., Pratt, A., & Geliebter, A. (2017). Sexual life after weight loss surgery. *Surgery for Obesity and Related Diseases, 13*(5), 855–861. doi: 10.1016/j.soard.2017.01.014

Corona, G., Giorda, C.B., Cucinotta, D., Guida, P., & Nada, E. (2014). Sexual dysfunction at the onset of type 2 diabetes: The interplay of depression, hormonal and cardiovascular factors. *Journal of Sexual Medicine, 11*(8), 2065–2073. doi: 10.1111/jsm.12601

Corona, G., Giorda, C.B., Cucinotta, D., Guida, P., & Nada, E. (2016). Sexual dysfunction in type 2 diabetes at diagnosis: Progression over time and drug and non-drug correlated factors. *PLOS ONE, 11*(10), e0157915. doi: 10.1371/journal.pone.0157915

Corona, G., Vignozzi, L., Sforza, A., Mannucci, E., & Maggi, M. (2015). Obesity and late-onset hypogonadism. *Molecular and Cellular Endocrinology, 418*(2), 120–133. doi: 10.1016/j.mce.2015.06.031

Corsini-Munt, S., Bergeron, S., & Rosen, N.O. (2020). Self-focused reasons for having sex: Associations between sexual goals and women's pain and sexual and psychological well-being for couples coping with provoked vestibulodynia. *Journal of Sexual Medicine, 17*(5), 975–984. doi: 10.1016/j.jsxm.2020.01.017

de Rooy, F.B.B., Buhmann, C., Schönwald, B., Martinez-Martin, P., Rodriguez-Blazquez, C., Putter, H., … van der Plas, A.A. (2019). Discussing sexuality with Parkinson's disease patients: A multinational survey among neurologists. *Journal of Neural Transmission (Vienna)*, *126*(10), 1273–1280. doi: 10.1007/s00702-019-02053-5

D'Eath, M., Byrne, M., Murphy, P., Jaarsma, T., McSharry, J., Murphy, A.W., … Casey, D. (2018). Participants' experiences of a sexual counseling intervention during cardiac rehabilitation: A nested qualitative study within the CHARMS pilot randomized controlled trial. *Journal of Cardiovascular Nursing*, *33*(5), E35–E45. doi: 10.1097/jcn.0000000000000482

Delaney, K.E., & Donovan, J. (2017). Multiple sclerosis and sexual dysfunction: A need for further education and interdisciplinary care. *NeuroRehabilitation*, *41*(2), 317–329. doi: 10.3233/nre-172200

Dorner, T.E., Berner, C., Haider, S., Grabovac, I., Lamprecht, T., Fenzl, K.H., & Erlacher, L. (2018). Sexual health in patients with rheumatoid arthritis and the association between physical fitness and sexual function: A cross-sectional study. *Rheumatology International*, *38*(6), 1103–1114. doi: 10.1007/s00296-018-4023-3

Dutton, G.R., Herman, K.G., Tan, F., Goble, M., Dancer-Brown, M., Van Vessem, N., & Ard, J.D. (2014). Patient and physician characteristics associated with the provision of weight loss counseling in primary care. *Obesity Research and Clinical Practice*, *8*(2), e123–e130. doi: 10.1016/j.orcp.2012.12.004

Egerod, I., Wulff, K., & Petersen, M.C. (2018). Experiences and informational needs on sexual health in people with epilepsy or multiple sclerosis: A focus group investigation. *Journal of Clinical Nursing*, *27*(13–14), 2868–2876. doi: 10.1111/jocn.14378

Eluri, S., Cross, R.K., Martin, C., Weinfurt, K.P., Flynn, K.E., Long, M.D., … Kappelman, M.D. (2018). Inflammatory bowel diseases can adversely impact domains of sexual function such as satisfaction with sex life. *Digestive Diseases and Sciences*, *63*(6), 1572–1582. doi: 10.1007/s10620-018-5021-8

Esteve-Ríos, A., Garcia-Sanjuan, S., Oliver-Roig, A., & Cabañero-Martínez, M.J. (2020). Effectiveness of interventions aimed at improving the sexuality of women with multiple sclerosis: A systematic review. *Clinical Rehabilitation*, *34*(4), 438–449. doi: 10.1177/0269215520901751

Faubion, S.S., Fairbanks, F., Kuhle, C.L., Sood, R., Kling, J.M., Vencill, J.A., … Kapoor, E. (2020). Association between body mass index and female sexual dysfunction: A cross-sectional study from the data registry on experiences of aging, menopause, and sexuality. *Journal of Sexual Medicine*, *17*(10), 1971–1980. doi: 10.1016/j.jsxm.2020.07.004

Ferrucci, R., Panzeri, M., Ronconi, L., Ardolino, G., Cogiamanian, F., Barbieri, S., … Priori, A. (2016). Abnormal sexuality in Parkinson's disease: Fact or fancy? *Journal of the Neurological Sciences*, *369*, 5–10. doi: 10.1016/j.jns.2016.07.058

Finn, E., Morrison, T.G., & McGuire, B.E. (2018). Correlates of sexual functioning and relationship satisfaction among men and women experiencing chronic pain. *Pain Medicine*, *19*(5), 942–954. doi: 10.1093/pm/pnx056

Franco, J.V., Turk, T., Jung, J.H., Xiao, Y.T., Iakhno, S., Garrote, V., & Vietto, V. (2018). Non-pharmacological interventions for treating chronic prostatitis/chronic pelvic pain syndrome. *Cochrane Database of Systematic Reviews*, *5*(5), Cd012551. doi: 10.1002/14651858.CD012551.pub3

Fugl-Meyer, K.S., Nilsson, M.I., von Koch, L., & Ytterberg, C. (2019). Closeness and life satisfaction after six years for persons with stroke and spouses. *Journal of Rehabilitation Medicine*, *51*(7), 492–498. doi: 10.2340/16501977-2566

Gao, Z., Liang, Y., Deng, W., Qiu, P., Li, M., & Zhou, Z. (2020). Impact of bariatric surgery on female sexual function in obese patients: A meta-analysis. *Obesity Surgery*, *30*(1), 352–364. doi: 10.1007/s11695-019-04240-5

Glina, F.P.A., de Freitas Barboza, J.W., Nunes, V.M., Glina, S., & Bernardo, W.M. (2017). What is the impact of bariatric surgery on erectile function? A systematic review and meta-analysis. *Sexual Medicine Reviews*, *5*(3), 393–402. doi: 10.1016/j.sxmr.2017.03.008

Goedel, W.C., Krebs, P., Greene, R.E., & Duncan, D.T. (2017). Associations between perceived weight status, body dissatisfaction, and self-objectification on sexual sensation seeking and sexual risk behaviors among men who have sex with men using Grindr. *Behavioral Medicine*, *43*(2), 142–150. doi: 10.1080/08964289.2015.1121130

Goetsch, M.L., & Caughey, A. (2015). A practical solution for dyspareunia in breast cnacer survivors: A randomized controlled trial. *Journal of Clinical Oncology*, *33*(30), 3394–3400. doi: 10.1200/ JCO.2014.60.7366

Goldstein, A.T., Pukall, C.F., Brown, C., Bergeron, S., Stein, A., & Kellogg-Spadt, S. (2016). Vulvodynia: Assessment and treatment. *Journal of Sexual Medicine*, *13*(4), 572–590. doi: 10.1016/j. jsxm.2016.01.020

Granero-Molina, J., Matarín Jiménez, T.M., Ramos Rodríguez, C., Hernández-Padilla, J.M., Castro-Sánchez, A.M., & Fernández-Sola, C. (2018). Social support for female sexual dysfunction in fibromyalgia. *Clinical Nursing Research*, *27*(3), 296–314. doi: 10.1177/1054773816676941

Green, J.M., Shields, M., Sevik, A., Palevsky, M., Fine, P., Arnold, M., & WeisbrodR. (2012). Renal provider perceptions and practice patterns regarding the management of pain, sexual dysfunction, and depression in hemodialysis patients. *Journal of Palliative Medicine*, *15*(2), 163–167. doi: 10.1089/jpm.2011.0284

Griffiths, S., Brennan, L., O'Gorman, B., Goedel, W.C., Sheffield, J., Bastian, B., & Barlow, F.K. (2018). Experiences of weightism among sexual minority men: Relationships with Body Mass Index, body dissatisfaction, and psychological quality of life. *Social Science and Medicine*, *214*, 35–40. doi: 10.1016/j.socscimed.2018.08.018

Gudzune, K.A., Beach, M.C., Roter, D.L., & Cooper, L.A. (2013). Physicians build less rapport with obese patients. *Obesity (Silver Spring, Md)*, *21*(10), 2146–2152. doi: 10.1002/oby.20384

Günzler, C., Kriston, L., Harms, A., & Berner, M.M. (2009). Association of sexual functioning and quality of partnership in patients in cardiovascular rehabilitation–A gender perspective. *Journal of Sexual Medicine*, *6*(1), 164–174. doi: 10.1111/j.1743-6109.2008.01039.x

Haapa, T., Suominen, T., Paavilainen, E., & Kylmä, J. (2018). Experiences of living with a sexually transmitted disease: An integrative review. *Scandinavian Journal of Caring Sciences*, *32*(3), 999–1011. doi: 10.1111/scs.12549

Hackett, G., Krychman, M., Baldwin, D., Bennett, N., El-Zawahry, A., Graziottin, A., … Incrocci, L. (2016). Coronary heart disease, diabetes, and sexuality in men. *Journal of Sexual Medicine*, *13*(6), 887–904. doi: 10.1016/j.jsxm.2016.01.023

Han, J.J., Beltran, T.H., Song, J.W., Klaric, J., & Choi, Y.S. (2017). Prevalence of genital human papillomavirus infection and human papillomavirus vaccination rates among US adult men: National Health and Nutrition Examination Survey (NHANES) 2013–2014. *JAMA Oncology*, *3*(6), 810–816. doi: 10.1001/jamaoncol.2016.6192

Harmsen, R.T.E., Nicolai, M.P.J., Den Oudsten, B.L., Putter, H., Haanstra, T.M., Nolte, P.A., … Elzevier, H. (2017). Patient sexual function and hip replacement surgery: A survey of surgeon attitudes. *International Orthopaedics*, *41*(12), 2433–2445. doi: 10.1007/s00264-017-3473-7

Helland, Y., Dagfinrud, H., Haugen, M.I., Kjeken, I., & Zangi, H. (2017). Patients' perspectives on information and communication about sexual and relational issues in Rheumatology Health Care. *Musculoskeletal Care*, *15*(2), 131–139. doi: 10.1002/msc.1149

Ho, J.H., Adam, S., Azmi, S., Ferdousi, M., Liu, Y., Kalteniece, A., … Soran, H. (2019). Male sexual dysfunction in obesity: The role of sex hormones and small fibre neuropathy. *PLOS ONE*, *14*(9), e0221992. doi: 10.1371/journal.pone.0221992

Ho, T.M., & Fernández, M. (2006). Patient's sexual health: Do we care enough? *Journal of Renal Care*, *32*(4), 183–186. doi: 10.1111/j.1755-6686.2006.tb00019.x

Holley, J.L., & Schmidt, R.J. (2010). Sexual dysfunction in CKD. *American Journal of Kidney Diseases*, *56*(4), 612–614. doi: 10.1053/j.ajkd.2010.07.006

Hösl, K.M., Deutsch, M., Wang, R., Roy, S., Winder, K., Niklewski, G., … Hilz, M.J. (2018). Sexual dysfunction seems to trigger depression in female multiple sclerosis patients. *European Neurology*, *80*(1–2), 34–41. doi: 10.1159/000492126

Jitkritsadakul, O., Jagota, P., & Bhidayasiri, R. (2015). Postural instability, the absence of sexual intercourse in the past month, and loss of libido are predictors of sexual dysfunction in Parkinson's disease. *Parkinsonism and Related Disorders*, *21*(1), 61–67. doi: 10.1016/j.parkreldis.2014.11.003

Jowett, A., Peel, E., & Shaw, R.L. (2012). Sex and diabetes: A thematic analysis of gay and bisexual men's accounts. *Journal of Health Psychology, 17*(3), 409–418. doi: 10.1177/1359105311412838

Kable, A., James, C., Snodgrass, S., Plotnikoff, R., Guest, M., Ashby, S., … Collins, C. (2015). Nurse provision of healthy lifestyle advice to people who are overweight or obese. *Nursing and Health Sciences, 17*, 451–459. doi: 10.1111/nhs.12214

Katz, A. (2017). Obesity and sexual dysfunction: Making the connection. *American Journal of Nursing, 117*(10), 45–50. doi: 10.1097/01.NAJ.0000525873.36360.5a

Kelly, R. (2007). Lesbian body image perceptions.*The context of body silence. Qualitative Health Research, 17*(7), 873–883. doi: 10.1177/1049732307306172

Khakbazan, Z., Daneshfar, F., Behboodi-Moghadam, Z., Nabavi, S.M., Ghasemzadeh, S., & Mehran, A. (2016). The effectiveness of the Permission, Limited Information, Specific suggestions, Intensive Therapy (PLISSIT) model based sexual counseling on the sexual function of women with multiple sclerosis who are sexually active. *Multiple Sclerosis and Related Disorders, 8*, 113–119. doi: 10.1016/j.msard.2016.05.007

Kim, S.J., Kim, J., & Yoon, H. (2019). Sexual pain and IC/BPS in women. *BMC Urology, 19*(1), 47. doi: 10.1186/s12894-019-0478-0

Kinsky, S., Stall, R., Hawk, M., & Markovic, N. (2016). Risk of the metabolic syndrome in sexual minority women: Results from the Esther study. *Journal of Women's Health (Larchmt), 25*(8), 784–790. doi: 10.1089/jwh.2015.5496

Kisic-Tepavcevic, D., Pekmezovic, T., Trajkovic, G., Stojsavljevic, N., Dujmovic, I., Mesaros, S., & Drulovic, J. (2015). Sexual dysfunction in multiple sclerosis: A 6-year follow-up study. *Journal of the Neurological Sciences, 358*(1–2), 317–323. doi: 10.1016/j.jns.2015.09.023

Kizilay, F., Gali, H.E., & Serefoglu, E.C. (2017). Diabetes and sexuality. *Sexual Medicine Reviews, 5*(1), 45–51. doi: 10.1016/j.sxmr.2016.07.002

Kogure, G.S., Ribeiro, V.B., Lopes, I.P., Furtado, C.L.M., Kodato, S., Silva de Sá, M.F., … Maria Dos Reis, R. (2019). Body image and its relationships with sexual functioning, anxiety, and depression in women with polycystic ovary syndrome. *Journal of Affective Disorders, 253*, 385–393. doi: 10.1016/j.jad.2019.05.006

Kolbe, N., Kugler, C., Schnepp, W., & Jaarsma, T. (2016). Sexual counseling in patients with heart failure: A silent phenomenon: Results from a convergent parallel mixed method study. *Journal of Cardiovascular Nursing, 31*(1), 53–61. doi: 10.1097/jcn.0000000000000215

Kotková, P., & Weiss, P. (2013). Psychiatric factors related to sexual functioning in patients with Parkinson's disease. *Clinical Neurology and Neurosurgery, 115*(4), 419–424. doi: 10.1016/j.clineuro.2012.06.020

Krychman, M.L. (2015). Obesity and sexual function. *Menopause, 22*(11), 1151–1152. doi: 10.1097/gme.0000000000000539

Kwon, S., & Schafer, M.H. (2017). Obesity and sexuality among older couples: Evidence from the national social life, health, and aging project. *Journal of Aging and Health, 29*(5), 735–768. doi: 10.1177/0898264316645541

Lake, J.E., Stanley, T.L., Apovian, C.M., Bhasin, S., Brown, T.T., Capeau, J., … Erlandson, K.M. (2017). Practical review of recognition and management of obesity and lipohypertrophy in human immunodeficiency virus infection. *Clinical Infectious Diseases, 64*(10), 1422–1429. doi: 10.1093/cid/cix178

Lavernia, C.J., & Villa, J.M. (2016). High rates of interest in sex in patients with hip arthritis. *Clinical Orthopaedics and Related Research, 474*(2), 293–299. doi: 10.1007/s11999-015-4421-8

Lee, Y., Dang, J.T., Switzer, N., Yu, J., Tian, C., Birch, D.W., & Karmali, S. (2019). Impact of bariatric surgery on male sex hormones and sperm quality: A systematic review and meta-analysis. *Obesity Surgery, 29*(1), 334–346. doi: 10.1007/s11695-018-3557-5

Leenhardt, R., Rivière, P., Papazian, P., Nion-Larmurier, I., Girard, G., Laharie, D., & Marteau, P. (2019). Sexual health and fertility for individuals with inflammatory bowel disease. *World Journal of Gastroenterology, 25*(36), 5423–5433. doi: 10.3748/wjg.v25.i36.5423

Lever, S., & Pryor, J. (2017). The impact of stroke on female sexuality. *Disability and Rehabilitation, 39*(20), 2011–2020. doi: 10.1080/09638288.2016.1213897

Levine, G.N., Steinke, E.E., Bakaeen, F.G., Bozkurt, B., Cheitlin, M.D., Conti, J.B., … Stewart, W.J. (2012). Sexual activity and cardiovascular disease. *Circulation, 125*(8), 1058–1072. doi: 10.1161/CIR.0b013e3182447787

Lin, M.C., Lu, M.C., Livneh, H., Lai, N.S., Guo, H.R., & Tsai, T.Y. (2017). Factors associated with sexual dysfunction in Taiwanese females with rheumatoid arthritis. *BMC Women's Health, 17*(1), 12. doi: 10.1186/s12905-017-0363-5

Loh, H.H., Yee, A., Loh, H.S., Kanagasundram, S., Francis, B., & Lim, L.-L. (2020). Sexual dysfunction in polycystic ovary syndrome: A systematic review and meta-analysis. *Hormones, 19*(3), 413–423. doi: 10.1007/s42000-020-00210-0

López-Medina, I.M., Gil-García, E., Sánchez-Criado, V., & Pancorbo-Hidalgo, P.L. (2016). Patients' experiences of sexual activity following myocardial ischemia. *Clinical Nursing Research, 25*(1), 45–66. doi: 10.1177/1054773814534440

Luo, L., Deng, T., Zhao, S., Li, E., Liu, L., Li, F., … Zhao, Z. (2017). Association between HIV infection and prevalence of erectile dysfunction: A systematic review and meta-analysis. *Journal of Sexual Medicine, 14*(9), 1125–1132. doi: 10.1016/j.jsxm.2017.07.001

Luo, L., Xiao, C., Xiang, Q., Zhu, Z., Liu, Y., Wang, J., … Zhao, Z. (2020). Significant increase of sexual dysfunction in patients with renal failure receiving renal replacement therapy: A systematic review and meta-analysis. *Journal of Sexual Medicine, 17*, 2382–2393. doi: 10.1016/j.jsxm.2020.08.019

Marck, C.H., Jelinek, P.L., Weiland, T.J., Hocking, J.S., De Livera, A.M., Taylor, K.L., … Jelinek, G.A. (2016). Sexual function in multiple sclerosis and associations with demographic, disease and lifestyle characteristics: An international cross-sectional study. *BMC Neurology, 16*(1), 210. doi: 10.1186/s12883-016-0735-8

Marín, L., Mañosa, M., Garcia-Planella, E., Gordillo, J., Zabana, Y., Cabré, E., & Domènech, E. (2013). Sexual function and patients' perceptions in inflammatory bowel disease: A case-control survey. *Journal of Gastroenterology, 48*(6), 713–720. doi: 10.1007/s00535-012-0700-2

McCaffery, K., Waller, J., Nazroo, J., & Wardle, J. (2006). Social and psychological impact of HPV testing in cervical screening: A qualitative study. *Sexually Transmitted Infections, 82*(2), 169–174. doi: 10.1136/sti.2005.016436

McGrath, M., Lever, S., McCluskey, A., & Power, E. (2019). Developing interventions to address sexuality after stroke: Findings from a four-panel modified Delphi study. *Journal of Rehabilitation Medicine, 51*(5), 352–360. doi: 10.2340/16501977-2548

Mercan, R., Mercan, S., Durmaz, B., Sur, H., Kilciksiz, C.M., Kacar, A.S., … Ata, B. (2019). Sexual dysfunction in women with human papilloma virus infection in the Turkish population. *Journal of Obstetrics and Gynaecology, 39*(5), 659–663. doi: 10.1080/01443615.2018.1547694

Miner, M., Esposito, K., Guay, A., Montorsi, P., & Goldstein, I. (2012). Cardiometabolic risk and female sexual health: The Princeton III summary. *Journal of Sexual Medicine, 9*(3), 641–651; quiz 652. doi: 10.1111/j.1743-6109.2012.02649.x

Miner, M., Parish, S.J., Billups, K.L., Paulos, M., Sigman, M., & Blaha, M.J. (2019). Erectile dysfunction and subclinical cardiovascular disease. *Sexual Medicine Reviews, 7*(3), 455–463. doi: 10.1016/j.sxmr.2018.01.001

Monaghan, M., Helgeson, V., & Wiebe, D. (2015). Type 1 diabetes in young adulthood. *Current Diabetes Reviews, 11*(4), 239–250. doi: 10.2174/1573399811666150421114957

Nackers, L.M., Appelhans, B.M., Segawa, E., Janssen, I., Dugan, S.A., & Kravitz, H.M. (2015). Associations between body mass index and sexual functioning in midlife women: The study of women's health across the nation. *Menopause, 22*(11), 1175–1181. doi: 10.1097/gme.0000000000000452

Nagele, E., Reich, O., Greimel, E., Dorfer, M., Haas, J., & Trutnovsky, G. (2016). Sexual activity, psychosexual distress, and fear of progression in women with human papillomavirus-related premalignant genital lesions. *Journal of Sexual Medicine, 13*(2), 253–259. doi: 10.1016/j.jsxm.2015.12.012

Narasimhan, M., Payne, C., Caldas, S., Beard, J.R., & Kennedy, C.E. (2016). Ageing and healthy sexuality among women living with HIV. *Reproductive Health Matters, 24*(48), 43–51. doi: 10.1016/j.rhm.2016.11.001

Nasimbera, A., Rosales, J., Silva, B., Alonso, R., Bohorquez, N., Lepera, S., ... Rodriguez, G.E. (2018). Everything you always wanted to know about sex and neurology: Neurological disability and sexuality. *Arquivos de Neuro-Psiquiatria, 76*(7), 430–435. doi: 10.1590/0004-282x20180061

Navaneethan, S.D., Vecchio, M., Johnson, D.W., Saglimbene, V., Graziano, G., Pellegrini, F., ... Strippoli, G.F.M. (2010). Prevalence and correlates of self-reported sexual dysfunction in CKD: A meta-analysis of observational studies. *American Journal of Kidney Diseases, 56*(4), 670–685. doi: 10.1053/j.ajkd.2010.06.016

Newlin Lew, K., Dorsen, C., & Long, T. (2018). Prevalence of obesity, prediabetes, and diabetes in sexual minority men: Results from the 2014 behavioral risk factor surveillance system. *Diabetes Educator, 44*(1), 83–93. doi: 10.1177/0145721717749943

Nilsson, M.I., Fugl-Meyer, K., von Koch, L., & Ytterberg, C. (2017). Experiences of sexuality six years after stroke: A qualitative study. *Journal of Sexual Medicine, 14*(6), 797–803. doi: 10.1016/j.jsxm.2017.04.061

Östlund, G., Björk, M., Valtersson, E., & Sverker, A. (2015). Lived experiences of sex life difficulties in men and women with early RA - The Swedish TIRA Project. *Musculoskeletal Care, 13*(4), 248–257. doi: 10.1002/msc.1105

Palefsky, J.M. (2010). Human papillomavirus-related disease in men: Not just a women's issue. *Journal of Adolescent Health, 46*(4), Suppl., S12–S19. doi: 10.1016/j.jadohealth.2010.01.010

Panza, E., Olson, K., Goldstein, C.M., Selby, E.A., & Lillis, J. (2020). Characterizing lifetime and daily experiences of weight stigma among sexual minority women with overweight and obesity: A descriptive study. *International Journal of Environmental Research and Public Health, 17*(13). doi: 10.3390/ijerph17134892

Pâquet, M., Rosen, N.O., Steben, M., Mayrand, M.H., Santerre-Baillargeon, M., & Bergeron, S. (2018). Daily anxiety and depressive symptoms in couples coping with vulvodynia: Associations with women's pain, women's sexual function, and both partners' sexual distress. *Journal of Pain, 19*(5), 552–561. doi: 10.1016/j.jpain.2017.12.264

Pereira, R., Margarida Oliveira, C., & Nobre, P. (2016). Sexual functioning and cognitions during sexual activity in men with genital pain: A comparative study. *Journal of Sex and Marital Therapy, 42*(7), 602–615. doi: 10.1080/0092623x.2015.1113582

Pereira, R., Oliveira, C.M., & Nobre, P.J. (2018). Pain intensity and sexual functioning in men with genital pain: The mediation role of sexually related thoughts. *Journal of Sex and Marital Therapy, 44*(3), 238–248. doi: 10.1080/0092623x.2017.1405298

Petersen, M., Kristensen, E., Giraldi, L., & Giraldi, A. (2020). Sexual dysfunction and mental health in patients with multiple sclerosis and epilepsy. *BMC Neurology, 20*(1), 41. doi: 10.1186/s12883-020-1625-7

Pinhas-Hamiel, O., Tisch, E., Levek, N., Ben-David, R.F., Graf-Bar-El, C., Yaron, M., ... Lerner-Geva, L. (2017). Sexual lifestyle among young adults with type 1 diabetes. *Diabetes/Metabolism Research and Reviews, 33*(2), e2837. doi: 10.1002/dmrr.2837

Polat Dunya, C., Tulek, Z., Uchiyama, T., Haslam, C., & Panicker, J.N. (2020). Systematic review of the prevalence, symptomatology and management options of sexual dysfunction in women with multiple sclerosis. *Neurourology and Urodynamics, 39*(1), 83–95. doi: 10.1002/nau.24232

Polland, A., Davis, M., Zeymo, A., & Venkatesan, K. (2018). Comparison of correlated comorbidities in male and female sexual dysfunction: Findings from the third national survey of sexual attitudes and lifestyles (Natsal-3). *Journal of Sexual Medicine, 15*(5), 678–686. doi: 10.1016/j.jsxm.2018.02.023

Pontiroli, A.E., Cortelazzi, D., & Morabito, A. (2013). Female sexual dysfunction and diabetes: A systematic review and meta-analysis. *Journal of Sexual Medicine, 10*(4), 1044–1051. doi: 10.1111/jsm.12065

Pool, A.C., Kraschnewski, J.L., Cover, L.A., Lehman, E.B., Stuckey, H.L., Hwang, K.O., ... Sciamanna, C.N. (2014). The impact of physician weight discussion on weight loss in US adults. *Obesity Research and Clinical Practice, 8*(2), e131–e139. doi: 10.1016/j.orcp.2013.03.003

Pöttgen, J., Rose, A., van de Vis, W., Engelbrecht, J., Pirard, M., Lau, S., ... Köpke, S. (2018). Sexual dysfunctions in MS in relation to neuropsychiatric aspects and its psychological treatment: A scoping review. *PLOS ONE, 13*(2), e0193381. doi: 10.1371/journal.pone.0193381

Puchner, R., Sautner, J., Gruber, J., Bragagna, E., Trenkler, A., Lang, G., ... Pieringer, H. (2019). High burden of sexual dysfunction in female patients with rheumatoid arthritis: Results of a cross-sectional study. *Journal of Rheumatology, 46*(1), 19–26. doi: 10.3899/jrheum.171287

Pukall, C.F. (2016). Primary and secondary provoked vestibulodynia: A review of overlapping and distinct factors. *Sexual Medicine Reviews, 4*(1), 36–44. doi: 10.1016/j.sxmr.2015.10.012

Rees, J., Abrahams, M., Doble, A., Cooper, A., & Prostatitis Expert Reference Group. (2015). Diagnosis and treatment of chronic bacterial prostatitis and chronic prostatitis/chronic pelvic pain syndrome: A consensus guideline. *BJU International, 116*(4), 509–525. doi: 10.1111/bju.13101

Restoux, L.J., Dasariraju, S.R., Ackerman, I.N., Van Doornum, S., Romero, L., & Briggs, A.M. (2020). Systematic review of the impact of inflammatory arthritis on intimate relationships and sexual function. *Arthritis Care and Research, 72*(1), 41–62. doi: 10.1002/acr.23857

Reyes, D., Kurako, K., & Galvez-Jimenez, N. (2014). Rasagiline induced hypersexuality in Parkinson's disease. *Journal of Clinical Neuroscience, 21*(3), 507–508. doi: 10.1016/j.jocn.2013.04.021

Richards, A., Dean, R., Burgess, G.H., & Caird, H. (2016). Sexuality after stroke: An exploration of current professional approaches, barriers to providing support and future directions. *Disability and Rehabilitation, 38*(15), 1471–1482. doi: 10.3109/09638288.2015.1106595

Romero-Alcalá, P., Hernández-Padilla, J.M., Fernández-Sola, C., Coín-Pérez-Carrasco, M.D.R., Ramos-Rodríguez, C., Ruiz-Fernández, M.D., & Granero-Molina, J. (2019). Sexuality in male partners of women with fibromyalgia syndrome: A qualitative study. *PLOS ONE, 14*(11), e0224990. doi: 10.1371/journal.pone.0224990

Rosen, R.C., Catania, J.A., Ehrhardt, A.A., Burnett, A.L., Lue, T.F., McKenna, K., ... Stoff, D.M. (2006). REPORTS: The Bolger conference on PDE-5 inhibition and HIV risk: Implications for health policy and prevention. *Journal of Sexual Medicine, 3*(6), 960–975. doi: 10.1111/j.1743-6109.2006.00323.x

Rosenbaum, T.Y., Barnard, E., & Wilhite, M. (2015). Psychosexual aspects of vulvar disease. *Clinics in Obstetrics and Gynaecology, 58*(3), 551–555. doi: 10.1097/grf.0000000000000136

Rowland, D.L., McNabney, S.M., & Mann, A.R. (2017). Sexual function, obesity, and weight loss in men and women. *Sexual Medicine Reviews, 5*(3), 323–338. doi: 10.1016/j.sxmr.2017.03.006

Rundblad, L., Zwisler, A.D., Johansen, P.P., Holmberg, T., Schneekloth, N., & Giraldi, A. (2017). Perceived sexual difficulties and sexual counseling in men and women across heart diagnoses: A nationwide cross-sectional study. *Journal of Sexual Medicine, 14*(6), 785–796. doi: 10.1016/j.jsxm.2017.04.673

Rutte, A., van Splunter, M.M., van der Heijden, A.A., Welschen, L.M., Elders, P.J., Dekker, J.M., ... Nijpels, G. (2015). Prevalence and correlates of sexual dysfunction in men and women with Type 2 diabetes. *Journal of Sex and Marital Therapy, 41*(6), 680–690. doi: 10.1080/0092623x.2014.966399

Ryan, D.H., & Yockey, S.R. (2017). Weight loss and improvement in comorbidity: Differences at 5%, 10%, 15%, and over. *Current Obesity Reports, 6*(2), 187–194. doi: 10.1007/s13679-017-0262-y

Sadeghi-Nejad, H., Wasserman, M., Weidner, W., Richardson, D., & Goldmeier, D. (2010). Sexually transmitted diseases and sexual function. *Journal of Sexual Medicine, 7*(1), 389–413. doi: 10.1111/j.1743-6109.2009.01622.x

Santana, L.M., Perin, L., Lunelli, R., Inácio, J.F.S., Rodrigues, C.G., Eibel, B., & Goldmeier, S. (2019). Sexual dysfunction in women with hypertension: A systematic review and meta-analysis. *Current Hypertension Reports, 21*(3), 25. doi: 10.1007/s11906-019-0925-z

Santerre-Baillargeon, M., Rosen, N.O., Steben, M., Pâquet, M., Macabena Perez, R., & Bergeron, S. (2018). Does self-compassion benefit couples coping with vulvodynia? Associations with psychological, sexual, and relationship adjustment. *Clinical Journal of Pain, 34*(7), 629–637. doi: 10.1097/ajp.0000000000000579

Santos, A.N., Pascoal, P.M., & Barros, L. (2020). Sexuality in emerging adults with type 1 diabetes mellitus: An exploratory study using thematic analysis. *Journal of Sex and Marital Therapy, 46*(3), 234–245. doi: 10.1080/0092623X.2019.1682730

Sayuk, G.S., Gott, B.M., Nix, B.D., & Lustman, P.J. (2011). Improvement in sexual functioning in patients with type 2 diabetes and depression treated with bupropion. *Diabetes Care, 34*(2), 332–334. doi: 10.2337/dc10-1714

Scheepe, J.R., Alamyar, M., Pastoor, H., Hintzen, R.Q., & Blok, B.F. (2017). Female sexual dysfunction in multiple sclerosis: Results of a survey among Dutch urologists and patients. *Neurourology and Urodynamics, 36*(1), 116–120. doi: 10.1002/nau.22884

Shallcross, R., Dickson, J.M., Nunns, D., Mackenzie, C., & Kiemle, G. (2018). Women's subjective experiences of living with vulvodynia: A systematic review and meta-ethnography. *Archives of Sexual Behavior*, *47*(3), 577–595. doi: 10.1007/s10508-017-1026-1

Smith, K.B., Pukall, C.F., Tripp, D.A., & Nickel, J.C. (2007). Sexual and relationship functioning in men with chronic prostatitis/chronic pelvic pain syndrome and their partners. *Archives of Sexual Behavior*, *36*(2), 301–311. doi: 10.1007/s10508-006-9086-7

Stapinska-Syniec, A., Grabowska, K., Szpotanska-Sikorska, M., & Pietrzak, B. (2018). Depression, sexual satisfaction, and other psychological issues in women with polycystic ovary syndrome. *Gynecological Endocrinology*, *34*(7), 597–600. doi: 10.1080/09513590.2018.1427713

Steffen, K.J., King, W.C., White, G.E., Subak, L.L., Mitchell, J.E., Courcoulas, A.P., … Huang, A.J. (2019). Changes in sexual functioning in women and men in the 5 years after bariatric surgery. *JAMA Surgery*, *154*(6), 487–498. doi: 10.1001/jamasurg.2018.1162

Stein, R., Sardinha, A., & Araújo, C.G. (2016). Sexual activity and heart patients: A contemporary perspective. *Canadian Journal of Cardiology*, *32*(4), 410–420. doi: 10.1016/j.cjca.2015.10.010

Steinke, E.E., Jaarsma, T., Barnason, S.A., Byrne, M., Doherty, S., Dougherty, C.M., … Professions, A. (2013). Sexual counselling for individuals with cardiovascular disease and their partners: A consensus document from the American Heart Association and the ESC Council on Cardiovascular Nursing and Allied Professions (CCNAP). *European Heart Journal*, *34*(41), 3217–3235. doi: 10.1093/eurheartj/eht270

Svatikova, A., & Kopecky, S.L. (2020). Why and how cardiovascular screening should be implemented in sexual medicine practice: Erectile dysfunction and cardiovascular disease. *Journal of Sexual Medicine*, *17*(6), 1045–1048. doi: 10.1016/j.jsxm.2020.01.024

Tagliabue, M., Gottero, C., Zuffranieri, M., Negro, M., Carletto, S., Picci, R.L., … Ostacoli, L. (2011). Sexual function in women with type 1 diabetes matched with a control group: Depressive and psychosocial aspects. *Journal of Sexual Medicine*, *8*(6), 1694–1700. doi: 10.1111/j.1743-6109.2011.02262.x

Tamam, Y., Tamam, L., Akil, E., Yasan, A., & Tamam, B. (2008). Post-stroke sexual functioning in first stroke patients. *European Journal of Neurology*, *15*(7), 660–666. doi: 10.1111/j.1468-1331.2008.02184.x

Tariq, S., Delpech, V., & Anderson, J. (2016). The impact of the menopause transition on the health and wellbeing of women living with HIV: A narrative review. *Maturitas*, *88*, 76–83. doi: 10.1016/j.maturitas.2016.03.015

Theofilou, P.A. (2012). Sexual functioning in chronic kidney disease: The association with depression and anxiety. *Hemodialysis International*, *16*(1), 76–81. doi: 10.1111/j.1542-4758.2011.00585.x

Thompson, H.S., & Ryan, A. (2009). The impact of stroke consequences on spousal relationships from the perspective of the person with stroke. *Journal of Clinical Nursing*, *18*(12), 1803–1811. doi: 10.1111/j.1365-2702.2008.02694.x

Thormann, A., Sørensen, P.S., Koch-Henriksen, N., Thygesen, L.C., Laursen, B., & Magyari, M. (2017). Chronic comorbidity in multiple sclerosis is associated with lower incomes and dissolved intimate relationships. *European Journal of Neurology*, *24*(6), 825–834. doi: 10.1111/ene.13297

Thylén, I., & Brännström, M. (2015). Intimate relationships and sexual function in partnered patients in the year before and one year after a myocardial infarction: A longitudinal study. *European Journal of Cardiovascular Nursing*, *14*(6), 468–477. doi: 10.1177/1474515115571061

Tran, A., Kaplan, J.A., Austin, S.B., Davison, K., Lopez, G., & Agénor, M. (2020). "It's all outward appearance-based attractions": A qualitative study of body image among a sample of young gay and bisexual men. *Journal of Gay and Lesbian Mental Health*, *24*(3), 281–307. doi: 10.1080/19359705.2019.1706683

Tudor, K.I., Eames, S., Haslam, C., Chataway, J., Liechti, M.D., & Panicker, J.N. (2018). Identifying barriers to help-seeking for sexual dysfunction in multiple sclerosis. *Journal of Neurology*, *265*(12), 2789–2802. doi: 10.1007/s00415-018-9064-8

Valvano, A.K., Rollock, M.J.D., Hudson, W.H., Goodworth, M.R., Lopez, E., & Stepleman, L. (2018). Sexual communication, sexual satisfaction, and relationship quality in people with multiple sclerosis. *Rehabilitation Psychology*, *63*(2), 267–275. doi: 10.1037/rep0000203

van Ek, G.F., Gawi, A., Nicolai, M.P.J., Krouwel, E.M., Den Oudsten, B.L., Den Ouden, M.E.M., … Elzevier, H.W. (2018). Sexual care for patients receiving dialysis: A cross-sectional study identifying the role of nurses working in the dialysis department. *Journal of Advanced Nursing*, *74*(1), 128–136. doi: 10.1111/jan.13386

van Ek, G.F., Krouwel, E.M., Nicolai, M.P., Bouwsma, H., Ringers, J., Putter, H., … Elzevier, H.W. (2015). Discussing sexual dysfunction with chronic kidney disease patients: Practice patterns in the Office of the Nephrologist. *Journal of Sexual Medicine*, *12*(12), 2350–2363. doi: 10.1111/jsm.13062

van Ek, G.F., Krouwel, E.M., van der Veen, E., Nicolai, M.P.J., Ringers, J., Den Oudsten, B.L., … Elzevier, H.W. (2017). The discussion of sexual dysfunction before and after kidney transplantation from the perspective of the renal transplant surgeon. *Progress in Transplantation*, *27*(4), 354–359. doi: 10.1177/1526924817731885

van Hees, P.J., van der Plas, A.A., van Ek, G.F., Putter, H., Den Oudsten, B.L., den Ouden, M.E., & Elzevier, H.W. (2017). Discussing sexuality with patients with Parkinson's disease: A survey among Dutch neurologists. *Journal of Neural Transmission (Vienna)*, *124*(3), 361–368. doi: 10.1007/s00702-016-1655-x

Varanda, S., Ribeiro da Silva, J., Costa, A.S., Amorim de Carvalho, C., Alves, J.N., Rodrigues, M., & Carneiro, G. (2016). Sexual dysfunction in women with Parkinson's disease. *Movement Disorders*, *31*(11), 1685–1693. doi: 10.1002/mds.26739

Vasconcelos, P., Oliveira, C., & Nobre, P. (2020). Self-compassion, emotion regulation, and female sexual pain: A comparative exploratory analysis. *Journal of Sexual Medicine*, *17*(2), 289–299. doi: 10.1016/j.jsxm.2019.11.266

Vikan, J.K., Nilsson, M.I., Bushnik, T., Deng, W., Elessi, K., Frost-Bareket, Y., … Fugl-Meyer, K.S. (2019). Sexual health policies in stroke rehabilitation: A multi national study. *Journal of Rehabilitation Medicine*, *51*(5), 361–368. doi: 10.2340/16501977-2552

Wang, G., Marrie, R.A., Fox, R.J., Tyry, T., Cofield, S.S., Cutter, G.R., & Salter, A. (2018). Treatment satisfaction and bothersome bladder, bowel, sexual symptoms in multiple sclerosis. *Multiple Sclerosis and Related Disorders*, *20*, 16–21. doi: 10.1016/j.msard.2017.12.006

Wright, T.M., & Kiropoulos, L.A. (2017). Intimate relationship quality, self-concept and illness acceptance in those with multiple sclerosis. *Psychology, Health and Medicine*, *22*(2), 212–226. doi: 10.1080/13548506.2016.1238492

Yodchai, K., Hutchinson, A.M., & Oumtanee, A. (2018). Nephrology nurses' perceptions of discussing sexual health issues with patients who have end-stage kidney disease. *Journal of Renal Care*, *44*(4), 229–237. doi: 10.1111/jorc.12257

Zeller, M.H., Brown, J.L., Reiter-Purtill, J., Sarwer, D.B., Black, L., Jenkins, T.M., … Noll, J.G. (2019). Sexual behaviors, risks, and sexual health outcomes for adolescent females following bariatric surgery. *Surgery for Obesity and Related Diseases*, *15*(6), 969–978. doi: 10.1016/j.soard.2019.03.001

Zhang, Q., Zhou, C., Chen, H., Zhao, Q., Li, L., Cui, Y., & Shen, B. (2018). Rheumatoid arthritis is associated with negatively variable impacts on domains of female sexual function: Evidence from a systematic review and meta-analysis. *Psychology, Health and Medicine*, *23*(1), 114–125. doi: 10.1080/13548506.2017.1338738

Zhao, B., Hong, Z., Wei, Y., Yu, D., Xu, J., & Zhang, W. (2019). Erectile dysfunction predicts cardiovascular events as an independent risk factor: A systematic review and meta-analysis. *Journal of Sexual Medicine*, *16*(7), 1005–1017. doi: 10.1016/j.jsxm.2019.04.004

Zhao, S., Li, E., Wang, J., Luo, L., Luo, J., & Zhao, Z. (2018). Rheumatoid arthritis and risk of sexual dysfunction: A systematic review and metaanalysis. *Journal of Rheumatology*, *45*(10), 1375–1382. doi: 10.3899/jrheum.170956

Zhao, S., Wang, J., Liu, Y., Luo, L., Zhu, Z., Li, E., & Zhao, Z. (2018). Association between multiple sclerosis and risk of female sexual dysfunction: A systematic review and meta-analysis. *Journal of Sexual Medicine*, *15*(12), 1716–1727. doi: 10.1016/j.jsxm.2018.09.016

Zhao, S., Wang, J., Xie, Q., Luo, L., Zhu, Z., Liu, Y., … Zhao, Z. (2019). Parkinson's disease is associated with risk of sexual dysfunction in men but not in women: A systematic review and meta-analysis. *Journal of Sexual Medicine*, *16*(3), 434–446. doi: 10.1016/j.jsxm.2018.12.017

Zona, S., Guaraldi, G., Luzi, K., Beggi, M., Santi, D., Stentarelli, C., … Rochira, V. (2012). Erectile dysfunction is more common in young to middle–aged HIV–infected men than in HIV–uninfected men. *Journal of Sexual Medicine*, *9*(7), 1923–1930. doi: 10.1111/j.1743-6109.2012.02750.x

6   How mental illness affects sexuality

People who experience alterations in their emotional/mental well-being often experience altered sexual functioning. In addition, many of the medications prescribed to treat depression and/or anxiety have a deleterious effect on sexual functioning and this is often the reason why individuals stop taking their medication. Serious mental illness such as schizophrenia has a profound effect on sexuality and sexual functioning, which in turn impacts social and romantic relationships. Dementia too has both inhibitory and excitatory impacts on sexuality and this is of special importance for those in residential care.

Depression

Depression is common in society today with an estimated prevalence of 14% in the general population (Lim et al., 2018). Depression is associated with sexual dysfunction as well as increased sexual risk taking (Field et al., 2016). There appears to be a bi-directional association with women who experience sexual problems also experiencing depression (Merwin, O'Sullivan, & Rosen, 2017); the same has been found in men who have erectile dysfunction (Liu et al., 2018). In women, depression is also related to subjective perception of physical attractiveness and the presence of scars, both affect sexual functioning (Cihan & Cihan, 2019).

Pregnancy and the post-partum period are also associated with depression. Women who experience post-partum depression and/or anxiety are at risk of experiencing a decrease in sexual activity excluding the anticipated decrease related to fatigue, etc. (Faisal-Cury, Menezes, Quayle, Matijasevich, & Diniz, 2015). Women with a vaginal birth injury such as laceration or episiotomy are also more likely to be depressed and experience sexual problems (Asselmann, Hoyer, Wittchen, & Martini, 2016). Women with sexual dysfunction are also more likely to experience post-partum depression in the 24 months after having a baby (Chang, Lin, Lin, Shyu, & Lin, 2018).

Sexual minority individuals access medical care to deal with depression with bisexual women reporting the highest risk for both depression and anxiety (Björkenstam, Björkenstam, Andersson, Cochran, & Kosidou, 2017). Adolescents with depression are more likely to experience alterations in desire, arousal, and orgasm (Deumic et al., 2016), and female adolescents who are depressed may have more sexual partners exposing them to the potential of acquiring sexually transmitted infections (STIs) or becoming pregnant due to less condom use (Foley et al., 2019).

This evidence points to the importance of assessing for sexual problems in both men and women who are depressed and for depression in those who report sexual problems.

DOI: 10.4324/9781003145745-6

Sexual side effects of anti-depressants

Selective-serotonin reuptake inhibitors (SSRIs) and serotonin-norepinephrine reuptake inhibitors (SNRIs) are the most common drugs used to treat depression; however, they have a range of sexual side effects. There are differences between agents with fluoxetine (Khazaie, Rezaie, Rezaei Payam, & Najafi, 2015) and paroxetine (Jacobsen, Zhong, Nomikos, & Clayton, 2019) causing more sexual problems in some individuals than other medications in the same class such as vortioxetine (Jacobsen, Mahableshwarkar, Chen, Chrones, & Clayton, 2015). Side effects increase with higher doses and individuals may stop taking these medications due to the sexual side effects. It is very important to discuss the risks of these side effects with patients prior to initiating treatment because ignoring them may result in distrust and non-adherence and potentially adverse events related to severe depression.

Men

Common sexual side effects of the SSRIs in men include delayed ejaculation (Segraves & Balon, 2014) as well as erectile dysfunction and decreased desire. The exact mechanism of these side effects is not known but it is thought that activation of serotonergic pathways is involved. Bupropion does not involve these pathways and is known to cause the least side effects (Segraves & Balon, 2014). Potential interventions are shown below.

Box 6.1 Management of treatment-related sexual dysfunction in men (Segraves, 2007)

Waiting for tolerance to develop (not effective)
Dose reduction (not therapeutic for depression)
Drug holiday (may result in withdrawal symptoms)
Switching agents (bupropion, mirtazapine, nefazodone)
Oral medications to treat ED (sildenafil, tadalafil)
Testosterone supplementation for hypogonadal men (Amiaz et al., 2011)

Women

Sexual side effects in women include loss of desire, problems with arousal, and also delayed or absent orgasm (Lorenz, Rullo, & Faubion, 2016). Some women report persistent genital arousal that is painful and distressing (Coskuner, Culha, Ozkan, & Kaleagasi, 2018). There is some preliminary evidence that SSRI use in childhood may cause decreased sexual desire in adult women (Lorenz et al., 2016). There are limited interventions to mitigate these side effects. Anticipatory guidance and counseling are essential before treatment starts to build a trusting relationship where the woman knows she can voice her concerns about the changes she experiences that may impact negatively on her self-image and relationship(s).

> ### Box 6.2 Management of treatment-related sexual dysfunction in women (Lorenz et al., 2016)
>
> Adding bupropion to the SSRI regimen
> Switching agents (bupropion, mirtazapine)
> Encouraging regular physical activity
> Using a vibrator to increase arousal
> Scheduling sexual activity three times a week
> Sildenafil or testosterone (not FDA approved in women)

The sexual side effects of these medications essentially multiply the inherent sexual problems caused by depression itself; alterations in sexual functioning, especially loss of desire, are hallmarks of depression. There is some limited evidence that neutraceuticals may provide some relief. Saffron in capsule form has been shown to improve arousal, pain, and lubrication in women (Kashani et al., 2013) and erectile function in men (Modabbernia et al., 2012) taking fluoxetine with minimal side effects.

Post-SSRI syndrome

There is increasing evidence that the sexual side effects of the SSRIs persist despite the discontinuation of the medication; this is known as the post-SSRI syndrome. The sexual problems seen with these medications may persist for years after discontinuation (Reisman, 2017).

The symptoms experienced by men include loss of desire, erectile dysfunction, weak or absent orgasm, and importantly, loss of genital sensation/genital numbing (Healy, Le Noury, & Mangin, 2018). Genital anesthesia is not often reported in studies; however, it has been shown to occur within 30 minutes of taking the first dose, but patients appear to ignore this or at least not report it to their health care provider. Sixty percent of women and 49% of men report this; however, the mechanism by which this occurs is not known. Persistent genital arousal has been reported in women after discontinuing SSRIs (Goldmeier & Leiblum, 2006). This is painful, not relieved by orgasm, and highly distressing.

Mitigation of the symptoms of post-SSRI syndrome is anecdotal and includes investigation of hormonal imbalances and correction. Lifestyle modification (avoiding alcohol and drug abuse) is also suggested and prescribing bupropion may also be helpful (Reisman, 2017). Studies of adding medications in the 5HT agonist and antagonist class have not shown improvement and may impose additional sexual problems (Bala, Nguyen, & Hellstrom, 2018). Counseling for the patient and importantly the partner as well is recommended to increase understanding and improve communication between the couple.

There is some evidence that nutraceuticals may help mitigate some of these sexual side effects; however, more research is needed. This syndrome may not be well known and thus it is important to ask about the previous SSRI use in both men and women who complain about sexual dysfunction.

Box 6.3 Case study

Heather is a 44-year old hairdresser who has recently purchased her own salon, something that has been a lifelong dream. She was so happy to quit her last job that she stayed in only for the money. She managed to save enough for a down payment on her new salon, but it came at a price. She had endured years of what she described as harassment by the owner of that salon. While from the outside it looked like a great place to work, Heather's experience was nothing like that. The owner, George, had built the place up over the years from a one-man show to a luxurious looking salon with 10 full-time stylists. But what went on in the background would have shocked the customers.

Staff were allowed only one 20-minute break per shift and if they needed the restroom, well that was just too bad. The staff lounge, if you could call it that, was a narrow space right in the back of the salon where the restroom was located. Staff sat on crates under which bottles of shampoo and conditioner were stored. There was no privacy for anyone using the restroom and staff constantly complained about having to eat their lunch or snack in the space. George didn't care. He also held monthly meetings that the stylists had to attend even though they were not paid for this time. At these meetings he doled out the shared tips and berated the staff for not earning more tips. It was not unusual for someone to leave the meeting in tears.

The ongoing stress of working there led Heather to go on anti-depressants. It took a while for her to find the one that worked the best for her and while she noticed that the medication seemed to decrease her desire for sex, she brushed this off. It was either sex or her mental state and she needed to save money to get out of there. But she felt better on the medication and was not as stressed or depressed every day.

About a month after opening her salon she was able to hire another stylist, a young woman who had just completed her training and she had plans to offer an apprenticeship to a student. She talked to her nurse practitioner about stopping the medication; she had never told her about the impact on her sex life but now she did.

"Yeah, remember we talked about that when you first started ..."

Heather had no recollection of any conversation about that, but she remained silent.

"So, you need to do this slowly. You don't want to go into withdrawal and you also need to monitor your mood carefully. Let me write down how you should do this ... ."

Heather followed the instructions carefully. After a month she was off the medication and felt fine. She even felt like sex again, but this is when she discovered something she did not expect. She felt nothing when she and her partner Ben were fooling around, her 'down there' felt like rubber or like her cheeks after going for a root canal. And it didn't just happen once, it was every single time. What was this and why was it happening?

She talked to her nurse practitioner again who had never heard of anyone experiencing this. She promised to talk to her colleagues about this. A week later she called Heather to report that none of her colleagues knew about this, but she had done some reading in the medical literature and had found one article about this.

"So, what can I do about it?" asked Heather, her voice rising with frustration, "I'm really not happy ... . Just when things were going well for me professionally and now my sex life is a bust ..."

"Hang in there, Heather, please. There was something in the article that I read that might help ... You can try to use a vibrator ... every day for 10 minutes or so ... that may help. But honestly, there is nothing that I found that might help. I'm really sorry ..."

Heather didn't respond; her phone lay on the table and she sat there, her hands covering her face.

Major mental illness

Individuals living with schizophrenia, severe anxiety or obsessive-compulsive disorder are known to experience sexual problems from the condition itself as well as iatrogenic effects of medications. Sexual dysfunction and mental illness appears to be bi-directional; global sexual problems are seen in both men and women and as the severity of the mental illness increases, so too do the frequency and the severity of sexual dysfunction (Clayton & Balon, 2009).

Schizophrenia is a severe mental illness with significant deleterious effects on social and relationship functioning. Individuals with this condition are often unable to form stable relationships, including sexual relationships. These social problems impact on the ability of the person to maintain good couple functioning and relationship breakdown is common (Aggarwal, Grover, & Chakrabarti, 2019). Despite desiring romantic and sexual relationships, many people living with schizophrenia report that these are out of reach (Östman, 2014) in part because they see themselves as poor sexual partners (Wainberg et al., 2016). Stigma is often experienced by this population and has a negative impact on self-esteem (Bonfils, Firmin, Salyers, & Wright, 2015) and the ability to be involved in a relationship (Boucher, Groleau, & Whitley, 2016). Other barriers to relationships include the symptoms of the condition such as delusions and hallucinations. However, these individuals also see the development of sexual and romantic relationships as a sign of recovery.

While some individuals experience increased sexual desire in the acute psychotic phase, most people experience decreased sexual function (Trovão & Serefoglu, 2018). The role that anti-psychotic medications play in sexual dysfunction is significant (de Boer, Castelein, Wiersma, Schoevers, & Knegtering, 2015); risperidone and haloperidol are the main culprits but olanzapine and quetiapine also cause sexual side effects while aripiprazole appears to have the lowest sexual impact but there is contradictory evidence of which medications cause the worst problems (Basson & Gilks, 2018). Sexual side effects of these medications are known to persist over time. It has been shown that men experience worse side effects than women. In one study, 36% of men versus 19% of women reported distress related to the sexual problems they were experiencing (Montejo et al., 2010).

Patients who are institutionalized experience significant negative experiences related to sexual function. In one study of this population, 71% of men and 57% of women with schizophrenia reported negative effects on all aspects of sexual functioning (Acuña, Martín, Graciani, Cruces, & Gotor, 2010). It is unclear if this is influenced by the institutional setting that is vastly different from the community. One study of mental health providers showed that there is a preponderance of concern about the risk to the patient of sexual harm. Institutionalized patients were subject to a 'no sex on site' rule with the net result that they had to find places outside the facility to be sexual; this in fact resulted in high-risk sex in unsafe locations (Evans, Holmes, & Quinn, 2020).

Treatment for sexual dysfunction associated with anti-psychotics

Education about the association of anti-psychotic medication and sexual dysfunction is important once the acute psychotic symptoms abate. Ongoing education and encouragement to disclose sexual problems to health care providers is also important. Changing medication to one that has a lower impact such as olanzapine on sexual functioning may be helpful but is not always possible; lowering the dose of anti-psychotics should be done with caution. For men, prescribing a phosphodiesterase 5 inhibitor such as sildenafil may help with erections (McMillan et al., 2017; Schmidt et al., 2012).

Face-to-face counseling and cognitive behavioral therapy may be considered for those with stable disease and social skills training focused on dating and relationships may also be useful (Helu-Brown & Aranda, 2016).

Communication with health care providers

Despite individuals with schizophrenia saying that they would talk to their primary care provider about sexual problems, they were aware that these providers were generally too busy to engage with them about this (McCann, 2010). Sixty eight percent of psychiatrists in one study said they were not comfortable talking about this with patients; 69% said that they would prefer that patients disclose sexual problems first. Eighty eight percent felt that sexual function was important to patients but just 17% felt competent to raise the topic (Nnaji & Friedman, 2018). In another study, 73% of physicians and other staff including nurses, psychologists, social workers, and occupational therapists, did not ask their patients about sexual functioning due to feelings of incompetence (Tharoor, Kaliappan, & Gopal, 2015). Sexuality may be seen as 'peripheral' in caring for patients with severe mental illness in addition to being hard to talk about and not seen as the responsibility of the practitioners caring for these patients (Urry, Chur-Hansen, & Khaw, 2019).

Dementia

The number of people living with dementia continues to grow and with that comes challenges for family care givers who may struggle with the effects of cognitive impairment in their loved ones. Sexuality does not disappear with the onset of this decline but there are instances where sexual activity is problematic. All humans need touch and this fundamental is present for all humans, from birth to death and for many elderly individuals and couples, sexual functioning in the later years is not focused on sexual intercourse but rather on touch and tenderness. There is evidence that elderly people living in the community are more likely to engage in acts of tenderness if they do not have cognitive impairment (Freak-Poli, Licher, Ryan, Ikram, & Tiemeier, 2018). Dementia has a significant impact on couples with changed roles, alterations in reciprocity, changes in self-identity, and displays of affection (Holdsworth & McCabe, 2018). While sexual activity may decline or end, verbal and non-verbal communication of love may take on a different meaning. When the person with dementia is not able to express affection, the consequences for the partner may be significant. If the partner with dementia is no longer able to recognize the other person, any form of physical connection may be difficult due to feelings of loss and loss of the relationship.

For sexual minority men and women, there are additional challenges. Older individuals in this population have lived through a period of history where they were vilified, persecuted, and even prosecuted for something that was not a choice. Dementia essentially takes away an individual's personhood and may become their primary identity. Being gay or lesbian may risk the double stigma of cognitive decline or dementia and belonging to a marginalized population. The individual or couple may feel the need to once again 'go back into the closet' or conceal their sexuality or the changes in cognition resulting in ignorance of their sexuality (McParland & Camic, 2018). For those in residential care, fear of stigma and/or discrimination, may force them to hide their sexual identity and relationship. The assumption that residents are heterosexual, called heteronormativity, may further compound the challenges of living in residential facilities (Westwood, 2016). Others have expressed concerns about being separated from their partner and because they were in a same-sex relationship, they would be viewed and treated differently than heterosexual couples (Waling et al., 2019).

Sexual disinhibition

Some individuals with dementia may experience disinhibition and act inappropriately to meet their needs for touch and closeness. Cipriani and colleagues (Cipriani, Ulivi, Danti, Lucetti, & Nuti, 2016) state that most often, individuals with dementia withdraw and appear indifferent or apathetic to sexual touch and activity. However, some will display verbal or physical behavior of a sexual nature that is disturbing to others. In one study of family caregivers of people with dementia, 26% reported sexual disinhibition (Chapman, Tremont, Malloy, & Spitznagel, 2019) described as unwanted sexual advances to a spouse or child, aggressive sexual touching of self or partner, attempts to kiss or touch other people, the use of foul language suggestive of sexual acts, and anger when rebuffed or told to stop. Men are more likely to act in this manner (Canevelli et al., 2017) and this behavior tends to influence institutionalization when spouses or other family caregivers cannot carry the burden of caring for the individual any longer (Chapman, Tremont, Malloy, & Spitznagel, 2020).

Residential care

The attitudes of staff towards sexual activity in residential care will be discussed in the next section but residents themselves have a positive attitude to all forms of sexual expression, including sexual intercourse (Mahieu & Gastmans, 2015). Residents may have a partner who is living in the community and the couple's need for closeness and sexual activity does not necessarily change when one is in a different location. The partners of individuals with dementia who live in residential care homes have described the challenges of having a spouse in residential care and the challenges of maintaining closeness in these circumstances (Roelofs, Luijkx, & Embregts, 2019). Institutional barriers include the presence of cameras and the complete lack of privacy, shared rooms and bathrooms, and the attitudes of staff towards displays of affection. In residential facilities where there is a 'special' room for couples to spend time, the knowledge that others would know what they were doing was also embarrassing.

In a study of women in residential care, participants described still feeling desire but were limited in expressing this by fear of the response by staff and other residents, but also by their spouse (Palacios-Ceña et al., 2016).

Box 6.4 Using the PLISSIT model to discuss sexual needs of resident with family members

Permission: Something we talk to family members about when a loved one is admitted to our facility is the issue of residents establishing a romantic relationship with another resident. What are your thoughts about this?

Limited Information: We have guidelines and policy about sexual activity between couples or singles who are residents. We try to accommodate this as much as possible; however, you may have different opinions about this and we find it better to talk about this with you as well as with the resident. What questions do you have at this time?

Specific Suggestion: We work with the residents all the time to assess whether they are able to consent as well as refuse attention from another resident. This is not always easy as you can imagine. But this is the resident's home and we want them to be happy and fulfilled and to have meaning in their lives while they are here. We get to know the residents really well, and we pride ourselves on respecting the wishes of the residents. But we also work very hard to protect them and ensure that they are safe. What are your feelings about your mom being romantically involved with another resident should that happen?

Intensive Therapy: We have an ethics consultant who works with staff, families, and the resident where possible if a situation arises that anyone is uncomfortable with. Would you like to meet with the consultant to discuss any concerns or to get answers to any questions?

Attitudes of family and staff

Sexual activity remains of interest to elderly individuals, including those in residential care and those with dementia (Bauer, Haesler, & Fetherstonhaugh, 2016). Nursing staff vary in their perspective of sexuality in residents of nursing homes with some seeing this as a basic human right to others who see the elderly and especially those with dementia as asexual (Vandrevala, Chrysanthaki, & Ogundipe, 2017). This perspective influences their actions and reactions that may be one of facilitation of sexual activity of any kind or reporting to the family of the resident to seek permission to allow or forbid the relationship. Others may try to distract the residents or prevent or forbid the relationship completely. Assessment of the resident's sexual needs and sexual health may not occur at all or only when inappropriate or disruptive behavior occurred (McAuliffe, Bauer, Fetherstonhaugh, & Chenco, 2015). This suggests a problem-based rather than affirmative approach and appears to negate the needs of the resident and instead focuses on prevention of litigation or other negative impacts on the facility.

For some residents, the ability to consent to sexual activity of any kind may have been removed due to the legal power given to family members. In a powerful description of this (Frankowski & Clark, 2009), residents in an assisted-living facility were not allowed to engage in a relationship with a member of the opposite sex without the express permission of the family. Residents in assisted-living facilities are usually there because they need help with activities of daily living and often do not have dementia. Staff overruled the wishes of the resident about something that is the right of every adult. Staff often see relationships between residents as inherently problematic especially if one of them has dementia (Villar, Celdrán, Serrat, Fabà, & Martínez, 2018). While staff may be accepting of non-physical contact between residents, they are likely to separate them if they think that the relationship is physical (Wiskerke & Manthorpe, 2018). Staff may rely on their own experiences and attitudes in their acceptance or rejection of sexual expression by residents and the presence of dementia in one or both of the potential couple to be a risk. The competence of one or both residents is seen as an ethical issue that has to be considered in permitting any relationship to continue (Thys et al., 2019).

Education of staff is essential to protect the personhood of the residents. Staff are generally willing to attend educational initiatives; however, these tend to be of low priority for administration (Jones & Moyle, 2018). It has been shown that person-centered care has a positive impact on staff attitudes to sexual expression in residential homes (Roelofs, Luijkx, Cloin, & Embregts, 2019). When policies exist in institutions, they may be restrictive and risk-aversive leading to more negative attitudes of staff. However, there are certainly ethical issues to be considered regarding the ability to consent to sexual touch or activity.

Ethical issues

Biomedical ethics rests on four principles: respect for autonomy, beneficence, non-maleficence, and justice (Kontos, Grigorovich, Kontos, & Miller, 2016). In the context of residential care for an individual with dementia, how are these principles enacted? Autonomy concerns not just informed consent but also self-determination and the right to privacy. These rights of the individual are often restricted for residents by formal or informal policies. These include 'open door' policies where doors cannot be locked or even kept closed that prevents any displays of affection, as well as informing family about romantic relationships. Beneficence in this context means doing and promoting good. A romantic or sexual relationship may be good for the self-esteem and need for connection for a resident. Non-maleficence concerns the duty to protect the individual and preventing harm. While protecting someone from unwanted sexual advances is important, preventing them from being happy and living a meaningful, if restricted, life constitutes harm. Of course, if the resident poses a risk to others, their right to safety comes into play. The last principle, justice, refers to equal treatment and freedom from violence and discrimination; the latter applies to treating women differently from men in residential care, something that happens frequently. Men are often 'allowed' to make romantic advances to female residents but women are seen to need protection. Once again, protection of others must be considered (Victor & Guidry-Grimes, 2019).

When dealing with people living with dementia, these ethical principles and actions are not always clear. Assessment of the ability to consent is often made in the moment when a staff person sees some activity that is sexual. The response of the staff person may be based more on their own cultural and personal values than on ethical principles or policy. Residents may get mixed messages about what is acceptable and what is not. It is often difficult to know if consent for sexual activity has been given or if the resident knows that they can refuse. Assessment of capacity to consent to sexual activity of any kind requires a deep knowledge of the resident(s) and what they understand and are capable of doing in that situation (Hillman, 2017). The need for staff to make decisions in the moment without guidance or policy may lead to moral distress (Cook, Schouten, Henrickson, & McDonald, 2017). Staff may know more about the day-to-day life of the residents, their wishes, and capacity than their families and this can lead to conflict when family members have legal power over what the resident can and cannot do.

Steps to accommodate sexual activity in residential facilities include reviewing laws that apply in the particular jurisdiction. Education of staff, clear guidelines and policies about sexual activity for residents, as well as support from clinical ethicists can help to ensure that residents are not only protected but also allowed to make personal choices and live a happy life. Families also need education and support as they deal with the wishes of their loved ones that may cause them discomfort or challenge their values. An expert in human sexuality such as a sex therapist or sexuality counselor can provide guidance about resources for residents such as lubricants and other sexual aids to promote physical safety and pleasure (Metzger, 2017).

Conclusions

Mental illness has a significant impact on sexuality and sexual functioning and there is an iatrogenic component to this; many of the medications to treat depression and psychosis themselves cause sexual dysfunction. Dementia presents unique ethical challenges in the care of residents in facilities and these can be a cause of stress and conflict to staff and family members. But sexuality is an essential part of personhood and this does not diminish or disappear when mental status is affected.

References

Acuña, M.J., Martín, J.C., Graciani, M., Cruces, A., & Gotor, F. (2010). A comparative study of the sexual function of institutionalized patients with schizophrenia. *Journal of Sexual Medicine, 7*(10), 3414–3423. doi: 10.1111/j.1743-6109.2010.01832.x

Aggarwal, S., Grover, S., & Chakrabarti, S. (2019). A comparative study evaluating the marital and sexual functioning in patients with schizophrenia and depressive disorders. *Asian Journal of Psychiatry, 39*, 128–134. doi: 10.1016/j.ajp.2018.12.021

Amiaz, R., Pope, H.G., Jr., Mahne, T., Kelly, J.F., Brennan, B.P., Kanayama, G., … Seidman, S.N. (2011). Testosterone gel replacement improves sexual function in depressed men taking serotonergic antidepressants: A randomized, placebo-controlled clinical trial. *Journal of Sex and Marital Therapy, 37*(4), 243–254. doi: 10.1080/0092623x.2011.582425

Asselmann, E., Hoyer, J., Wittchen, H.-U., & Martini, J. (2016). Sexual problems during pregnancy and after delivery among women with and without anxiety and depressive disorders prior to pregnancy: A prospective-longitudinal study. *Journal of Sexual Medicine, 13*(1), 95–104. doi: 10.1016/j.jsxm.2015.12.005

Bala, A., Nguyen, H.M.T., & Hellstrom, W.J.G. (2018). Post-SSRI sexual dysfunction: A literature review. *Sexual Medicine Reviews, 6*(1), 29–34. doi: 10.1016/j.sxmr.2017.07.002

Basson, R., & Gilks, T. (2018). Women's sexual dysfunction associated with psychiatric disorders and their treatment. *Women's Health (Lond), 14*, 1745506518762664. doi: 10.1177/1745506518762664

Bauer, M., Haesler, E., & Fetherstonhaugh, D. (2016). Let's talk about sex: Older people's views on the recognition of sexuality and sexual health in the health-care setting. *Health Expectations, 19*(6), 1237–1250. doi: 10.1111/hex.12418

Björkenstam, C., Björkenstam, E., Andersson, G., Cochran, S., & Kosidou, K. (2017). Anxiety and depression among sexual minority women and men in Sweden: Is the risk equally spread within the sexual minority population? *Journal of Sexual Medicine, 14*(3), 396–403. doi: 10.1016/j.jsxm.2017.01.012

Bonfils, K.A., Firmin, R.L., Salyers, M.P., & Wright, E.R. (2015). Sexuality and intimacy among people living with serious mental illnesses: Factors contributing to sexual activity. *Psychiatric Rehabilitation Journal, 38*(3), 249–255. doi: 10.1037/prj0000117

Boucher, M.E., Groleau, D., & Whitley, R. (2016). Recovery and severe mental illness: The role of romantic relationships, intimacy, and sexuality. *Psychiatric Rehabilitation Journal, 39*(2), 180–182. doi: 10.1037/prj0000193

Canevelli, M., Lucchini, F., Garofalo, C., Talarico, G., Trebbastoni, A., D'Antonio, F., ... Bruno, G. (2017). Inappropriate sexual behaviors among community-dwelling patients with dementia. *American Journal of Geriatric Psychiatry, 25*(4), 365–371. doi: 10.1016/j.jagp.2016.11.020

Chang, S.R., Lin, W.A., Lin, H.H., Shyu, M.K., & Lin, M.I. (2018). Sexual dysfunction predicts depressive symptoms during the first 2 years postpartum. *Women and Birth, 31*(6), e403–e411. doi: 10.1016/j.wombi.2018.01.003

Chapman, K.R., Tremont, G., Malloy, P., & Spitznagel, M.B. (2019). Identification of sexual disinhibition in dementia by family caregivers. *Alzheimer Disease and Associated Disorders, 33*(2), 154–159. doi: 10.1097/wad.0000000000000302

Chapman, K.R., Tremont, G., Malloy, P., & Spitznagel, M.B. (2020). The role of sexual disinhibition to predict caregiver burden and desire to institutionalize among family dementia caregivers. *Journal of Geriatric Psychiatry and Neurology, 33*(1), 42–51. doi: 10.1177/0891988719856688

Cihan, A., & Cihan, E. (2019). Interrelation between appearance anxiety and sexual functions in women: The role of surgical scars, morphologic features, and accompanying depression. *Journal of Sexual Medicine, 16*(11), 1769–1778. doi: 10.1016/j.jsxm.2019.08.004

Cipriani, G., Ulivi, M., Danti, S., Lucetti, C., & Nuti, A. (2016). Sexual disinhibition and dementia. *Psychogeriatrics, 16*(2), 145–153. doi: 10.1111/psyg.12143

Clayton, A.H., & Balon, R. (2009). Continuing medical education: The impact of mental illness and psychotropic medications on sexual functioning: The evidence and management (CME). *Journal of Sexual Medicine, 6*(5), 1200–1211. doi: 10.1111/j.1743-6109.2009.01255.x

Cook, C., Schouten, V., Henrickson, M., & McDonald, S. (2017). Ethics, intimacy and sexuality in aged care. *Journal of Advanced Nursing, 73*(12), 3017–3027. doi: 10.1111/jan.13361

Coskuner, E.R., Culha, M.G., Ozkan, B., & Kaleagasi, E.O. (2018). Post-SSRI sexual dysfunction: Preclinical to clinical. Is it fact or fiction? *Sexual Medicine Reviews, 6*(2), 217–223. doi: 10.1016/j.sxmr.2017.11.004

de Boer, M.K., Castelein, S., Wiersma, D., Schoevers, R.A., & Knegtering, H. (2015). The facts about sexual (dys)function in schizophrenia: An overview of clinically relevant findings. *Schizophrenia Bulletin, 41*(3), 674–686. doi: 10.1093/schbul/sbv001

Deumic, E., Butcher, B.D., Clayton, A.D., Dindo, L.N., Burns, T.L., & Calarge, C.A. (2016). Sexual functioning in adolescents with major depressive disorder. *Journal of Clinical Psychiatry, 77*(7), 957–962. doi: 10.4088/JCP.15m09840

Evans, A.M., Holmes, D., & Quinn, C. (2020). Madness, sex, and risk: A poststructural analysis. *Nursing Inquiry, 27*(4), e12359. doi: 10.1111/nin.12359

Faisal-Cury, A., Menezes, P.R., Quayle, J., Matijasevich, A., & Diniz, S.G. (2015). The relationship between mode of delivery and sexual health outcomes after childbirth. *Journal of Sexual Medicine, 12*(5), 1212–1220. doi: 10.1111/jsm.12883

Field, N., Prah, P., Mercer, C.H., Rait, G., King, M., Cassell, J.A., ... Sonnenberg, P. (2016). Are depression and poor sexual health neglected comorbidities? Evidence from a population sample. *BMJ, (Open), 6*(3), e010521. doi: 10.1136/bmjopen-2015-010521

Foley, J.D., Vanable, P.A., Brown, L.K., Carey, M.P., DiClemente, R.J., Romer, D., & Valois, R.F. (2019). Depressive symptoms as a longitudinal predictor of sexual risk behaviors among African-American adolescents. *Health Psychology, 38*(11), 1001–1009. doi: 10.1037/hea0000780

Frankowski, A.C., & Clark, L.J. (2009). Sexuality and intimacy in assisted living: Residents' perspectives and experiences. *Sexuality Resaerch and Social Policy, 6*(4), 25–37.

Freak-Poli, R., Licher, S., Ryan, J., Ikram, M.A., & Tiemeier, H. (2018). Cognitive impairment, sexual activity and physical tenderness in community-dwelling older adults: A cross-sectional exploration. *Gerontology, 64*(6), 589–602. doi: 10.1159/000490560

Goldmeier, D.L., & Leiblum, S.R. (2006). Persistent genital arousal in women – A new syndrome entity. *International Journal of STD and AIDS, 17*(4), 215–216.

Healy, D., Le Noury, J., & Mangin, D. (2018). Enduring sexual dysfunction after treatment with antidepressants, 5α-reductase inhibitors and isotretinoin: 300 Cases. *International Journal of Risk and Safety in Medicine, 29*(3–4), 125–134. doi: 10.3233/jrs-180744

Helu-Brown, P., & Aranda, M. (2016). Psychosocial approaches for sexual health and intimate relationships among patients with serious mental illness. *Sexual Medicine Reviews, 4*(1), 26–35. doi: 10.1016/j.sxmr.2015.10.010

Hillman, J. (2017). Sexual consent capacity: Ethical issues and challenges in long-term care. *Clinical Gerontologist, 40*(1), 43–50. doi: 10.1080/07317115.2016.1185488

Holdsworth, K., & McCabe, M. (2018). The impact of dementia on relationships, intimacy, and sexuality in later life couples: An integrative qualitative analysis of existing literature. *Clinical Gerontologist, 41*(1), 3–19. doi: 10.1080/07317115.2017.1380102

Jacobsen, P., Zhong, W., Nomikos, G., & Clayton, A. (2019). Paroxetine, but not vortioxetine, impairs sexual functioning compared with placebo in healthy adults: A randomized, controlled trial. *Journal of Sexual Medicine, 16*(10), 1638–1649. doi: 10.1016/j.jsxm.2019.06.018

Jacobsen, P.L., Mahableshwarkar, A.R., Chen, Y., Chrones, L., & Clayton, A.H. (2015). Effect of vortioxetine vs. escitalopram on sexual functioning in adults with well-treated major depressive disorder experiencing SSRI-induced sexual dysfunction. *Journal of Sexual Medicine, 12*(10), 2036–2048. doi: 10.1111/jsm.12980

Jones, C., & Moyle, W. (2018). Are gerontological nurses ready for the expression of sexuality by individuals with dementia? *Journal of Gerontological Nursing, 44*(5), 2–4. doi: 10.3928/00989134-20180413-01

Kashani, L., Raisi, F., Saroukhani, S., Sohrabi, H., Modabbernia, A., Nasehi, A.-A., … Akhondzadeh, S. (2013). Saffron for treatment of fluoxetine-induced sexual dysfunction in women: Randomized double-blind placebo-controlled study. *Human Psychopharmacology: Clinical and Experimental, 28*(1), 54–60. doi: 10.1002/hup.2282

Khazaie, H., Rezaie, L., Rezaei Payam, N., & Najafi, F. (2015). Antidepressant-induced sexual dysfunction during treatment with fluoxetine, sertraline and trazodone; a randomized controlled trial. *General Hospital Psychiatry, 37*(1), 40–45. doi: 10.1016/j.genhosppsych.2014.10.010

Kontos, P., Grigorovich, A., Kontos, A.P., & Miller, K.L. (2016). Citizenship, human rights, and dementia: Towards a new embodied relational ethic of sexuality. *Dementia (London), 15*(3), 315–329. doi: 10.1177/1471301216636258

Lim, G.Y., Tam, W.W., Lu, Y., Ho, C.S., Zhang, M.W., & Ho, R.C. (2018). Prevalence of depression in the community from 30 countries between 1994 and 2014. *Scientific Reports, 8*(1), 2861–2861. doi: 10.1038/s41598-018-21243-x

Liu, Q., Zhang, Y., Wang, J., Li, S., Cheng, Y., Guo, J., … Zhu, Z. (2018). Erectile dysfunction and depression: A systematic review and meta-analysis. *Journal of Sexual Medicine, 15*(8), 1073–1082. doi: 10.1016/j.jsxm.2018.05.016

Lorenz, T., Rullo, J., & Faubion, S. (2016). Antidepressant-induced female sexual dysfunction. *Mayo Clinic Proceedings, 91*(9), 1280–1286. doi: 10.1016/j.mayocp.2016.04.033

Mahieu, L., & Gastmans, C. (2015). Older residents' perspectives on aged sexuality in institutionalized elderly care: A systematic literature review. *International Journal of Nursing Studies, 52*, 1891–1905. doi: 10.1016/j.ijnurstu.2015.07.007

McAuliffe, L., Bauer, M., Fetherstonhaugh, D., & Chenco, C. (2015). Assessment of sexual health and sexual needs in residential aged care. *Australasian Journal on Ageing, 34*(3), 183–188. doi: 10.1111/ajag.12181

McCann, E. (2010). Investigating mental health service user views regarding sexual and relationship issues. *Journal of Psychiatric and Mental Health Nursing, 17*(3), 251–259. doi: 10.1111/j.1365-2850.2009.01509.x

McMillan, E., Adan Sanchez, A., Bhaduri, A., Pehlivan, N., Monson, K., Badcock, P., … O'Donoghue, B. (2017). Sexual functioning and experiences in young people affected by mental health disorders. *Psychiatry Research, 253*, 249–255. doi: 10.1016/j.psychres.2017.04.009

McParland, J., & Camic, P.M. (2018). How do lesbian and gay people experience dementia? *Dementia (London), 17*(4), 452–477. doi: 10.1177/1471301216648471

Merwin, K.E., O'Sullivan, L.F., & Rosen, N.O. (2017). We need to talk: Disclosure of sexual problems is associated with depression, sexual functioning, and relationship satisfaction in women. *Journal of Sex and Marital Therapy, 43*(8), 786–800. doi: 10.1080/0092623x.2017.1283378

Metzger, E. (2017). Ethics and intimate sexual activity in long-term care. *AMA Journal of Ethics, 19*(7), 640–648. doi: 10.1001/journalofethics.2017.19.7.ecas1-1707

Modabbernia, A., Sohrabi, H., Nasehi, A.-A., Raisi, F., Saroukhani, S., Jamshidi, A., ... Akhondzadeh, S. (2012). Effect of saffron on fluoxetine-induced sexual impairment in men: Randomized double-blind placebo-controlled trial. *Psychopharmacology (Berlin), 223*(4), 381–388. doi: 10.1007/s00213-012-2729-6

Montejo, Á.L., Majadas, S., Rico-Villademoros, F., Llorca, G., De La Gándara, J., Franco, M., ... for the Spanish Working Group for the Study of Psychotropic-Related Sexual, D. (2010). Frequency of sexual dysfunction in patients with a psychotic disorder receiving antipsychotics. *Journal of Sexual Medicine, 7*(10), 3404–3413. doi: 10.1111/j.1743-6109.2010.01709.x

Nnaji, R.N., & Friedman, T. (2018). Sexual dysfunction and schizophrenia: Psychiatrists' attitudes and training needs. *Psychiatric Bulletin, 32*(6), 208–210. doi: 10.1192/pb.bp.107.016162

Östman, M. (2014). Low satisfaction with sex life among people with severe mental illness living in a community. *Psychiatry Research, 216*(3), 340–345. doi: 10.1016/j.psychres.2014.02.009

Palacios-Ceña, D., Martínez-Piedrola, R.M., Pérez-de-Heredia, M., Huertas-Hoyas, E., Carrasco-Garrido, P., & Fernández-de-Las-Peñas, C. (2016). Expressing sexuality in nursing homes. The experience of older women: A qualitative study. *Geriatric Nursing, 37*(6), 470–477. doi: 10.1016/j.gerinurse.2016.06.020

Reisman, Y. (2017). Sexual consequences of post-SSRI syndrome. *Sexual Medicine Reviews, 5*(4), 429–433. doi: 10.1016/j.sxmr.2017.05.002

Roelofs, T.S., Luijkx, K.G., & Embregts, P.J. (2019). Love, intimacy and sexuality in residential dementia care: A spousal perspective. *Dementia (London), 18*(3), 936–950. doi: 10.1177/1471301217697467

Roelofs, T.S.M., Luijkx, K.G., Cloin, M.C.M., & Embregts, P. (2019). The influence of organizational factors on the attitudes of residential care staff toward the sexuality of residents with dementia. *BMC Geriatrics, 19*(1), 8. doi: 10.1186/s12877-018-1023-9

Schmidt, H.M., Hagen, M., Kriston, L., Soares-Weiser, K., Maayan, N., & Berner, M.M. (2012). Management of sexual dysfunction due to antipsychotic drug therapy. *Cochrane Database of Systematic Reviews, 11*(11), Cd003546. doi: 10.1002/14651858.CD003546.pub3

Segraves, R.T. (2007). Sexual dysfunction associated with antidepressant therapy. *Urologic Clinics of North America, 34*(4), 575–579. doi: 10.1016/j.ucl.2007.08.003

Segraves, R.T., & Balon, R. (2014). Antidepressant-induced sexual dysfunction in men. *Pharmacology, Biochemistry, and Behavior, 121*, 132–137. doi: 10.1016/j.pbb.2013.11.003

Tharoor, H., Kaliappan, A., & Gopal, S. (2015). Sexual dysfunctions in schizophrenia: Professionals and patients perspectives. *Indian Journal of Psychiatry, 57*(1), 85–87. doi: 10.4103/0019-5545.148532

Thys, K., Mahieu, L., Cavolo, A., Hensen, C., Dierckx de Casterlé, B., & Gastmans, C. (2019). Nurses' experiences and reactions towards intimacy and sexuality expressions by nursing home residents: A qualitative study. *Journal of Clinical Nursing, 28*(5–6), 836–849. doi: 10.1111/jocn.14680

Trovão, J.N., & Serefoglu, E.C. (2018). Neurobiology of male sexual dysfunctions in psychiatric disorders: The cases of depression, anxiety, mania and schizophrenia. *International Journal of Impotence Research, 30*(6), 279–286. doi: 10.1038/s41443-018-0077-8

Urry, K., Chur-Hansen, A., & Khaw, C. (2019). 'It's just a peripheral issue': A qualitative analysis of mental health clinicians' accounts of. (Not) addressing sexuality in their work. *International Journal of Mental Health Nursing, 28*(6), 1278–1287. doi: 10.1111/inm.12633

Vandrevala, T., Chrysanthaki, T., & Ogundipe, E. (2017). "Behind closed doors with open minds?": A qualitative study exploring nursing home staff's narratives towards their roles and duties within the context of sexuality in dementia. *International Journal of Nursing Studies, 74*, 112–119. doi: 10.1016/j.ijnurstu.2017.06.006

Victor, E., & Guidry-Grimes, L. (2019). Relational autonomy in action: Rethinking dementia and sexuality in care facilities. *Nursing Ethics, 26*(6), 1654–1664. doi: 10.1177/0969733018780527

Villar, F., Celdrán, M., Serrat, R., Fabà, J., & Martínez, T. (2018). Staff's reactions towards partnered sexual expressions involving people with dementia living in long-term care facilities. *Journal of Advanced Nursing*, *74*(5), 1189–1198. doi: 10.1111/jan.13518

Wainberg, M.L., Cournos, F., Wall, M.M., Norcini Pala, A., Mann, C.G., Pinto, D., … McKinnon, K. (2016). Mental illness sexual stigma: Implications for health and recovery. *Psychiatric Rehabilitation Journal*, *39*(2), 90–96. doi: 10.1037/prj0000168

Waling, A., Lyons, A., Alba, B., Minichiello, V., Barrett, C., Hughes, M., … Edmonds, S. (2019). Experiences and perceptions of residential and home care services among older lesbian women and gay men in Australia. *Health and Social Care in the Community*, *27*(5), 1251–1259. doi: 10.1111/hsc.12760

Westwood, S. (2016). Dementia, women and sexuality: How the intersection of ageing, gender and sexuality magnify dementia concerns among lesbian and bisexual women. *Dementia (London)*, *15*(6), 1494–1514. doi: 10.1177/1471301214564446

Wiskerke, E., & Manthorpe, J. (2018). New relationships and intimacy in long-term care: The views of relatives of residents with dementia and care home staff. *Dementia (London)*, *17*(4), 405–422. doi: 10.1177/1471301216647814

7 Trauma and sexual dysfunction

Trauma, physical and/or mental, has a profound effect on sexual functioning for both men and women. Since the wars in Iraq and Afghanistan, sexual problems have been recognized as a direct result of physical and mental trauma experienced by combat veterans. Genito-urinary damage from improvised explosive devices (IEDs) has obvious repercussions for sexual functioning. The ubiquitous experience of post-traumatic stress syndrome (PTSD) as well as traumatic brain injury (TBI) also affect sexuality by altering personality; this has a significant impact on the veteran's sexual partner(s).

Sexual assault is another kind of trauma that affects all aspects of sexuality; this includes military sexual trauma that has been recognized as having far-reaching implications. Childhood sexual abuse has long-lasting effects on sexual development and adult sexual functioning. Sexual assault affects women more than men, but the consequences for both are far reaching in the impact on the individuals' and couple's sexual relationship.

PTSD and sexual function

Post-traumatic stress disorder (PTSD) is a complex condition that may occur after experiencing or witnessing a traumatic event such as a serious accident, combat, or sexual assault. It is characterized by intrusive thoughts, avoidance of reminders of the initial trauma, negative emotions and thoughts, and altered reactions to a variety of stimuli (Benedek, 2020). Yehuda and colleagues (Yehuda, Lehrner, & Rosenbaum, 2015) suggest that sexual dysfunction is mediated by PTSD through biological, cognitive, and emotional processes. Sexual behavior is controlled by hormonal and neurologic networks and these are the same that are involved in PTSD. Both sexual activity and PTSD are arousal states, but sexual activity requires the inhibition of fear and threats. If the brain is not able to differentiate between fear/threats and sexual arousal, persistence of PTSD-related hypervigilance may be experienced, and this has a negative impact on sexual activity. For example, sexual sensations causing arousal are interpreted as a threat and the 'fight or flight' response is engaged (Yehuda et al., 2015).

The symptoms of PTSD run counter to the vulnerability and loss of control that are the key aspects of healthy sexuality. Individuals with PTSD who avoid sex, something that is not uncommon, may be exhibiting a sub-conscious avoidance of physical and emotional vulnerability that is essential for the experience of emotional connection. Loss of control is essential to the experience of orgasm and if the individual is hypervigilant, a symptom of PTSD, then the person may be unable to experience orgasm. Sexual pleasure is replaced by feelings of helplessness and lack of control, something that is experienced as negative. Another symptom of PTSD, emotional numbing, has a significant impact on relationships. Emotional numbing is characterized by detachment from others, a limited range of emotions, and loss

DOI: 10.4324/9781003145745-7

of interest in life in general (Nunnink, Goldwaser, Afari, Nievergelt, & Baker, 2010). The individual who experiences this will have difficulty in feeling and expressing love, joy, and connection and this has a negative effect on relationships.

PTSD and sexual dysfunction in the military

Studies have been conducted investigating the prevalence and symptoms of sexual dysfunction among combat veterans who served in Afghanistan and Iraq. Most of the studies involved men; however, there is some limited data on female service members. It is recognized that combat veterans are at risk for sexual dysfunction due to physical injury, traumatic brain injury, and PTSD.

In one study (Beaulieu et al., 2015), 18% of veterans who attended a routine post-deployment clinic reported sexual difficulties. Of note is that in this study, 10% of the veterans were women. Other factors associated with sexual dysfunction were depression and PTSD that was identified in 56% of the sample. Alcohol abuse was reported by 27% and depression by 31%. Another study (Badour, Gros, Szafranski, & Acierno, 2015) found that 12% of the male veterans who presented for treatment of PTSD symptoms reported erectile dysfunction (ED). This is noteworthy as the population of veterans is young, with a mean age of 34.9 years. In another study (Wilcox, Redmond, & Hassan, 2014), 33% of veterans reported erectile problems. The men in this study were 36–40 years old and the rate of ED was twice that seen in civilian men over 40 years of age. Veterans who reported poor mental health and who had experienced traumatic life events and/or relationship distress were more likely to report sexual problems.

Loss of sexual desire is also common in veterans with PTSD (Bentsen, Giraldi, Kristensen, & Andersen, 2015); this may be associated with the erectile dysfunction as a reaction to not being able to be aroused. It may also reflect the use of anti-depressants, anti-psychotics, and other medications prescribed for the management of PTSD that are known to cause sexual dysfunction. A qualitative study of male combat veterans describes global sexual problems in addition to ED and loss of desire (Helmer et al., 2015). These include early- and delayed ejaculation and distraction that contributes to both ED and orgasm disorders. The men described that their sexual problems negatively impacted on how they saw themselves and also had an impact on their romantic partners. Some of the men said that it was just easier to masturbate than engage in partnered sexual activity. Most men had tried to resolve their sexual problems by using medication or herbal remedies, viewing pornography, or using sex toys, usually with little effect.

When one member of a couple experiences PTSD that affects sexual functioning, the partner is going to be affected (Bachem, Levin, & Solomon, 2020). Alcohol use, anti-social behavior, PTSD, and depression are known to influence the partner relationship. While not clearly described, all of these will affect the couple's sexual relationship and may be linked to infidelity and relationship breakdown (Riviere, Merrill, Thomas, Wilk, & Bliese, 2012). Emotional numbing and emotional detachment is common with PTSD and this can cause relationship stress (Richardson et al., 2019). The partner may interpret this distancing as something that they caused and attempts to connect emotionally and/or physically may be met with anger and verbal or physical aggression.

Female veterans experience unique challenges on deployment including lack of social support, sexual trauma, and lack of privacy for personal hygiene. They also report PTSD symptoms, depression, and poor mental health that affect sexual functioning. In one study, 27% reported painful intercourse (Sadler, Mengeling, Fraley, Torner, & Booth, 2012). Female veterans are more likely to use health care services for mental health problems including depression and PTSD than their male counterparts and are also more likely to be hospitalized for mental illness (Sairsingh, Solomon, Helstrom, & Treglia, 2017).

Many veterans experience depression in addition to PTSD and the 'invisible' wounds of war, primarily traumatic brain injury (TBI). Polytrauma is common with explosive devices that result in loss of limb(s), burns, and traumatic brain injury in addition to the potential for loss of vision and/or hearing and PTSD. Tepper (2014) describes the multiple sexual difficulties experienced as a result of these injuries. Amputations not only cause functional challenges for sexual intercourse but also ongoing pain and alternations in body image. Burns may result in contractures and limited mobility as well as significant scarring that alters body image. Spinal cord injuries (see Chapter 8) and genital trauma have significant consequences for global aspects of sexual functioning.

In a review of over 12,000 injured veterans from the Department of Defense Trauma Registry (Nnamani et al., 2018), 4.6% of the injuries recorded were to the genito-urinary complex. Thirteen percent of those with these injuries experienced sexual dysfunction and half of these veterans also were diagnosed with TBI that compounds the effects of the physical injuries to the pelvis. Pelvic fractures are also associated with genito-urinary trauma, affecting the penis, testicles, and prostate gland. These injuries are related not just to the blast from improvised explosive devices but also to penetrating fragments. These injuries are also related to post-traumatic fistulae that are associated with significant sepsis and sexual dysfunction (Kucera, Jezior, & Duncan, 2017).

Female service members have also experienced genito-urinary injuries in combat with vulvar, vaginal, and perineal wounds being the most common. Lower limb amputation and colorectal injuries were also associated with these injuries that occurred from improvised explosive devices (Reed, Janak, Orman, & Hudak, 2018). It is suggested that because the female sexual organs are mostly internal, the risk of traumatic injury to the area is less than in males whose genital organs are external. However, internal injuries may be missed when triaging injuries in the field and ultimately lead to more serious complications.

There is underreporting of sexual dysfunction in veterans (Helmer et al., 2013) and also a discrepancy between veterans reporting problems and treatment prescribed, particularly for medications that treat erectile dysfunction (Hosain, Latini, Kauth, Goltz, & Helmer, 2013). Underreporting may be due to reluctance on the part of men to disclose sexual dysfunction, particularly in the military where masculinity is prized and admitting to something that relates to decreased virility is embarrassing.

Interventions should start with a thorough assessment of all physical and emotional symptoms as well as a medication review. Assessment of pain and medications used to treat it is also important as is a review of alcohol and recreational drugs. Vitamins and 'natural' remedies should also be reviewed as they may interact with prescribed medication. It is not enough to prescribe medications to treat erectile dysfunction without the cooperation of the partner who needs to understand the psychological and emotional processes involved with PTSD and combat trauma. A multi-disciplinary approach to both PTSD and sexual dysfunction treatment is necessary and acceptable to veterans (Malaktaris et al., 2018). Equine-assisted therapy for veterans with PTSD has shown some efficacy in the short-term for depression and PTSD symptoms (Arnon et al., 2020). There is some evidence that for female veterans, group exposure therapy is effective for PTSD symptoms and a 12-week exercise program showed promising results for depression and PTSD.

The military uses the Skills Training for Affective and Interpersonal Regulation (STAIR) program to treat individuals with PTSD. This is a cognitive behavioral therapy that has been shown to improve emotional management and interpersonal skills in the areas of social support and healthy relationships (Cloitre, Jackson, & Schmidt, 2016). Further, PTSD therapy in the military includes prolonged exposure therapy and cognitive processing therapy; this is regarded as the first line treatment but it has not shown to be effective for the treatment of sexual dysfunction (Tran, Dunckel, & Teng, 2015).

Traumatic brain injury

Individuals with traumatic brain injury (TBI) experience a range of cognitive, physical, behavioral, and social changes, all of which may affect sexuality. The injury is usually caused by some form of external force such as a motor vehicle accident, sports injury, or in the case of the military, the force of an explosive device. Sexuality is affected in different ways as shown in Box 7.1.

Box 7.1 Causes of sexual dysfunction in individuals with TBI (Sander & Maestas, 2014)

Hormonal changes
Medication side effects
Mobility problems
Cognitive changes
Changes in social relationships
Emotional changes
Side effects of medication
Fatigue

The global effects of TBI have a significant effect on romantic relationships or the ability to form a connection with a potential partner. Fifty seven percent of affected individuals in one study reported decreased sexual functioning; factors contributing to this included low confidence (32%), feelings of unattractiveness (24%), pain (26%), and difficulties communicating (17%) (Downing, Stolwyk, & Ponsford, 2013). Hormonal changes are associated with decreased arousal in women (O'Reilly, Wilson, & Peters, 2018) and men (Yang et al., 2018). Depression is also common as well as low self-esteem and lack of opportunity for social contact (Ponsford, Downing, & Stolwyk, 2013). Experiencing a TBI in adolescence has been shown to have long-term negative impacts with the potential for poor mental and social functioning, increased vulnerability, and sexual exploitation or abuse (Wiseman-Hakes et al., 2019). In the year following TBI, both women and men report sexual problems with almost a third reporting dissatisfaction with their sex life (Sander et al., 2012). Problematic sexual behavior occurs infrequently (less than 10%), but this poses a problem for family members and health care providers who may be the target of unwanted touch. Problematic sexual behavior is associated with younger age at the time of injury and a more severe or prior head injury (Turner, Schöttle, Krueger, & Briken, 2015).

Various aspects of sexual function are impacted including alterations in desire, hypersexuality, decreased arousal, and difficulty achieving orgasm. Emotional and behavioral dysregulation, manifested as apathy, agitation, depression, or irritability, can have a significant effect on relationships (Bivona et al., 2016) and partners of individuals with TBI report a broad range of sexual changes including dissatisfaction with sexual functioning, decreases in desire and frequency of sexual activity (Sander, Maestas, Pappadis, Hammond, & Hanks, 2016).

Individuals with TBI and their partner report unmet needs in the areas of sexuality education (Moreno, Gan, Zasler, & McKerral, 2015). Twenty six percent of participants in one study reported that they wanted information about sexuality, 15% said they had sexual problems and 21% wanted to be told about the sexual side effects of the medications they were prescribed. Seventy two percent of the sample said they almost never had discussions about sexual problems with a health care provider. This is confirmed by a study of health care professionals, the majority of whom were neuropsychologists (Arango-Lasprilla et al., 2017) where 36% reported talking to some of their patients and partners about sexuality and 29% said they would engage in a discussion if it was brought up by the patient/partner. Just 53% of these professionals felt comfortable talking about sexuality despite 97% stating that this should be discussed during rehabilitation. The person responsible for the discussion was thought to be a sex therapist, physiatrist, or family therapist. These are all specialists, and in most instances, would require referral and cost to the patient. Ideally a multi-disciplinary team should provide information, education, and support during the early phase of rehabilitation (Marier Deschênes, Lamontagne, Gagnon, & Moreno, 2019).

Sexual trauma

Sexual abuse in childhood, a form of sexual trauma, has far-reaching consequences and is regarded as a betrayal trauma. Abuse by a caregiver or a trusted older sibling, people that children trust, leads to damage in multiple domains of functioning. Sexual trauma in childhood impacts on adult sexuality by causing problems with communication about sex as well as dissociation during sexual activity (Rosenthal & Freyd, 2017). Some childhood sexual abuse survivors experience post-traumatic growth such as coping, personal strength, and enhanced intimacy with a partner. However, negative experiences are more likely to occur and include the perception of low competence, decreased trust and intimacy, and compromised identity (Simon, Smith, Fava, & Feiring, 2015). Childhood sexual trauma is associated with the development of PTSD (Gewirtz-Meydan & Lahav, 2020) that is seen to occur more frequently when the abuse happened repeatedly, at a younger age, and involved a family member. Childhood sexual abuse may lead to hypersexuality in both men and women; men are more likely to engage in compulsive sexual activity than women (Slavin et al., 2020).

The negative effects of sexual assault in women, another form of sexual trauma, include changes in attitude towards sexual activity as well as changes in sexual behavior with some female survivors avoiding sex while others have multiple partners. Some survivors turn to alcohol and drugs to cope; this is related to some women becoming sex workers to support their addiction. Some women may feel safer with a female sexual partner if their sexual trauma was related to a male perpetrator (O'Callaghan, Shepp, Ullman, & Kirkner, 2019). PTSD symptoms, including having flashbacks, contribute to sexual difficulties (O'Loughlin & Brotto, 2020), poor relationship satisfaction, and poor sexual communication (DiMauro & Renshaw, 2019). Physical effects of the sexual trauma may also lead to future sexual problems with vaginal trauma as well as anal trauma, particularly in male victims (Hendriks, Vandenberghe, Peeters, Roelens, & Keygnaert, 2018). Women who have been sexually assaulted experience problems with arousal and men may experience loss of desire, erectile dysfunction and premature ejaculation (Laumann, Paik, & Rosen, 1999). Women are also more likely to experience dyspareunia and chronic pelvic pain

(Weaver, 2009). Sexual trauma is also associated with bipolar and obsessive-compulsive disorder and importantly with suicidality, the risk of which is higher than in other forms of trauma; this may be related to the stigma and shame that survivors experience (Dworkin, Menon, Bystrynski, & Allen, 2017). This experience is also associated with depression and low sexual self-esteem, both of which are risk factors for future sexual victimization (Krahé & Berger, 2017).

Male-on-male sexual assault, which accounts for 5–10% of sexual assaults (McLean, 2013), remains a taboo and is under-reported to both the authorities and sexual assault clinics. Men also tend to seek help later than women (Larsen & Hilden, 2016). Male victims are more likely to be assaulted by a stranger, assaults often include multiple perpetrators, and drug use is often involved. This form of sexual trauma has significant social and cultural meaning; men are supposed to be physically strong and able to ward off the assault. The perception is that this happens only in prisons and not in general society. This also has implications for the sexual identity of the man who may think that others are going to think that he is homosexual and masculine identity may be diminished; this adds to the psychological distress that the man experiences. If the victim experienced an erection or ejaculation during the assault, this may further cast doubt on his masculinity despite the fact that these are both not fully under physiological control and do not imply consent (McLean, 2013). Sexual trauma is not relegated to male-on-male assault; forced sexual activity by a female perpetrator is also known to occur (Rubio-Aurioles, 2018). There is a paucity of literature about sexual trauma in sexual minority populations, including intimate partner sexual violence.

Box 7.2 Sexual symptoms from sexual trauma (Wendy Maltz, 2002)

Avoiding or fearing sex

Loss of sexual interest

Seeing sex as an obligation

Negative feelings (anger, disgust, guilt) in response to touch

Difficulty becoming aroused

Feeling distant during sex

Intrusive or disturbing images and thoughts

Inappropriate or compulsive sexual activity

Vaginal pain or difficulty with orgasms in women

Erectile, orgasmic, or ejaculatory problems in men

Difficulty establishing or maintaining romantic relationships

---

The partner of the person who has experienced sexual trauma may also experience challenges. For the male partner, this may include difficulty talking about what happened, not being able to provide support to his partner, as well as sexual changes (Connop & Petrak, 2004). But responses may be positive such as the man appreciating and valuing his partner and/or challenging his own sexual behaviors that might be coercive. However, changes tend to be more negative including less frequent sexual activity, erectile problems, and premature ejaculation and even hostile thoughts towards the partner who had sexual contact with another man. In one study, partners recognized that sexual activity could trigger flashbacks and one man said that he was not sure if his partner engaged in sex willingly or out of a sense of obligation (O'Callaghan et al., 2019). All of these effects may result in relationship distress and eventual breakdown.

Disclosing sexual trauma to a partner, family member, friend, or a professional can be difficult and some may be reluctant to do so and may mis-label what happened. It is not uncommon for women to suggest that they had too much alcohol and that resulted in the sexual assault or that they had initially consented to kissing and then things 'went too far' (Dardis, Kraft, & Gidycz, 2017). Disclosing sexual trauma to a partner, friend, or family member may elicit a positive or negative response (Therriault, Bigras, Hébert, & Godbout, 2020). Those who report a positive response on disclosure do not experience negative effects but those who experience a negative response are reported to experience sexual problems and distress. There is preliminary evidence that disclosing sexual trauma to a partner may be protective by decreasing symptoms of the trauma. This is theorized to occur by a process of learning that the sexual cues (for example feelings of arousal) are not dangerous and repeated exposure to these sexual cues may extinguish the triggers usually experienced (Staples et al., 2016).

Box 7.3 Case study

Brad and James have lived together for six months, having met at a conference and fallen instantly in love. They were both born and raised in small towns in the mid-West and came out during college. This was a first serious relationship for them both and they loved entertaining their friends in their small apartment.

The first New Year's eve that they were together they held a party and invited all their friends to celebrate with them. They cooked and cleaned and decorated for days before the big event and the apartment sparkled when the guests arrived. Brad was a little concerned when more people than expected showed up. It appeared that some of their friends had brought their own guests, but James told him to just go with the flow and enjoy himself. The wine flowed and someone took charge of making the cocktails; before long there was dancing and one of James's friends fell over the couch, taking down a string of fairy lights.

In all the frivolity James lost sight of Brad but figured that he must be somewhere in the apartment. The celebrations went on well past midnight and eventually the last person left close to 3 am. James started to clean up the glasses and bottles that were spread all over the kitchen and living room. He had had quite a bit to drink and as his buzz lifted, he realized that he had not seen Brad for ages. He called out his name as he went to the bathroom to brush his teeth. The sight of the blood spatters on the floor sobered him up immediately. What had happened? There was no broken glass and the bathroom looked okay other than a blood-stained towel on the floor.

The only other room in the apartment was the bedroom and James rushed there, calling for Brad. The room was dark, and James stood in the doorway for a moment as his eyes adjusted. The bed looked untouched and he saw Brad on the floor, his arms wrapped around his knees and his shoulders shaking.

"What happened? Are you okay?"

His voice was too loud as he leapt towards Brad who put out his arms to keep James away.

"There's blood in the bathroom and ... are you hurt? Did someone do something to you?"

Brad just shook his head and now that James's eyes had adjusted to the dark, he could see that Brad was in shock. His eyes were wide, his face pale, and there was a scratch along his jaw line.

"I'm calling the cops!" James was still talking too loudly.

"Don't, just please don't," whispered Brad, "I just want to go to sleep ... ."

He helped Brad get into their bed and he went to the couch, ignoring the mess around him, and spent the next few hours in the dark, staring at the window as the sky lightened. Brad woke just after 8 am by which time James had cleaned up most of the mess. They sat in their tiny kitchen and Brad slowly described what had happened. James bit the inside of his lip as he listened. His impulse was to call their invited guests to ask who had brought someone who had done this to Brad. As his partner haltingly went over what had happened, the tears poured down James's cheeks.

Later that day they went to the Emergency Room at the hospital down the block from where they lived. Brad was seen by a junior physician who was gentle and kind and spent a long time talking to them. Brad's physical injuries were minor, and he would heal within the week. But the emotional damage to them both would take months to resolve. They stopped seeing most of the people who had been at their party and they never did find out who raped Brad, or why. They didn't talk about that night ever again, but they stopped having sex. The first time James tried Brad pushed him away. The second time, on their anniversary they started kissing but for the first time in their relationship, Brad did not get an erection. James reassured him and suggested it was the wine, but Brad just shook his head. It was as if a switch had been turned off. He felt nothing, not in his body or mind. James insisted that it would pass, that it was just a one-time thing. It made no difference to Brad; he was changed, and they would never be the same again. Three months later, Brad moved out. It took James two years before he was able to date and he never saw Brad again.

Treatment for survivors of sexual trauma

The usual treatment approaches for addressing PTSD are not effective when dealing with the sexual problems that are a consequence of sexual trauma (O'Driscoll & Flanagan, 2016). Rape crisis centers deal with the immediate trauma as well as mental health issues but they often do not talk about sexual functioning (Voth Schrag & Edmond, 2018). Sexual problems may only appear later, and survivors may not know how to access counseling or may not be able to afford it. A patient education pamphlet published by the *Journal of Sexual Medicine* may be helpful in explaining the sexual problems experienced after sexual assault (Daglieri & Andelloux, 2013). By not addressing sexual problems during counseling for the survivor, the perception that sexuality is not important may be felt by the survivor. Baggett and colleagues (Baggett et al., 2017) suggest that a sex-positive approach may be more effective than the traditional cognitive behavioral and prolonged exposure frameworks. Both of these interventions expose the survivor to stimuli that are distressing and may elicit responses that are negative; they also do not address the sexual dysfunctions that are consequences of the sexual trauma. A sex-positive approach as suggested by Baggett focuses on sexual pleasure and not just the absence of harm. This has been shown to help survivors reclaim a sense of healthy sexuality.

Wendy Maltz (2002) is a well-regarded expert on sexual trauma and its effects on sexuality and provides direction for what needs to be accomplished in providing survivors with a road map to recovery, something she calls sexual healing. Key elements of this are presented in Box 7.4.

Box 7.4 Sexual healing (Maltz, 2001)

1. Understand the nature and consequences of abuse
2. Reframe sexual dysfunctions as functional and helping to avoid negative feelings and memories
3. Avoid negative transference by the therapist/counselor doing the opposite of what happened in the abuse (kindness, maintaining boundaries, etc.)
4. Improve sexual attitudes and thoughts by encouraging survivors to feel good about their body parts, etc.
5. Stop negative sexual behaviors and identify triggers
6. Include the partner in the process
7. New skills for approaching touch
8. Use standard sex therapy to address specific sexual problems
9. Address survivor concerns about sexual fantasies that they find problematic
10. The therapist should practice good self-care to address the challenges of therapy with survivors

---

Each survivor needs to be treated as an individual with unique values and reactions to their trauma. The symptoms of PTSD they experience may need to be addressed before attempting to address sexual problems. A multi-disciplinary team-based approach may be the most comprehensive approach for these individuals and couples.

It is important to remember that individuals who have experienced sexual trauma may avoid health care for a variety of reasons including fear of physical and intrusive examinations including pelvic and/or rectal exams (Ades, Goddard, Pearson Ayala, & Greene, 2019). They may also have difficulty with imaging studies where they need to keep very still or hold their breath; this may relate to the sexual trauma they experienced and cause flashbacks. Routine dental care may be neglected if going to the dentist reminds them of being orally assaulted.

All patients presenting for care should be asked if they have a history of sexual assault. If the response is in the affirmative, special care needs to be taken to avoid re-traumatizing the individual. Ades and colleagues (Ades, Wu, Stephanie, et al., 2019) recommend that the health care provider use open and accepting body language with hands in view, arms uncrossed and eye contact. All physical contact should be prefaced by asking for permission to touch the patient and each step of any examination needs to be clearly explained. Language is important too and avoidance of the word 'victim' is discouraged and 'survivor' used instead. Looking for signs of emotional distress and/or physical response such as trembling or self-protective posture should precipitate a pause and allow for de-escalation.

Military sexual assault

The experience of sexual harassment and sexual assault during military service, called military sexual trauma (MST), is concerning. The US Department of Defense defines sexual violence or sexual assault as sexual contact that uses force, threats, intimidation or the abuse of power or authority when the victim cannot or does not consent (Arbeit, 2017). It is estimated that up to 33% of female military service members have experienced this and 4% of men (Pulverman, Christy, & Kelly, 2019). Because there are 20 times more men than women in the military, the prevalence in both sexes is almost the same. Risk for sexual harassment and assault includes being of lower rank than the perpetrator and having completed fewer years of service. A previous history of assault or abuse is also noted as a risk factor and the dominant male culture in the military, including allegiance to the team, provides additional risk (Bell, Dardis, Vento, & Street, 2018). Many women in the military have a history of childhood sexual trauma, another risk factor for additional sexual trauma (Parnell et al., 2018). Additional risk factors include living in mixed-sex dormitories during training and under close conditions when deployed as well as the use of alcohol (Silber Ashley et al., 2019). It may also be difficult to report the assault due to fear of retribution, being revictimized, and having to continue to work with or be under the command of the perpetrator (Dardis, Reinhardt, Foynes, Medoff, & Street, 2018).

The consequences of experiencing sexual trauma in the military are wide ranging and include physical symptoms such as headaches, insomnia, substance use, and chronic pain. Psychological side effects include depression, PTSD, and anxiety (Pulverman et al., 2019). Sexual dysfunction is a significant result of this trauma; at least one sexual symptom was reported in 81.5% of male and 74.4% of female veterans (Garneau-Fournier, Habarth, & Turchik, 2018). Among men, 56% reported loss of desire, 48.2% erectile dysfunction, and problems with ejaculation were experienced by 26% of men. Female veterans reported low desire (64.6%), absence of orgasms (32.7%), and pain with sex (23.6%). Having PTSD and depression was associated with sexual problems in female veterans with the most common problem identified as sexual pain (Pulverman & Creech, 2019). Other chronic pain conditions such as fibromyalgia, joint- and back pain are also associated with the experience of assault or harassment in this population and may interfere with sexual function (Cichowski et al., 2017).

The Veterans Administration routinely screens veterans for military sexual trauma; however, screening for sexual dysfunction is not included, so the prevalence among both men and women is likely underestimated (Pulverman et al., 2019). While the priority for the military is treatment of PTSD, cognitive behavioral and exposure therapies have not shown positive results in the treatment of MST-related sexual dysfunction in women. Treatments for sexual dysfunction should address physical symptoms; estrogen therapy may improve sexual pain but the use of testosterone is not recommended or FDA approved (Pulverman et al., 2019). Mindfulness-based stress reduction has been shown to be effective in the treatment of depression and anxiety as well as PTSD and may prove to be effective for MST (Gallegos, Cross, & Pigeon, 2015).

Conclusions

Sexual trauma in the form of sexual abuse or military sexual trauma is a challenging condition to address. Sexual trauma impacts on the development of healthy sexual functioning in children and adolescents, and trauma in later life may impact negatively on physical, mental, and emotional health as well as on relationships. There are limited treatments for sexual trauma and survivors often do not report the event for multiple reasons so the consequences may be long lasting and devastating to the physical and emotional health of the survivor.

References

Ades, V., Goddard, B., Pearson Ayala, S., & Greene, J.A. (2019). Caring for long term health needs in women with a history of sexual trauma. *BMJ, 367*, l5825. doi: 10.1136/bmj.l5825

Ades, V., Wu, S., Rabinowitz, E., Chemouni Bach, S., Goddard, B., Pearson Ayala, S., & Greene, J. (2019). An integrated, trauma-informed care model for female survivors of sexual violence: The engage, motivate, protect, organize, self-worth, educate, respect (EMPOWER) clinic. *Obstetrics and Gynecology, 133*(4), 803–809. doi: 10.1097/AOG.0000000000003186.

Arango-Lasprilla, J.C., Olabarrieta-Landa, L., Ertl, M.M., Stevens, L.F., Morlett-Paredes, A., Andelic, N., & Zasler, N. (2017). Provider perceptions of the assessment and rehabilitation of sexual functioning after traumatic brain injury. *Brain Injury, 31*(12), 1605–1611. doi: 10.1080/02699052.2017.1332784

Arbeit, M.R. (2017). "Make sure you're not getting yourself in trouble:" Building sexual relationships and preventing sexual violence at the U.S. Military Academy at West Point. *Journal of Sex Research, 54*(8), 949–961. doi: 10.1080/00224499.2016.1207055

Arnon, S., Fisher, P.W., Pickover, A., Lowell, A., Turner, J.B., Hilburn, A., ... Neria, Y. (2020). Equine-assisted therapy for veterans with PTSD: Manual development and preliminary findings. *Military Medicine, 185*(5–6), e557–e564. doi: 10.1093/milmed/usz444

Bachem, R., Levin, Y., & Solomon, Z. (2020). Posttraumatic stress and sexual satisfaction in husbands and wives: A dyadic analysis. *Archives of Sexual Behavior, 49*(5), 1533–1543. doi: 10.1007/s10508-020-01680-4

Badour, C.L., Gros, D.F., Szafranski, D.D., & Acierno, R. (2015). Problems in sexual functioning among male OEF/OIF veterans seeking treatment for posttraumatic stress. *Comprehensive Psychiatry, 58*, 74–81. doi: 10.1016/j.comppsych.2014.12.012

Baggett, L.R., Eisen, E., Gonzalez-Rivas, S., Olson, L.A., Cameron, R.P., & Mona, L.R. (2017). Sex-positive assessment and treatment among female trauma survivors. *Journal of Clinical Psychology, 73*(8), 965–974. doi: 10.1002/jclp.22510

Beaulieu, G.R., Latini, D.M., Helmer, D.A., Powers-James, C., Houlette, C., & Kauth, M.R. (2015). An exploration of returning veterans' sexual health issues using a brief self-report measure. *Sexual Medicine, 3*(4), 287–294. doi: 10.1002/sm2.92

Bell, M.E., Dardis, C.M., Vento, S.A., & Street, A.E. (2018). Victims of sexual harassment and sexual assault in the military: Understanding risks and promoting recovery. *Military Psychology, 30*(3), 219–228. doi: 10.1037/mil0000144

Benedek, D.M. (2020). PTSD care and "getting better" what does that mean? *Military Medicine, 185*(9–10), e1376–e1377. doi: 10.1093/milmed/usz477

Bentsen, I.L., Giraldi, A.G.E., Kristensen, E., & Andersen, H.S. (2015). Systematic review of sexual dysfunction among veterans with post-traumatic stress disorder. *Sexual Medicine Reviews, 3*(2), 78–87. doi: 10.1002/smrj.47

Bivona, U., Antonucci, G., Contrada, M., Rizza, F., Leoni, F., Zasler, N.D., & Formisano, R. (2016). A biopsychosocial analysis of sexuality in adult males and their partners after severe traumatic brain injury. *Brain Injury, 30*(9), 1082–1095. doi: 10.3109/02699052.2016.1165867

Cichowski, S.B., Rogers, R.G., Clark, E.A., Murata, E., Murata, A., & Murata, G. (2017). Military sexual trauma in female veterans is associated with chronic pain conditions. *Military Medicine, 182*(9–10), e1895–e1899. doi: 10.7205/milmed-d-16-00393

Cloitre, M., Jackson, C., & Schmidt, J.A. (2016). Case reports: STAIR for strengthening social support and relationships among veterans with military sexual trauma and PTSD. *Military Medicine, 181*(2), e183–e187. doi: 10.7205/milmed-d-15-00209

Connop, V., & Petrak, J. (2004). The impact of sexual assault on heterosexual couples. *Sexual and Relationship Therapy, 19*(1), 29–38. doi: 10.1080/14681990410001640817

Daglieri, T., & Andelloux, M. (2013). Sexuality and sexual pleasure after sexual assault. *Journal of Sexual Medicine, 10*(10), 2611–2612. doi: 10.1111/jsm.12317

Dardis, C.M., Kraft, K.M., & Gidycz, C.A. (2017). "Miscommunication" and undergraduate women's conceptualizations of sexual assault: A qualitative analysis. *Journal of Interpersonal Violence, 36*(1–2), 33–61. doi: 10.1177/0886260517726412

Dardis, C.M., Reinhardt, K.M., Foynes, M.M., Medoff, N.E., & Street, A.E. (2018). "Who are you going to tell? Who's going to believe you?":Women's experiences disclosing military sexual trauma. *Psychology of Women Quarterly, 42*(4), 414–429. doi: 10.1177/0361684318796783

DiMauro, J., & Renshaw, K.D. (2019). PTSD and relationship satisfaction in female survivors of sexual assault. *Psychological Trauma, 11*(5), 534–541. doi: 10.1037/tra0000391

Downing, M.G., Stolwyk, R., & Ponsford, J.L. (2013). Sexual changes in individuals with traumatic brain injury: A control comparison. *Journal of Head Trauma Rehabilitation, 28*(3), 171–178. doi: 10.1097/HTR.0b013e31828b4f63

Dworkin, E.R., Menon, S.V., Bystrynski, J., & Allen, N.E. (2017). Sexual assault victimization and psychopathology: A review and meta-analysis. *Clinical Psychology Review, 56*, 65–81. doi: 10.1016/j.cpr.2017.06.002

Gallegos, A.M., Cross, W., & Pigeon, W.R. (2015). Mindfulness-based stress reduction for veterans exposed to military sexual trauma: Rationale and implementation considerations. *Military Medicine, 180*(6), 684–689. doi: 10.7205/milmed-d-14-00448

Garneau-Fournier, J., Habarth, J., & Turchik, J.A. (2018). Factors associated with sexual dysfunction symptoms among veterans who have experienced military sexual trauma. *International Journal of Sexual Health, 30*(1), 28–41. doi: 10.1080/19317611.2017.1404541

Gewirtz-Meydan, A., & Lahav, Y. (2020). Sexual dysfunction and distress among childhood sexual abuse survivors: The role of post-traumatic stress disorder. *Journal of Sexual Medicine, 17*(11), 2267–2278. doi: 10.1016/j.jsxm.2020.07.016

Helmer, D.A., Beaulieu, G.R., Houlette, C., Latini, D., Goltz, H.H., Etienne, S., & Kauth, M. (2013). Assessment and documentation of sexual health issues of recent combat veterans seeking VHA care. *Journal of Sexual Medicine, 10*(4), 1065–1073. doi: 10.1111/jsm.12084

Helmer, D.A., Beaulieu, G., Powers, C., Houlette, C., Latini, D., & Kauth, M. (2015). Perspectives on sexual health and function of recent male combat veterans of Iraq and Afghanistan. *Sexual Medicine, 3*(3), 137–146. doi: 10.1002/sm2.62

Hendriks, B., Vandenberghe, A.M.A., Peeters, L., Roelens, K., & Keygnaert, I. (2018). Towards a more integrated and gender-sensitive care delivery for victims of sexual assault: Key findings and recommendations from the Belgian sexual assault care centre feasibility study. *International Journal for Equity in Health, 17*(1), 152. doi: 10.1186/s12939-018-0864-3

Hosain, G.M.M., Latini, D.M., Kauth, M., Goltz, H.H., & Helmer, D.A. (2013). Sexual dysfunction among male veterans returning from Iraq and Afghanistan: Prevalence and correlates. *Journal of Sexual Medicine, 10*(2), 516–523. doi: 10.1111/j.1743-6109.2012.02978.x

Krahé, B., & Berger, A. (2017). Longitudinal pathways of sexual victimization, sexual self-esteem, and depression in women and men. *Psychological Trauma, 9*(2), 147–155. doi: 10.1037/tra0000198

Kucera, W.B., Jezior, J.R., & Duncan, J.E. (2017). Management of post-traumatic rectovesical/rectourethral fistulas: Case series of complicated injuries in wounded warriors and review of the literature. *Military Medicine, 182*(3–4), e1835–e1839. doi: 10.7205/milmed-d-16-00148

Larsen, M.-L., & Hilden, M. (2016). Male victims of sexual assault: 10 years' experience from a Danish Assault Center. *Journal of Forensic and Legal Medicine, 43*, 8–11. doi: 10.1016/j.jflm.2016.06.007

Laumann, E.O., Paik, A., & Rosen, R.C. (1999). Sexual dysfunction in the united StatesPrevalence and predictors. *JAMA, 281*(6), 537–544. doi: 10.1001/jama.281.6.537

Malaktaris, A.L., Buzzella, B.A., Siegel, M.E., Myers, U.S., Browne, K.C., Norman, S.B., & Angkaw, A.C. (2018). OEF/OIF/OND veterans seeking PTSD treatment: Perceptions of partner involvement in trauma-focused treatment. *Military Medicine, 184*(3–4), e263–e270. doi: 10.1093/milmed/usy231

Maltz, W. (2001). Sex therapy with survivors of sexual abuse. In P.J. Kleinplatz (Ed.), *New directions in sex therapy: Innovations and alternatives* (pp. 258–278). Philadelphia, PA: Brunner-Routledge.

Maltz, W. (2002). Treating the sexual intimacy concerns of sexual abuse survivors. *Sexual and Relationship Therapy, 17*(4), 321–327. doi: 10.1080/1468199021000017173

Marier Deschênes, P., Lamontagne, M.-E., Gagnon, M.-P., & Moreno, J.A. (2019). Talking about sexuality in the context of rehabilitation following traumatic brain injury: An integrative review of operational aspects. *Sexuality and Disability, 37*(3), 297–314. doi: 10.1007/s11195-019-09576-5

McLean, I.A. (2013). The male victim of sexual assault. *Best Practice and Research: Clinical Obstetrics and Gynaecology, 27*(1), 39–46. doi: 10.1016/j.bpobgyn.2012.08.006

Moreno, A., Gan, C., Zasler, N., & McKerral, M. (2015). Experiences, attitudes, and needs related to sexuality and service delivery in individuals with traumatic brain injury. *NeuroRehabilitation, 37*(1), 99–116. doi: 10.3233/nre-151243

Nnamani, N.S., Pugh, M.J., Amuan, M.E., Eapen, B.C., Hudak, S.J., Liss, M.A., & Orman, J.A. (2018). Outcomes of genitourinary injury in U.S. Iraq and Afghanistan war veterans receiving care from the veterans health administration. *Military Medicine, 184*(3–4), e297–e301. doi: 10.1093/milmed/usy196

Nunnink, S.E., Goldwaser, G., Afari, N., Nievergelt, C.M., & Baker, D.G. (2010). The role of emotional numbing in sexual functioning among veterans of the Iraq and Afghanistan wars. *Military Medicine, 175*(6), 424–428. doi: 10.7205/milmed-d-09-00085

O'Callaghan, E., Shepp, V., Ullman, S.E., & Kirkner, A. (2019). Navigating sex and sexuality after sexual assault: A qualitative study of survivors and informal support providers. *Journal of Sex Research, 56*(8), 1045–1057. doi: 10.1080/00224499.2018.1506731

O'Driscoll, C., & Flanagan, E. (2016). Sexual problems and post-traumatic stress disorder following sexual trauma: A meta-analytic review. *Psychology and Psychotherapy: Theory, Research and Practice, 89*(3), 351–367. doi: 10.1111/papt.12077

O'Loughlin, J.I., & Brotto, L.A. (2020). Women's sexual desire, trauma exposure, and posttraumatic stress disorder. *Journal of Traumatic Stress, 33*(3), 238–247. doi: 10.1002/jts.22485

O'Reilly, K., Wilson, N., & Peters, K. (2018). Narrative literature review: Health, activity and participation issues for women following traumatic brain injury. *Disability and Rehabilitation, 40*(19), 2331–2342. doi: 10.1080/09638288.2017.1334838

Parnell, D., Ram, V., Cazares, P., Webb-Murphy, J., Roberson, M., & Ghaed, S. (2018). Sexual assault and disabling PTSD in active duty service women. *Military Medicine, 183*(9–10), e481–e488. doi: 10.1093/milmed/usy048

Ponsford, J.L., Downing, M.G., & Stolwyk, R. (2013). Factors associated with sexuality following traumatic brain injury. *Journal of Head Trauma Rehabilitation, 28*(3), 195–201. doi: 10.1097/HTR.0b013e31828b4f7b

Pulverman, C.S., Christy, A.Y., & Kelly, U.A. (2019). Military sexual trauma and sexual health in women veterans: A systematic review. *Sexual Medicine Reviews, 7*(3), 393–407. doi: 10.1016/j.sxmr.2019.03.002

Pulverman, C.S., & Creech, S.K. (2019). The impact of sexual trauma on the sexual health of women veterans: A comprehensive review. *Trauma, Violence, and Abuse,* 1524838019870912. doi: 10.1177/1524838019870912

Reed, A.M., Janak, J.C., Orman, J.A., & Hudak, S.J. (2018). Genitourinary injuries among female U.S. Service members during operation Iraqi freedom and operation enduring freedom: Findings from the trauma outcomes and urogenital health (TOUGH) project. *Military Medicine, 183*(7–8), e304–e309. doi: 10.1093/milmed/usx079

Richardson, J.D., Ketcheson, F., King, L., Forchuk, C.A., Hunt, R., St. Cyr, K., … Elhai, J.D. (2019). Sexual dysfunction in male Canadian Armed Forces members and veterans seeking mental health treatment. *Military Medicine, 185*(1–2), 68–74. doi: 10.1093/milmed/usz163

Riviere, L.A., Merrill, J.C., Thomas, J.L., Wilk, J.E., & Bliese, P.D. (2012). 2003–2009 Marital functioning trends among U.S. enlisted soldiers following combat deployments. *Military Medicine, 177*(10), 1169–1177. doi: 10.7205/milmed-d-12-00164

Rosenthal, M.N., & Freyd, J.J. (2017). Silenced by betrayal: The path from childhood trauma to diminished sexual communication in adulthood. *Journal of Aggression, Maltreatment and Trauma, 26*(1), 3–17. doi: 10.1080/10926771.2016.1175533

Rubio-Aurioles, E. (2018). Is male sexual abuse a topic for sexual medicine? *Journal of Sexual Medicine, 15*(7), 933–934. doi: 10.1016/j.jsxm.2018.02.022

Sadler, A.G., Mengeling, M.A., Fraley, S.S., Torner, J.C., & Booth, B.M. (2012). Correlates of sexual functioning in women veterans: Mental health, gynecologic health, health status, and sexual assault history. *International Journal of Sexual Health, 24*(1), 60–77. doi: 10.1080/19317611.2011.640388

Sairsingh, H., Solomon, P., Helstrom, A., & Treglia, D. (2017). Depression in female veterans returning from deployment: The role of social factors. *Military Medicine, 183*(3–4), e133–e139. doi: 10.1093/milmed/usx065

Sander, A.M., & Little Maestas, K. (2014). Sexuality after traumatic brain injury. *Archives of Physical Medicine and Rehabilitation, 95*(9), 1801–1802. doi: 10.1016/j.apmr.2013.06.004

Sander, A.M., & Maestas, K. (2014). Information/education page. Sexuality after traumatic brain injury. *Archives of Physical Medicine and Rehabilitation, 95*(9), 1801–1802. doi: 10.1016/j.apmr.2013.06.004

Sander, A.M., Maestas, K.L., Pappadis, M.R., Hammond, F.M., & Hanks, R.A. (2016). Multicenter study of sexual functioning in spouses/partners of persons with traumatic brain injury. *Archives of Physical Medicine and Rehabilitation, 97*(5), 753–759. doi: 10.1016/j.apmr.2016.01.009

Sander, A.M., Maestas, K.L., Pappadis, M.R., Sherer, M., Hammond, F.M., & Hanks, R. (2012). Sexual functioning 1 year after traumatic brain injury: Findings from a prospective traumatic brain injury model systems collaborative study. *Archives of Physical Medicine and Rehabilitation, 93*(8), 1331–1337. doi: 10.1016/j.apmr.2012.03.037

Silber Ashley, O., Lane, M.E., Morgan, J.K., Charm, S., Tharp, A., & Brown, M. (2019). Perceptions of high-risk situations for sexual assault: Gender differences in the U.S. Air Force. *Military Medicine, 184*(Supplement_1), 443–450. doi: 10.1093/milmed/usy350

Simon, V.A., Smith, E., Fava, N., & Feiring, C. (2015). Positive and negative posttraumatic change following childhood sexual abuse are associated with youths' adjustment. *Child Maltreatment, 20*(4), 278–290. doi: 10.1177/1077559515590872

Slavin, M.N., Blycker, G.R., Potenza, M.N., Bőthe, B., Demetrovics, Z., & Kraus, S.W. (2020). Gender-related differences in associations between sexual abuse and hypersexuality. *Journal of Sexual Medicine, 17*(10), 2029–2038. doi: 10.1016/j.jsxm.2020.07.008

Staples, J.M., Eakins, D., Neilson, E.C., George, W.H., Davis, K.C., & Norris, J. (2016). Sexual assault disclosure and sexual functioning: The role of trauma symptomatology. *Journal of Sexual Medicine, 13*(10), 1562–1569. doi: 10.1016/j.jsxm.2016.08.001

Tepper, M.S. (2014). Sexual healthcare for wounded warriors with serious combat-related injuries and disabilities. *Sexual Medicine Reviews, 2*(2), 64–74. doi: 10.1002/smrj.24

Therriault, C., Bigras, N., Hébert, M., & Godbout, N. (2020). All involved in the recovery: Disclosure and social reactions following sexual victimization. *Journal of Aggression, Maltreatment and Trauma, 29*(6), 661–679. doi: 10.1080/10926771.2020.1725210

Tran, J.K., Dunckel, G., & Teng, E.J. (2015). Sexual dysfunction in veterans with post-traumatic stress disorder. *Journal of Sexual Medicine, 12*(4), 847–855. doi: 10.1111/jsm.12823

Turner, D., Schöttle, D., Krueger, R., & Briken, P. (2015). Sexual behavior and its correlates after traumatic brain injury. *Current Opinion in Psychiatry, 28*(2), 180–187. doi: 10.1097/yco.0000000000000144

Voth Schrag, R., & Edmond, T.E. (2018). Treatment goals, assessment, and evaluation practices in rape crisis centers. *Violence and Victims, 33*(6), 1055–1071. doi: 10.1891/0886-6708.33.6.1055

Weaver, T. (2009). Impact of rape on female sexuality: Review of selected literature. *Clinical Obstetrics and Gynecology, 52*(4), 702–711. doi: 10.1097/GRF.0b013e3181bf4bfb.

Wilcox, S.L., Redmond, S., & Hassan, A.M. (2014). Sexual functioning in military personnel: Preliminary estimates and predictors. *Journal of Sexual Medicine, 11*(10), 2537–2545. doi: 10.1111/jsm.12643

Wiseman-Hakes, C., Saleem, M., Poulin, V., Nalder, E., Balachandran, P., Gan, C., & Colantonio, A. (2019). The development of intimate relationships in adolescent girls and women with traumatic brain injury: A framework to guide gender specific rehabilitation and enhance positive social outcomes. *Disability and Rehabilitation, 42*(24), 3559–3565.– doi: 10.1080/09638288.2019.1597180

Yang, Y.J., Chien, W.C., Chung, C.H., Hong, K.T., Yu, Y.L., Hueng, D.Y., … Tzeng, N.S. (2018). Risk of erectile dysfunction after traumatic brain injury: A nationwide population-based cohort study in Taiwan. *American Journal of Men's Health, 12*(4), 913–925. doi: 10.1177/1557988317750970

Yehuda, R., Lehrner, A., & Rosenbaum, T.Y. (2015). PTSD and sexual dysfunction in men and women. *Journal of Sexual Medicine, 12*(5), 1107–1119. doi: 10.1111/jsm.12856

Recommended books

Effective Treatment for PTSD, 3rd Edition (2020)
  David Forbes, Jonathan Bisson, Candice Monson & Lucy Berliner (Eds).
  Guilford Press
Treating Complex Traumatic Stress Disorders in Adults 2nd Edition (2020)
  Julian Ford & Christine Courtois (Eds)
  Guilford Press
Military Stress Reaction: Rethinking Trauma and PTSD (2020)
  Carrie Kennedy
  Guilford Press
Developmental Couple Therapy for Complex Trauma: A Manual for Therapists (2019)
  Heather B. MacIntosh
  Routledge

Patient education resources

Sexuality After Traumatic Brain Injury: Information Education Page (Angelle M. Sander & Little Maestas, 2014).
  Sexuality and Sexual Pleasure after Sexual Assault.
Daglieri, T., & Andelloux, M. (2013). Sexuality and Sexual Pleasure after Sexual Assault. *The journal of sexual medicine, 10*(10), 2611-2612. doi:10.1111/jsm.12317

8   Disability and sexuality

Individuals with disabilities have the same rights to love, relationships, sexual pleasure, and choice (Addlakha, Price, & Heidari, 2017). But disability is also a source of shame for some as well as discrimination, and there is a lack of specialized services to support sexuality in this population. These challenges may begin in adolescence when the need for knowledge about healthy sexuality may be neglected (Holland-Hall & Quint, 2017). Persons with disabilities may be viewed as asexual despite having the same desire for romantic and sexual relationships in young and older adulthood.

Persons with disabilities may be stigmatized, infantilized, socially excluded, and/or seen as less than their able-bodied counterparts (Agmon, Sa'ar, & Araten-Bergman, 2016). They may also be seen as in need of protection, and while some may be at risk due to mobility issues, they are still capable of consent and participation in pleasurable sexual activities.

Spinal cord injury

Spinal cord injury (SCI) is more common in men due to motor vehicle accidents and other trauma. The vast majority of the evidence regarding sexual problems in those who have experienced SCI is found in men, particularly young men. The impact on physical sexual functioning depends on the level of the cord injury; however, the psychological impact is a significant factor in overall sexual functioning.

Spinal cord injury in men

The physical side effects of SCI affect erections, ejaculation, and orgasm and depend on the level of the spinal cord injury. Erections are dependent on the S2–S4 reflex arc in addition to functioning blood vessels (Kasum et al., 2018). Tactile sensation from the penis causes a reflex arc that sends signals to the blood vessels to dilate, resulting in an erection. This is a reflex and not the same as a psychogenic erection that involves the brain. Injury above this level does not impact on the ability to achieve erections; however, maintaining an erection may be difficult (Latella, Maggio, Manuli, Militi, & Calabrò, 2019) and while this may have no physical cause, psychological factors play an important role in many aspects of sexual functioning. These physical changes contribute to overall dissatisfaction with life (D'Andrea et al., 2020). Sleep deprivation and hypertension are associated with more severe erectile dysfunction (Khak et al., 2016).

Ejaculation is controlled by nerves in the T10–L2 area of the spinal cord (Kasum et al., 2018). Ejaculation is a complex process involving multiple centers in the spinal cord and brain; ejaculation itself is a spinal cord reflex and damage at and below the T10–L2 area of

DOI: 10.4324/9781003145745-8

the spinal cord will result in the inability to ejaculate (Latella et al., 2019). The sensations of orgasm may not be felt so SCI at this level may result in sexual dissatisfaction due to the loss of sensation. This is also important for fertility due to the lack of emission. Despite these changes, sexual desire may not be impacted and is seen to remain high in most men with SCI (Miranda et al., 2016).

Reactive loss of desire may occur when men experience sexual difficulties and/or relationship changes. Having a partner and engaging in regular masturbation as well as sexual intercourse have been shown to be protective of sexual desire (Ferro et al., 2019) however men should be aware that masturbation may require more time and focus to achieve orgasm (Alexander, Courtois, Elliott, & Tepper, 2017).

Autonomic dysregulation is common in men with a spinal injury above T6 (Soler et al 2018). This is experienced as a rise in blood pressure and spasticity during arousal and/or orgasm/ejaculation. Ejaculation and/or orgasm may cause hyperventilation, sweating, and tachycardia as well as increased muscle tone (Alexander et al., 2017). These same sensations are experienced normally during sex, but autonomic dysregulation is distressing and regarded as dangerous when severe.

Loss of masculine self-image may impact negatively on the man's perception that he can attract a partner and his motivation to date may decrease (Ferro 2019). Because SCI is frequently seen in younger men, the repercussions may be significant. Psychological distress and difficulties adjusting to life after SCI are common (Barbonetti, Cavallo, Felzani, Francavilla, & Francavilla, 2012) and may contribute to substance abuse, depression and anxiety, and potentially suicidality. Men who adhere to masculine scripts that favor potency and sexual prowess may suffer more negative psychological impacts and have more difficulty adjusting to life after SCI (Burns, Hough, Boyd, & Hill, 2010). Men report that return of sexual function is a priority (Simpson et al., 2012) and remains an ongoing problem for years after the injury occurred (van der Meer et al., 2017).

Other factors impact on sexual function in these men. Both bladder- and bowel incontinence have a negative impact on sexuality (Park et al., 2017) with embarrassment potentially leading to avoidance of sexual activity. Pain and changes to mobility may make sexual activity difficult as may the partner's willingness and attraction to the man. Medications to treat depression as discussed in Chapter 6 cause sexual dysfunction; medications such as pregabalin and gabapentin, used to treat neuropathic pain, as well as baclofen to treat spasticity also impact negatively on sexual function.

The impact on the partner of the man with an SCI is important as it relates not only on relationship satisfaction but also on the emotional health of the partner. In a qualitative study of female partners (Eglseder & Demchick, 2017), a rich description of the impact of the SCI on the partner and sexual relationship was presented. The women described role changes from that of a romantic partner to a caregiver who often has to attend to bladder and bowel care; they reported taking on a maternal role and/or saw their partner as a patient rather than a lover. Caregiving resulted in loss of sexual desire and the physical changes to the man's body led to a decrease in sexual attraction. In terms of the sexual relationship, the women felt guilty because they could not please their partner anymore while at the same time recognizing that the man was no longer as sexually capable as they had been before the SCI. These experiences highlight the significant impact of the changes caused by the SCI on global aspects of the partnered relationship.

Men are able to experience sexual satisfaction (Soler, Navaux, & Previnaire, 2018) and sexual dysfunction is related to the level but not the severity of the injury. In this study, 32 of 33 men enjoyed lengthy foreplay and 90% said that they experienced pleasure with intercourse and they also reported a sense of fulfillment and relaxation afterwards. Their female partner was responsible for initiating sex. Of note is that all of the men in the study had attended an in-patient rehabilitation program and were seeing a sex therapist as out-patients.

There is a paucity of evidence about the experience of sexual minority individuals in the literature.

Box 8.1 Five As Assessment

Imagine that you are a nurse assigned to take care of Joel, a 26-year old man with a spinal cord injury at the T12 level. He was injured in motor bike accident and is due to transfer to a rehabilitation facility at the end of the week. When you came on duty the night staff tell you that he has been 'sexually inappropriate' with one of the janitorial staff, a young woman who is new to the facility.

The following is an example of how you might address the situation:

Ask what the patient needs or wants to talk about: "Good morning Joel. My name is XXXX and I am going to be taking care of you today. This morning when I came on duty, I was told that there was an incident last night with one of the housekeepers. Can you tell me what happened?"

Joel: "Okay, so this is how it went … . I was alone and well, you know … I couldn't get to sleep and, you know, I was … . okay, I was jerking off or trying to … . And this person, this woman, walks into my room and I guess she saw what I was doing, or trying to do, and she freaked out!"

Assess what the problem or issue is: "That probably was a little scary for her, and maybe a bit embarrassing for you. So how can we help prevent something like this happening again?"

Joel: "Well, maybe people should not just barge into my room, like!"

Advise the patient about what can be done: "Yes of course, I understand. I can talk to the rest of the staff about them closing your door after your late-night meds. The housekeeping staff know that they should knock before entering, and perhaps they shouldn't try to come into your room if the door is closed. That might help too. What do you think about that?"

Joel: "That sounds okay … but is it alright if I ask you something? So another reason for me doing that … you know what I'm talking about? What I was doing last night … . well, it's not just about getting to sleep … It's, well it's really embarrassing to you about this … but, well, my … um … it's not working you know? Like I try every damn night … and nothing. Nothing works and if I don't have that, well, what's the point of going on, you know?"

Assist the patient in resolving the issue: "So let's talk about exactly what's going on. Is the problem with erections or orgasms? Don't look so horrified, it's part of my job to talk about these things. And yes, I have talked about it before with lots of patients and I survived and so will you … . It's really not a big deal to me. Your injury is above the level where there's an impact on erections. There could be other reasons for you having trouble with that. But at the level where your injury is, it means you won't have any ejaculate, you remember the doctor telling you that? I'll ask the clinical nurse specialist to come and see you before you transfer to the rehab hospital. If he can't help you, we can organize for you to see a urologist, either here or at the rehab place. How does that sound?"

Joel: "You said the other nurse, the specialist one, is a guy, right? Okay, I'll talk to him. Might be easier … but you did a good job just now. For a girl, I mean …"

Arrange follow-up: "Well, thanks for the compliment; at least I think it was a compliment! The clinical nurse specialist's name is Jonathan and he'll be around later this morning. I'll ask him to see you. And I'm going to check in with you later to hear what he told you. Maybe I can learn something … ."

Interventions

Oral medications to treat erectile dysfunction such as sildenafil, tadalafil and vardenafil have shown to be effective in men with SCI (Kovac & Lipshultz, 2016). Of note is the results of a study that showed sildenafil to increase intercourse success and ejaculation frequency (Ohl, Carlsson, Stecher, & Rippon, 2017). There is little evidence of the effectiveness of other interventions such as the vacuum pump, intra-urethral alprostadil (Lombardi, Musco, Wyndaele, & Del Popolo, 2015) but intra-cavernosal injections, particularly the combination of papaverine and phentolamine, have been shown to be highly effective (Chochina et al., 2016). If men choose to use the vacuum pump, they should be warned that the constriction ring can only be left in place for 30 minutes before it poses a problem to perfusion of the penile tissues.

Willingness to experiment sexually is important; neural plasticity allows for new areas of the body to respond to touch in a sexually pleasurable way (Ferro et al., 2019). Men may need to focus on the sensations that they are aware of, including those experienced during masturbation, as this may attune their bodies to these and enhance arousal and the sexual experience, alone or with a partner. This may help them to reframe their sexual experience by reinforcing what their sexual response is after the SCI. The use of sexual fantasy to increase arousal may be helpful as well as erotic stimuli such as pornography. The use of a vibrator to increase genital sensation has been shown to be effective; however, the man must have an intact lumbosacral complex for this to be effective (Alexander et al., 2017). While men may use any external vibrator to help with arousal and ejaculation, the Ferticare™ personal device is recommended and has been shown to be effective in clinical studies. It can be placed anywhere on the shaft of the penis and provides transcutaneous mechanical nerve stimulation (https://medicalvibrator.com/product/the-ferticare-personal/) and is FDA approved; however, it is expensive.

Prevention of autonomic dysregulation is important and this can be achieved by stopping sexual activity when symptoms appear, sitting up and lowering the legs to allow blood to flow to the lower extremities, and loosening or removing any constricting clothing (Alexander et al., 2017).

As with all conditions, treatment should begin with assessment of physical, emotional, and relationship function. A multi-disciplinary approach is necessary to consider the multiple facets of rehabilitation and ongoing recovery after SCI (Aikman, Oliffe, Kelly, & McCuaig, 2018). However, the same barriers to addressing concerns about sexual functioning exist in the care of individuals with SCI. These include lack of knowledge and time, inadequate or absent remuneration, and the perception that another member of the health care team should address sexual concerns (Elliott, Hocaloski, & Carlson, 2017; New, Seddon, Redpath, Currie, & Warren, 2016; Pieters, Kedde, & Bender, 2018). The expectation that the patient will ask for help also influences the reasons for not initiating the conversation, but the patient may be embarrassed or not sure that their health care provider will be comfortable talking about.

An interesting review of topics included in social media discussions (Latack & Samplaski, 2020) found that people ask about how others manage erectile dysfunction and urinary tract infections after sexual intercourse as well as where and how to find information about vibrators and medications. The negative impact of sexual problems on quality of life was also found to be a common discussion point and how long it took for things to improve. Suggestions for the use of alternative therapies such as hypnosis and cannabis were also posted. This suggests that education and anticipatory guidance for patients is not optimal and more is needed (Eglseder & Demchick, 2017).

Sex therapy may provide additional support for those who require more than education; however, assessment and treatment are within the expertise of the primary care provider in the community. It is suggested that a framework such as the PLISSIT model (Annon, 1974) can be helpful in addressing the need for education and support in these men with or without the partner (Aikman et al., 2018).

Spinal cord injury in women

There is less evidence about the effects of SCI on women, mainly due to the lower prevalence of women participating in high-risk activities leading to physical trauma. However, as discussed in Chapter 7, genito-urinary trauma experienced in combat conveys risk for spinal cord injury. Courtois and associates (Courtois, Alexander, & McLain, 2017) describe three major impacts from SCI. The first is the neurological damage that causes changes in arousal and lubrication. The second impact is from the secondary changes such as alterations in mobility, pain, spasticity, contractures, incontinence, and side effects of medication used to treat these symptoms. Finally, psychosocial sequelae such as depression and anxiety as well as alcohol and substance abuse also impact on sexuality and relationships.

Loss of desire is common and associated with medications to treat depression, as well as fatigue and pain (Stoffel, Van der Aa, Wittmann, Yande, & Elliott, 2018). Arousal is reported to be very difficult for women after SCI and this is made worse if the woman feels unattractive or fears incontinence during sexual activity (Kreuter, Taft, Siösteen, & Biering-Sørensen, 2011). A study of women from the United Kingdom showed that sexuality is important for feeling feminine and sexual activity remains satisfying and pleasurable despite the changes after SCI (Thrussell et al., 2018). The women in this study reported pelvic floor dysfunction, decreased lubrication and loss of vaginal sensation as well as bladder and bowel incontinence. In particular, women stated that pressure felt in the abdomen from penetration caused a bowel movement and this was devastating to the woman. Autonomic dysregulation was tolerated to a degree but if the symptoms were severe, intercourse was stopped. Psychological changes included low self-esteem and negative body image. The preparation for sexual activity, including emptying the bladder and bowel, was seen as something that 'killed the mood.' Some women reported feeling detached during sex while others worried about whether they were pleasing their partner or not. Feeling dependent on the partner and experiencing changes in the relationship were distressing for some of the women. For those who were partnered, the sexual changes were easy to adapt to in some cases while some relationships ended. For women who were single, deciding when and how much to disclose to a potential partner was another stressor. The partners of some women were negatively impacted but for those who were in supportive relationships, security and love were described. The loss of spontaneity was mentioned but using sex toys and pornography helped to enhance sex for some.

Interventions

Assessment of the degree and severity of sexual changes is necessary to identify what needs to be addressed as well as assessment of the woman's emotional and relationship health. Because there are a limited number of approved medications for sexual dysfunction in women, treatments focus on alleviating symptoms such as lack of lubrication; various psychological interventions are also recommended. Attention to bladder and bowel hygiene is recommended to prevent incontinence during sexual activity and pillows and foam wedges can be used to enhance comfort during sex. A key to sexual recovery, limited as it may be, is for the woman to discover for herself what feels good and what increases arousal. The use of a vibrator or the Eros Clitoral Therapy Device can be helpful. Exploring other areas of the body can increase the woman's erogenous zones. Massage, fantasy, role play, and erotic literature or movies can also increase arousal. As in men, it may take longer for the woman to become aroused and both she and her partner need to adapt to this change. Arousal may cause some spasticity and this should be recognized as a sign of sexual responsiveness. Similarly, signs of autonomic dysregulation, when mild, may signal the onset of an orgasm rather than something dangerous (Courtois et al., 2017).

Vaginal and vulvar moisturizers may provide comfort to women who experience dryness of the genitalia but they are not the same as lubricants that are used for sexual activity (see Chapter 14). Any sexual aids that the woman likes can be used to enhance the sexual experience. Hormone therapy, local or systemic, will alleviate vaginal dryness (Stoffel et al., 2018) but caution is needed due to concerns about long-term use.

Women report that health care providers do not address their needs for information and support regarding sexuality. The lack of attention to this is distressing and adds to the woman's experience of loss of confidence and self-esteem. Peer support may be very helpful as well as counseling provided by knowledgeable professionals (Thrussell et al., 2018).

Box 8.2 Resources for men and women with SCI

SCIRE Community Spinal Cord Injury Research Evidence
https://scireproject.com/community/
Sexual Medicine Society of North America
https://www.smsna.org/V1/index.php
VCH, GF Strong – Sexual Health Rehabilitation Servicehttps://www.brainstreams
.ca/resources/returning-to-life/sexual-health-rehabilitation-service-gf-strong/

Amputation

Evidence from a limited number of studies of individuals with lower limb amputation present a picture of overall adaptation to the consequences of loss of a limb. Many of the individuals in these studies have diabetes and the long-term consequences of the disease resulted in amputation. Changes in sexual functioning for these individuals may exist before the surgery and some may have not been sexually active for some time. In one study of both men and women, half of the participants were not sexually active at the time of amputation and of those who were sexually active, 60% met the clinical definition for sexual dysfunction. Sixty nine percent of the men reported erectile difficulties, 59% premature ejaculation, 40% avoided sex, and overall, 40% were dissatisfied with their sex life. Seventy five percent of the women reported infrequent sexual activity and 63% reported vaginismus or contraction of the muscles at the entrance to the vagina. Fifty percent of the women reported avoidance of sex (Woods, Hevey, Ryall, & O'Keeffe, 2018). Many of the sexual difficulties in men in particular are associated with the psychological effects of amputation and not with any organic cause. The level of the amputation and pain affects sexual positions and men with sexual problems experience depression as a result (Em et al., 2019). In another study, 56% of individuals reported a sexual problem; men were more likely to report at least one problem and having a recent amputation was more likely to result in developing a sexual problem (Verschuren, Geertzen, Enzlin, Dijkstra, & Dekker, 2016). A qualitative study reflected a similar picture (Verschuren, Geertzen, Enzlin, Dijkstra, & Dekker, 2015). Poor body image as a result of the surgery and a sense of not being 'complete' was described. Some participants said they felt ashamed and limited their activities as a result as well as the clothes they wore. Men reported erectile dysfunction associated with prescribed medication that was resolved with a change in dose. The reaction of the sexual partner to the stump was also mentioned as contributing to changes in sexuality. When partners were asked about the changes in their sexual relationship, a different reaction is seen (Verschuren, Zhdanova, et al., 2013). Only minor changes were described that were resolved by the couple; these included using different positions for sex. Some of the sexual changes were thought to be as a result of growing older or because of the disease that resulted in the loss of limb.

Communication with health care providers about sexual changes was limited in all of the studies cited. While participants in these studies said that it would have been helpful, there was recognition that during the early stages of rehabilitation, the focus was on mobility and healing from surgery and not on sexuality (Verschuren et al., 2015). When asked, 78% of health care providers working in rehabilitation programs said that they had not been asked about sexual changes by patients (Verschuren, Enzlin, Geertzen, Dijkstra, & Dekker, 2013).

Implications for health care providers

Inclusion of assessment of sexual functioning, education about healthy sexuality and adaptation to sexual changes, and referral to a specialist when needed are essential to the provision of care to anyone living with a spinal cord injury or amputation. This is especially important for health care providers working in rehabilitation teams where unfortunately, sexual health is often omitted in programming. Men are more likely to receive information about this than women and partners are not always included. This has led to general dissatisfaction with the information provided (New et al., 2016). When sexuality is addressed as part of rehabilitation, participants are generally satisfied with the information received (Rodger, 2019) and staff who provide the service find it enjoyable (Rodger, 2019). A sexuality training program for rehabilitation staff developed in the Netherlands, the Team Training Sexual Health Care (TTSHC), provides education based on the core themes of using a bio-psycho-social approach, identifying and understanding sexual health, talking about sex, and using multi-disciplinary teams to address sexuality as part of rehabilitation (Pieters, Kedde, & Bender, 2018).

A framework created for psychologists has application for all health care providers interacting with persons with a disability; the Disability and Sexuality Health Care Competency Model (DASH-CM) presents five competencies that are important for the comprehensive care of this population (Mona, Cameron, & Clemency Cordes, 2017). These competencies include critical awareness, knowledge about sexuality, a set of skills related to communication about sexuality, the use of acceptable language for the individual client/patient, and the ability to assess sexuality and sexual functioning including sexual diversity. This framework acknowledges that disability is a culture of its own and cultural competence must be part of any interactions with people living with a disability.

Conclusion

People who live with disability experience challenges in everyday life that may feel overwhelming at first but with expert help, most people adapt. One area that is unfortunately neglected is that of sexuality and sexual functioning. Rehabilitation after spinal cord injury or limb amputation should include assessment of sexual functioning, alterations to body image, and information and anticipatory guidance about expected changes. A baseline level of knowledge about these changes and how to adapt to them and/or where to find other health care providers with expertise in the area should be within the scope of practice of all health care providers who care for this population.

References

Addlakha, R., Price, J., & Heidari, S. (2017). Disability and sexuality: Claiming sexual and reproductive rights. *Reproductive Health Matters*, *25*(50), 4–9. doi: 10.1080/09688080.2017.1336375

Agmon, M., Sa'ar, A., & Araten-Bergman, T. (2016). The person in the disabled body: A perspective on culture and personhood from the margins. *International Journal for Equity in Health*, *15*(1), 147. doi: 10.1186/s12939-016-0437-2

Aikman, K., Oliffe, J.L., Kelly, M.T., & McCuaig, F. (2018). Sexual health in men with traumatic spinal cord injuries: A review and recommendations for primary health-care providers. *American Journal of Men's Health*, *12*(6), 2044–2054. doi: 10.1177/1557988318790883

Alexander, M., Courtois, F., Elliott, S., & Tepper, M. (2017). Improving sexual satisfaction in persons with spinal cord injuries: Collective wisdom. *Topics in Spinal Cord Injury Rehabilitation*, *23*(1), 57–70. doi: 10.1310/sci2301-57

Annon, J. (1974). *The behavioral treatment of sexual problems*. Honolulu: Enabling Systems.

Barbonetti, A., Cavallo, F., Felzani, G., Francavilla, S., & Francavilla, F. (2012). Erectile dysfunction is the main determinant of psychological distress in men with spinal cord injury. *Journal of Sexual Medicine*, *9*(3), 830–836. doi: 10.1111/j.1743-6109.2011.02599.x

Burns, S.M., Hough, S., Boyd, B.L., & Hill, J. (2010). Men's adjustment to spinal cord injury: The unique contributions of conformity to masculine gender norms. *American Journal of Men's Health*, *4*(2), 157–166. doi: 10.1177/1557988309332690

Chochina, L., Naudet, F., Chéhensse, C., Manunta, A., Damphousse, M., Bonan, I., & Giuliano, F. (2016). Intracavernous injections in spinal cord injured men with erectile dysfunction, a systematic review and meta-analysis. *Sexual Medicine Reviews*, *4*(3), 257–269. doi: 10.1016/j.sxmr.2016.02.005

Courtois, F., Alexander, M., & McLain, A.B.J. (2017). Women's sexual health and reproductive function after SCI. *Topics in Spinal Cord Injury Rehabilitation, 23*(1), 20–30. doi: 10.1310/sci2301-20

D'Andrea, S., Minaldi, E., Castellini, C., Cavallo, F., Felzani, G., Francavilla, S., & Barbonetti, A. (2020). Independent association of erectile dysfunction and low testosterone levels with life dissatisfaction in men with chronic spinal cord injury. *Journal of Sexual Medicine, 17*(5), 911–918. doi: 10.1016/j.jsxm.2020.01.018

Eglseder, K., & Demchick, B. (2017). Sexuality and spinal cord injury: The lived experiences of intimate partners. *OTJR (Thorofare N J), 37*(3), 125–131. doi: 10.1177/1539449217701394

Elliott, S., Hocaloski, S., & Carlson, M. (2017). A multidisciplinary approach to sexual and fertility rehabilitation: The sexual rehabilitation framework. *Topics in Spinal Cord Injury Rehabilitation, 23*(1), 49–56. doi: 10.1310/sci2301-49

Em, S., Karakoc, M., Sariyildiz, M.A., Bozkurt, M., Aydin, A., Cevik, R., & Nas, K. (2019). Assessment of sexual function and quality of life in patients with lower limb amputations. *Journal of Back and Musculoskeletal Rehabilitation, 32*(2), 277–285. doi: 10.3233/bmr-170873

Ferro, J.K.O., Lemos, A., Silva, C.P.D., Lima, C., Raposo, M.C.F., Cavalcanti, G.A., & Oliveira, D.A. (2019). Predictive factors of male sexual dysfunction after traumatic spinal cord injury. *Spine (Phila Pa 1976), 44*(17), 1228–1237. doi: 10.1097/brs.0000000000003049

Holland-Hall, C., & Quint, E.H. (2017). Sexuality and disability in adolescents. *Pediatric Clinics of North America, 64*(2), 435–449. doi: 10.1016/j.pcl.2016.11.011

Kasum, M., Orešković, S., Kordić, M., Čehić, E., Hauptman, D., Ejubović, E., Lila, A., & Smolčić, G. (2018). Improvement of sexual and reproductive function in men with spinal cord lesion. *Acta Clinica Croatica, 57*(1), 149–156. doi: 10.20471/acc.2018.57.01.19

Khak, M., Hassanijirdehi, M., Afshari-Mirak, S., Holakouie-Naieni, K., Saadat, S., Taheri, T., & Rahimi-Movaghar, V. (2016). Evaluation of sexual function and its contributing factors in men with spinal cord injury using a self-administered questionnaire. *American Journal of Men's Health, 10*(1), 24–31. doi: 10.1177/1557988314555122

Kovac, J.R., & Lipshultz, L.I. (2016). The importance of sexual function in men with spinal cord injuries. *Asian Journal of Andrology, 18*(3), 391. doi: 10.4103/1008-682x.179247

Kreuter, M., Taft, C., Siösteen, A., & Biering-Sørensen, F. (2011). Women's sexual functioning and sex life after spinal cord injury. *Spinal Cord, 49*(1), 154–160. doi: 10.1038/sc.2010.51

Latack, K., & Samplaski, M. (2020). Thematic analysis of sexual function conversations on a spinal cord injury social media platform. *Journal of Sexual Medicine, 17*(1), S33. doi: 10.1016/j.jsxm.2019.11.069

Latella, D., Maggio, M.G., Manuli, A., Militi, D., & Calabrò, R.S. (2019). Sexual dysfunction in male individuals with spinal cord iniury: What do we know so far? *Journal of Clinical Neuroscience, 68*, 20–27. doi: 10.1016/j.jocn.2019.07.038

Lombardi, G., Musco, S., Wyndaele, J.J., & Del Popolo, G. (2015). Treatments for erectile dysfunction in spinal cord patients: Alternatives to phosphodiesterase type 5 inhibitors? *Spinal Cord, 53*(12), 849–854. doi: 10.1038/sc.2015.116

Miranda, E.P., Gomes, C.M., de Bessa, J., Jr., Najjar Abdo, C.H., Suzuki Bellucci, C.H., de Castro Filho, J.E., de Carvalho, F., de Souza, D., Battistella, L., Scazufca, M., Bruschini, H., Barros Filho, T., & Srougi, M. (2016). Evaluation of sexual dysfunction in men with spinal cord injury using the male sexual quotient. *Archives of Physical Medicine and Rehabilitation, 97*(6), 947–952. doi: 10.1016/j.apmr.2016.01.005

Mona, L.R., Cameron, R.P., & Clemency Cordes, C. (2017). Disability culturally competent sexual healthcare. *American Psychology, 72*(9), 1000–1010. doi: 10.1037/amp0000283

New, P.W., Seddon, M., Redpath, C., Currie, K.E., & Warren, N. (2016). Recommendations for spinal rehabilitation professionals regarding sexual education needs and preferences of people with spinal cord dysfunction: A mixed-methods study. *Spinal Cord, 54*(12), 1203–1209. doi: 10.1038/sc.2016.62

Ohl, D.A., Carlsson, M., Stecher, V.J., & Rippon, G.A. (2017). Efficacy and safety of sildenafil in men with sexual dysfunction and spinal cord injury. *Sexual Medicine Reviews, 5*(4), 521–528. doi: 10.1016/j.sxmr.2017.01.007

Park, S.E., Elliott, S., Noonan, V.K., Thorogood, N.P., Fallah, N., Aludino, A., & Dvorak, M.F. (2017). Impact of bladder, bowel and sexual dysfunction on health status of people with thoracolumbar spinal cord injuries living in the community. *Journal of Spinal Cord Medicine*, *40*(5), 548–559. doi: 10.1080/10790268.2016.1213554

Pieters, R., Kedde, H., & Bender, J. (2018). Training rehabilitation teams in sexual health care: A description and evaluation of a multidisciplinary intervention. *Disability and Rehabilitation*, *40*(6), 732–739. doi: 10.1080/09638288.2016.1271026

Rodger, S. (2019). Evaluating sexual function education for patients after a spinal cord injury. *British Journal of Nursing*, *28*(21), 1374–1378. doi: 10.12968/bjon.2019.28.21.1374

Simpson, L.A., Hsieh, J., Wolfe, D. and the Spinal Cord Injury Rehabilitation Evidee (SCIRE) Team (2012). The health and life priorities of individuals with spinal cord injury: A systematic review. *Journal of Neurotrauma*, *29*(8), 1548–1555. doi: 10.1089/neu.2011.2226

Soler, J.M., Navaux, M.A., & Previnaire, J.G. (2018). Positive sexuality in men with spinal cord injury. *Spinal Cord*, *56*(12), 1199–1206. doi: 10.1038/s41393-018-0177-9

Stoffel, J.T., Van der Aa, F., Wittmann, D., Yande, S., & Elliott, S. (2018). Fertility and sexuality in the spinal cord injury patient. *World Journal of Urology*, *36*(10), 1577–1585. doi: 10.1007/s00345-018-2347-y

Thrussell, H., Coggrave, M., Graham, A., Gall, A., Donald, M., Kulshrestha, R., & Geddis, T. (2018). Women's experiences of sexuality after spinal cord injury: A UK perspective. *Spinal Cord*, *56*(11), 1084–1094. doi: 10.1038/s41393-018-0188-6

van der Meer, P., Post, M.W.M., van Leeuwen, C.M.C., van Kuppevelt, H.J.M., Smit, C.A.J., & van Asbeck, F.W.A. (2017). Impact of health problems secondary to SCI one and five years after first inpatient rehabilitation. *Spinal Cord*, *55*(1), 98–104. doi: 10.1038/sc.2016.103

Verschuren, J.E., Enzlin, P., Geertzen, J.H., Dijkstra, P.U., & Dekker, R. (2013). Sexuality in people with a lower limb amputation: A topic too hot to handle? *Disability and Rehabilitation*, *35*(20), 1698–1704. doi: 10.3109/09638288.2012.751134

Verschuren, J.E., Geertzen, J.H., Enzlin, P., Dijkstra, P.U., & Dekker, R. (2015). People with lower limb amputation and their sexual functioning and sexual well-being. *Disability and Rehabilitation*, *37*(3), 187–193. doi: 10.3109/09638288.2014.913704

Verschuren, J.E., Geertzen, J.H., Enzlin, P., Dijkstra, P.U., & Dekker, R. (2016). Sexual functioning and sexual well-being in people with a limb amputation: A cross-sectional study in the Netherlands. *Disability and Rehabilitation*, *38*(4), 368–373. doi: 10.3109/09638288.2015.1044029

Verschuren, J.E., Zhdanova, M.A., Geertzen, J.H., Enzlin, P., Dijkstra, P.U., & Dekker, R. (2013). Let's talk about sex: Lower limb amputation, sexual functioning and sexual well-being: A qualitative study of the partner's perspective. *Journal of Clinical Nursing*, *22*(23–24), 3557–3567. doi: 10.1111/jocn.12433

Woods, L., Hevey, D., Ryall, N., & O'Keeffe, F. (2018). Sex after amputation: The relationships between sexual functioning, body image, mood and anxiety in persons with a lower limb amputation. *Disability and Rehabilitation*, *40*(14), 1663–1670. doi: 10.1080/09638288.2017.1306585

Resources

BOOKS

The Ultimate Guide to Sex and Disability: For All of Us Who Live with Disabilities, Chronic Pain, & Illness (2010). Miriam Kaufman, Corey Silverberg, and Fran Odette. Cleis Press; San Fransisco, CA

Sex and Disability (2012) by Robert Mcruer and Anna Mollow. Duke University Press: Durham, NC

A Quick & Easy Guide to Sex & Disability (2020) by A. Andrews. Limerance Press; Portland, OR

9   Cancer in women

Breast cancer is the most common solid tumor in women, closely followed by gynecologic cancer. Both these cancers affect organs that are connected to body image and femininity for many women and, as a result, have significant risks to sexuality and sexual function.

Breast cancer

The most common cancer in women is breast cancer with more than 1.7 million cases annually worldwide; breast cancer represents 25% of all cancers in women. It is the fifth most common cause of cancer-related deaths with more than half a million deaths per year worldwide (World Cancer Research Fund) (https://www.wcrf.org/dietandcancer/breast-cancer). While rates of survival continue to rise with early diagnosis and effective treatments, the long- and late-term effects impact on quality of life, one aspect of which is sexuality and sexual functioning. Cancers affecting women include gynecologic cancers comprising cervical, endometrial, ovarian, and vulvar cancer.

Sexual side effects of breast cancer treatments

Treatment for breast cancer depends on the pathology of the tumor and whether it has spread to the lymph nodes and beyond. Most women receive multi-modality treatment with one or more strategies including surgery, radiation, chemotherapy, and adjuvant endocrine manipulating therapy. These treatments cause a number of side effects including altered body image, and sexual dysfunction. Sexual problems may be more acute for women under the age of 35 years, with 50% in one study reporting a decrease in sexual frequency and altered or absent orgasms (Blouet et al., 2019) and relationship difficulties (Congard et al., 2019).

1. Body image

Surgery for breast cancer, both mastectomy and lumpectomy, impact on body image and perception of femininity (Fallbjork, Salander, & Rasmussen, 2012). Women who undergo mastectomy report worse sexual function than women who have a lumpectomy, but the notion that body image is not or is minimally affected after lumpectomy is inaccurate. Any surgery will alter the physical appearance of the breast after lumpectomy and women may struggle to find a bra that fits correctly, they may find that their clothes don't fit properly or struggle with thoughts of what others see. This is highlighted in a study asking women about their satisfaction with the surgical scar from lumpectomy or mastectomy (Gass, Mitchell, & Hanna, 2019). When asked, 64% of women who had a lumpectomy and 67% of women who

DOI: 10.4324/9781003145745-9

had mastectomy disliked the location of the surgical scar. Only 26% of women who had a lumpectomy and 14% of women who had a mastectomy reported that they experienced minimal or no negative impact from the scars. The women also reported that they had to change the style of clothing they wore to hide the scar and they were also embarrassed if someone saw them undressed; they also felt uncomfortable when undressed, even if alone.

Mastectomy is associated with shame for some women (Moreira & Canavarro, 2010) and younger women appear to have more difficulty with body image after this surgery (Paterson, Lengacher, Donovan, Kip, & Tofthagen, 2016). While surgery is associated with worse body image, adjuvant radiation therapy and changes in weight add to the negative impact on body image (Rosenberg et al., 2013). If the woman is also depressed, something that is common in individuals with cancer during treatment, she may find it difficult to accept the changes in her body (Zimmermann, Scott, & Heinrichs, 2010) and this may further increase her depression. Changes to body image are associated with stress, guilt, avoidance of the partner, and for some, feeling deformed and unattractive (Rezaei, Elyasi, Janbabai, Moosazadeh, & Hamzehgardeshi, 2016). Some women report feeling uncomfortable during sex; this is especially pertinent to the woman who has not had reconstruction after mastectomy where being naked exposes an empty space and scar where her breast used to be (Fallbjörk, Rasmussen, Karlsson, & Salander, 2013).

Women who had a poor body image before treatment experience significant distress after surgery (Dahl, Reinertsen, Nesvold, Fosså, & Dahl, 2010). Reconstruction is reported to increase self-confidence and a sense of femininity (Hart, Pinell-White, & Losken, 2016) as well as attractiveness (Schmidt, Wetzel, Lange, Heine, & Ortmann, 2017). Those who have reconstruction experience better sexual function than women who have mastectomy without reconstruction (Archangelo, Sabino Neto, Veiga, Garcia, & Ferreira, 2019).

Immediate reconstruction is suggested to have a lesser impact on body image however this is not always the case. Women have described being shocked by the appearance of the scars after reconstruction (Herring, Paraskeva, Tollow, & Harcourt, 2019). Others report disappointment in the difference between their contralateral unaffected breast and the reconstructed one both in appearance and response to touch (Fallbjork et al., 2012). For those who have a breast implant rather than autologous tissue transfer, the breast may feel hard or "not even part of [my] body." There is variation in response; some women may be happy with the loss of lower abdominal fat after autologous tissue reconstruction or with firmer, smaller, or bigger breasts if they had bilateral mastectomy and reconstruction. Some women may expect an outcome that does not match with the reality and they are likely to be dissatisfied or even angry at the outcome of reconstruction (Hart, Pinell-White, Egro, & Losken, 2015).

Another factor impacting on body image is lymphedema resulting from axillary node dissection or removal (Alcorso & Sherman, 2016). The swelling leads to difficulty finding clothes that fit properly and the woman may be very sensitive to others commenting or asking about this. Sexual functioning is impacted by lymphedema depending on how much swelling there is, the need to wear a compression sleeve, and the partner's response to this (Winch et al., 2015) as well as feeling unattractive. Women also report that wearing a compression sleeve made undressing as part during sexual activity difficult. (Radina, Fu, Horstman, & Kang, 2015).

African American (AA) women may have different values related to body image; while health care providers may encourage AA women to undergo reconstruction with breast implants after mastectomy, some AA women may prefer autologous tissue procedures as it feels more natural to use their own tissue for reconstruction. Some may have a mistrust of the medical profession for historical reasons and refuse reconstruction after mastectomy.

Access to breast prostheses and financial concerns as well as the finding a prosthesis to match their skin color are also cited as factors in decisions about post-surgery intervention (Rubin, Chavez, Alderman, & Pusic, 2013). Latinix women describe a host of changes incurred with treatment including feeling incomplete, distress with weight gain, and alopecia having a profound effect on body image. Fear of rejection coupled with shame and embarrassment when undressing in front of their (male) partner accompanied concerns about the partner's response to lack of sex during treatment (Buki, Reich, & Lehardy, 2016).

2. Sexual functioning

Breast cancer treatment results in global sexual problems for women including loss of desire, lack of arousal and orgasm, and loss of sexual pleasure. This is in addition to the body image changes cited above resulting in changes to sexual self-image and sexual self-esteem. No matter the type of surgery – mastectomy with or without reconstruction or breast-conserving surgery (lumpectomy) – women experience sexual changes (Cornell et al., 2017).

An important aspect of female sexual functioning is the role that breast sensuality plays in the sexual response. The breast and nipple-areola complex is a sensual organ recognized as playing a role in desire, arousal, and orgasm (Levin & Meston, 2006; Levin, 2006). Gass and colleagues (Gass et al., 2017) report that 86.2% of the women in their study agreed that their breasts played an important role during sexual activity before surgery. Of those treated with any surgery (lumpectomy, mastectomy with- or without reconstruction), 42% had significant sexual dysfunction. Women who had lumpectomy reported greater pleasure from breast caressing, an important aspect of sexual arousal. An important finding from this study is that nipple-sparing mastectomy, while esthetically more pleasing to women, does not result in better sexual functioning. Hypoesthesia, loss of sensation over part of or the whole breast, as well as phantom breast pain after mastectomy, also contribute to sexual changes (Lovelace, McDaniel, & Golden, 2019).

Chemotherapy has a profound effect on sexual functioning because of its impact on ovarian production of estrogen as well as causing alopecia, including loss of pubic hair. The loss of estrogen results in vulvo-vaginal atrophy, leading to pain with genital touch and dyspareunia (Tat, Doan, Yoo, & Levine, 2018). Chemically-induced menopause has global effects on sexuality including fatigue, loss of libido, anorgasmia, and loss of pleasurable sexual sensations (Emilee, Ussher, & Perz, 2010). Another side effect of loss of estrogen is a weakened pelvic floor; the loss of tone in the pelvic floor musculature results in incontinence that also has a negative impact on sexuality and sexual activity (Ghizzani, Bruni, & Luisi, 2018).

Endocrine therapy, used as long-term adjuvant therapy for women with hormone-dependant breast cancer, is recommended by the National Comprehensive Cancer Network (NCCN) (https://www.nccn.org/professionals/physician_gls/pdf/breast.pdf). Women who are premenopausal at diagnosis should take tamoxifen for at least 5 years and when menopausal, take an aromatase inhibitor (AI) for another 5 years (Saha et al., 2017). Women who are post-menopausal at diagnosis should take an AI for at least 5 years. These recommendations are updated regularly with new evidence, but adjuvant therapy remains an important strategy in preventing recurrence and mortality from breast cancer.

It is also recommended that pre-menopausal women with high-risk breast cancer who need chemotherapy should also be prescribed ovarian suppression in addition to endocrine therapy to reduce the risk of recurrence (Burstein et al., 2016). This multi-modal adjuvant therapy has been shown to increase the severity of side effects including sexual side effects

(Colleoni & Munzone, 2015). Tamoxifen plus ovarian suppression causes increased vaginal dryness and/or loss of desire.

In early clinical trials the sexual side effects of these medications were underreported (Zhu, Cohen, Rosenzweig, & Bender, 2019). Subsequent studies have shown that sexual side effects are common. Thirty one percent of women on tamoxifen reported dyspareunia in one study (Baumgart et al., 2013) and 63% reached the threshold for sexual dysfunction in another (Daldoul et al., 2017). The latter study also found an increase in anxiety and depression and low relationship satisfaction. In pre-menopausal women under the age of 39 years, 36% cited vaginal dryness as the reason for avoiding sexual intercourse (Ljungman et al., 2018). Vulvar symptoms are among the most common sexual side effects encompassing dryness and discomfort in the labia and clitoris. Women who are not sexually active while on endocrine therapy cite loss of interest/libido (78%) as well as not feeling attractive (Marino, Saunders, & Hickey, 2017).

The aromatase inhibitors are known to cause the worst side effects; 64.7% of women taking this form of endocrine therapy experienced sexual dysfunction compared to 33.8% of women who were prescribed tamoxifen (Gandhi et al., 2019). In the first 2 years of AI use, only 52% of the women in a study were sexually active and a further 79% developed a new sexual problem. Twenty four percent of these women stopped having sex and 13% switched to another therapy. Three-quarters of the total sample were distressed about these problems (Schover, Baum, Fuson, Brewster, & Melhem-Bertrandt, 2014).

Changes to the vulvar structure of women on AI therapy are noticeable on physical examination and include decreased fat on the mons pubis, retracted clitoris, decreased volume of the labia, and dry, shiny, and pale introital tissues (Lester, Pahouja, Andersen, & Lustberg, 2015). These result in dyspareunia and fear of pain during sexual activity leading to loss of libido (Robinson, Bell, Christakis, Ivezic, & Davis, 2017). Assessment of these changes can be conducted using the Vaginal Assessment Scale (VAS) and the Vulvar Assessment Scale (VuAS) (Eaton et al., 2017). These 4-item scales are administered by a health care provider and measure the woman's perception of dryness, soreness, irritation, and pain (dyspareunia or touch).

Urinary incontinence is also not uncommon in these women (Soldera, Ennis, Lohmann, & Goodwin, 2018). Fecal incontinence has also been shown to occur (Robinson, Bell, Christakis, Ivezic, & Davis, 2017) and these both have negative impacts on sexual activity as well as body image (Sousa et al., 2018) and decreased sexual satisfaction (Landi et al., 2016).

Impact on partner and the couple

The diagnosis and treatment of breast cancer precipitates a change of role for the partner of the woman that ultimately affects the relationship dynamic (Ussher & Perz, 2010). The sexual relationship changes too, and couples may experience a decrease in physical and emotional closeness. The physical changes after surgery result in both the woman and her partner needing to re-establish their response to her altered body (de Boer, Zeiler, & Slatman, 2019). This is not just about how her body looks but also about how she responds to sexual touch; this can be a minefield where the partner may not understand her responses to what was pleasurable and is now painful or numb. Sexual adjustment involves experiencing sexual changes as a loss and the importance of mourning what has been lost. Adjusting to these changes is a cognitive process, influenced by social and cultural factors while rehabilitation requires treatment of physical changes and sexual behaviors (Benoot, Saelaert, Hannes, & Bilsen, 2017). Non-sexual affection is seen to improve satisfaction for couples

(Rottmann et al., 2017). Kissing and caressing are important in maintaining emotional connection for both partners and increase satisfaction with their sex life, even when it is different from what they experienced before.

Cancer itself is an experience of uncertainty about the future and this uncertainty plays out in the couple's sexual and affectional relationship. Partners often make assumptions about how each other is thinking and feeling and this is highlighted in a qualitative study exploring changes in the sexual relationship related to uncertainty (Canzona, Fisher, & Ledford, 2019). The partners described what they saw as the woman's preoccupation with the changes in her body. When the woman hid her body during sexual activity, the partner was uncertain if she would continue to do this. They felt guilty about wanting sex and guilty about being angry about the changed sexual relationship. These men (all partners in this study were male) also struggled with how to show support. Some talked about avoiding looking at the woman's chest during sex to prevent her from feeling bad. This affected their communication as well; they avoided any mention of their feelings about the altered sexual relationship. These descriptions were contradicted by the women who felt afraid that men felt rejected due to her loss of interest. The women questioned whether their partner was telling the truth when they said that they were not bothered by her physical changes. The one aspect of this that both individuals agreed on was the belief that there was nothing that would help their situation and that talking about this was futile.

Communication is an important aspect of relationship satisfaction; when one or both members of the couple attempt to buffer their communication about how they are feeling to protect the other, the emotional bond between them may be negatively impacted, despite the intent of protecting the other (Perndorfer, Soriano, Siegel, & Laurenceau, 2019). When the partner's communication does not meet the expectations of the woman with cancer, conflict, and relationship dissatisfaction may result (Borstelmann et al., 2015).

Breast cancer in sexual minority women

Much like their heterosexual counterparts, sexual minority women describe a connection between their physical body and sexuality (Brown & McElroy, 2018). The side effects of mastectomy for sexual minority women also result in loss of breast sensuality and sensation, loss of libido, and a negative impact on their sexual relationship. They also experience sexual pain, difficulties with orgasm, and less frequent sexual activity (Boehmer, Ozonoff, Timm, Winter, & Potter, 2014). Endocrine therapy has a similar effect on sexual minority women as it does on heterosexual women with decreased desire, loss of breast sensation, and absence of sexual activity (Brown & McElroy, 2018). An area of unmet needs for this population is the provision of information about sexuality and relationships as well as information about treatment choices including the option for women undergoing mastectomy to decline reconstruction (Lisy, Peters, Schofield, & Jefford, 2018). The care of sexual minority women with breast cancer remains an understudied topic and this lack of evidence may influence the care they receive (Cathcart-Rake, 2018).

Interventions for women with breast cancer

Women may not seek help for sexual problems, perhaps believing that they should live with them and be glad to be alive. Less than half (49%) of women in one study sought help of any kind, and of those, only 24% talked to a health care provider (Reese et al., 2020). They primarily talked to their gynecologist, followed by an oncologist or oncology nurse or nurse practitioner. They also talked to their partner, friends, and looked for information online. Finding help can be difficult and it may be embarrassing to talk about sexual problems (Sousa et al., 2018). Women want to be forewarned about sexual changes when taking endocrine therapy; 68% wanted written information about physical changes including changes to body image and sexual response (Ussher, Perz, & Gilbert, 2012). Just 41% had received information about these side effects and of these, only 39% had talked to their oncologist. The information that women receive may not always meet their needs or be provided by the health care provider of their choice. Some women may prefer to talk to a nurse or their primary care provider rather than a specialist and the partner should be part of the conversation (Den Ouden, Pelgrum-Keurhorst, Uitdehaag, & De Vocht, 2019). Young women may be particularly in need of timely information related to sexual changes (Recio-Saucedo, Gerty, Foster, Eccles, & Cutress, 2016). There is evidence that a group-based intervention about vulvo-vaginal dryness is acceptable to women (Millman et al., 2020). This is important because lack of resources is often cited as a barrier to treating sexual problems in women. A brief 2-hour group-based intervention was found to be acceptable to those who attended and allowed for peer support.

A detailed description of moisturizers, lubricants, and other sexual aids can be found in Chapter 14. A multi-disciplinary approach including both physical and psycho-sexual interventions is considered the most effective in providing assistance to the woman as an individual and as part of a couple (Krychman & Millheiser, 2013). Both hormonal and non-hormonal medications may be helpful in relieving vulvo-vaginal symptoms; a step-wise approach is recommended starting with identification of where the irritation or pain is experienced. This is important because women will often state that they are dry 'down there' and a different approach is needed to treat vulvar versus vaginal atrophy. Non-hormonal moisturizers and/or lubricants can initially be recommended and, if pelvic floor involvement is suspected, a referral to a pelvic floor physiotherapist should be made. A sexuality counselor or sex therapist can provide valuable support for more specialized individuals and couples.

The use of local estrogen is a controversial topic and one that has generated much discussion. The North American Menopause Society (NAMS), the International Society for the Study of Women's Sexual Health (ISSWSH) (Faubion et al., 2018) and the American College of Obstetricians and Gynecologists (ACOG) ("Committee Opinion No. 659: The Use of Vaginal Estrogen in Women With a History of Estrogen-Dependent Breast Cancer.," 2016) recommend that the use of local estrogen should only be undertaken after non-hormonal interventions are insufficient and should include discussion with the treating oncologist and informed consent of the woman.

Topical or local estrogen is the only treatment that addresses the problem (Eden, 2016) – lack of estrogen – while moisturizers and lubricants provide temporary relief at best. Low-dose estrogen is absorbed in very small amounts; blood levels are in the normal range for post-menopausal women (Santen et al., 2017). Both low-dose estradiol (E2) and estriol (E3) are effective in treating vulvo-vaginal atrophy with minimal absorption (Donders, Ruban, Bellen, & Grinceviciene, 2019). Conjugated equine estrogen (CEE) in cream form results in higher absorption but a small amount massaged into the tissues at the vaginal introitus can be helpful for women who experience acute pain in that area (Faubion et al., 2018).

It is suggested that using local estrogen is safer in women taking tamoxifen than an aromatase inhibitor because tamoxifen blocks estrogen receptors while the AIs reduce estrogen in the blood (Faubion et al., 2018). For women taking an AI who do not find relief from non-hormonal products, switching to tamoxifen and using ultra-low dose local estrogen may be considered (Sassarini et al., 2018). In a meta-analysis of studies investigating the safety of local estrogen for women on AIs, Pavlović and associates (Pavlović et al., 2019) concluded that local estrogen was not associated with systemic absorption of sex hormones and thus may be regarded as safe. A product that contains estriol and lyophillized *Lactobacillus acidophilus* (Gynoflor™) has been shown to be safe for women taking AIs (Donders et al., 2014).

Other strategies include ospemifene, a selective estrogen receptor modulator (SERM) similar to tamoxifen that has no effect on breast tissue. Dehydroepiandrosterone (DHEA) also has been shown to be effective in the treatment of vulvo-vaginal atrophy and in small studies, vaginal testosterone has been shown to reduce symptoms in post-menopausal women on AIs (Lemke et al., 2017). It has been suggested that vaginal laser treatment may be effective for these women and early studies showed improvements in vulvo-vaginal symptoms (Jha, Wyld, & Krishnaswamy, 2019; Pearson, Booker, Tio, & Marx, 2019), but women reported severe pain during the treatment (Pitsouni, Grigoriadis, Falagas, Salvatore, & Athanasiou, 2017). While approved for other indications, the FDA has issued a warning about the use of laser therapies for the treatment of vulvo-vaginal atrophy (https://www.fda.gov/medical-de vices/safety-communications/fda-warns-against-use-energy-based-devices-perform-vaginal -rejuvenation-or-vaginal-cosmetic).

Physician comfort in prescribing local hormonal therapy for women after breast cancer is generally low (Kingsberg et al., 2019). In one study, 21% of oncologists prescribed local estrogen to their patients with breast cancer and 25% said this should only be for women with breast cancer that is not hormone dependent (Biglia et al., 2017). Some prescribed this only after the cessation of endocrine therapy while others would prescribe for women on tamoxifen. Just 15% of those surveyed thought that local estrogen therapy was safe. In another study, 84% of physicians felt comfortable prescribing local estrogen to women with non-hormone-dependent breast cancer (Richter et al., 2019).

Couple-based interventions

It is important for the partner of the woman to be involved in treatment decision-making so that they understand what lies ahead and to mitigate challenges to communication (Miaja, Platas, & Martinez-Cannon, 2017). Attention should be paid to how the partner is coping and to offer psychosocial support even when they deny difficulties. A small pilot program of a 5-session educational intervention showed positive impacts on partners' depression, anxiety, and adjustment (Lewis et al., 2008). While the focus was not on sexuality, the partners reported that after attending the program, they found ways of connecting with their spouse. The female partners reported that the men were more compassionate, and they felt closer to them. Reese et al. (2016) conducted a study of an intimacy enhancement intervention for couples affected by breast cancer. The 4-session, telephone-based program focuses on communication and sexuality and included exercises to be done between sessions. The intervention had good results, especially in the areas of sexual functioning and related distress. The education included content about breast touching that was reinforced in the sensate focus exercises that were included as homework.

In a review of couple-based interventions, excluding the Reese study cited above, six interventions were assessed (Carroll, Baron, & Carroll, 2016). The programs included psychoeducation about cancer treatments and side effects and the impact on couples and comprised three to six sessions, each lasting 60–120 minutes. Improvements were seen in all domains of sexual functioning, sexual self-image, and sexual relationships but not in physical symptoms. Of note is that women experienced an increase in sexual desire and body image, two factors that impact on the couple's sexual relationship. In a systematic review of couple-based interventions for all cancers, the role of reframing negative thoughts about sexual activity was noted as a benefit (Jonsdottir, Jonsdottir, & Klinke, 2018).

Couple-based interventions improve communication and sexual as well as relationship functioning (Regan et al., 2012); however, partners are sometimes reluctant to attend joint counseling, thinking that this is the woman's problem to solve. It may be difficult for the couple to discuss sexual problems and they may actively avoid the topic (Yu & Sherman, 2015). Men may struggle to maintain closeness to their partner in the absence of sex (Fergus & Gray, 2009) and if communication about this is avoided, the relationship itself may suffer from inaccurate assumptions about emotions and desire. Couple counseling can be helpful in addressing negative or inaccurate assumptions; encouraging the couple to talk freely about their thoughts and feelings can bring them closer together (Moreira & Canavarro, 2013).

Box 9.1 Using the BETTER model with a woman with breast cancer

B: Bring up the topic

"Women taking the same medication to prevent a recurrence of breast cancer often experience some sexual problems. What has been your experience since you started treatment?"

E: Explain that sexuality is important for quality of life

"Many women stop having sex because of pain and loss of desire. But sex is important for your relationship and general well-being."

T: Tell the patient that resources will be found to answer her questions

"We have books and videos that explain some of the things you can do to make sex more comfortable. Let me show you where you can find these."

T: While the timing may not be right, there is always help available if she needs it

"We also have a sexual medicine specialist who sees many of our patients. If you need to see her at any point during or after your treatment, I can arrange a referral."

E: Educate about the sexual side effects of treatment

"Because the medication you are taking essentially removes any estrogen in your body, women experience big change in their vulva and vagina. Lubricants and moisturizers can provide some relief as you will read in the pamphlet I have given you. But you can always ask for more information from me or any other member of your health care team."

R: Record the discussion in the patient's chart

"Patient informed about changes to sexuality and offered a referral to Dr XXXXX when needed."

Gynecologic cancer

Gynecologic cancer affects the uterus, ovaries, cervix, or vulva and has a profound impact on sexual functioning, physically as well as psychologically. Treatment involves multi-modality interventions depending on the location, grade, and stage of the cancer; these include surgery, radiation (external and internal), and chemotherapy. Surgery has a major impact on sexual functioning due to disruption of nerves and blood vessels supplying the pelvic organs. Anatomical changes including the loss of the upper third of the vagina (Iavazzo et al., 2015) are theorized to play an important role in arousal and accommodating the penis during penetration. Radiation causes alterations in the elasticity of the vaginal tissues as well as making blood vessels friable (Rodrigues et al., 2012).

Sexual problems experienced after treatment tend to persist over time, and with increasing age, women are less likely to be sexually active (Grimm et al., 2015). Women describe feeling empty; this eventually fades but their experience of their own body is unpredictable. The impact on sexuality is profound with the loss of what was once pleasurable now being problematic (Sekse, Gjengedal, & Raheim, 2013). Similar to women treated for other cancers, loss of libido and pain with sexual activity are common (Sekse, Hufthammer, & Vika, 2017). It is important to note that radiation to the pelvis is associated not only with vaginal stenosis and pain (Lind et al., 2011) but also with urinary and fecal incontinence (Pieterse et al., 2013); these are associated with social and psychological consequences as well as with sexual problems (Dunberger et al., 2010). The psychological impact of these cancers is important to consider. For some women, the removal of part or all of the sexual organs has a profoundly negative impact on femininity and sexual identity (Rowlands, Lee, Beesley, & Webb, 2014). It is important to remember that survivors of gynecologic cancers are first and foremost women with a comprehensive context to their lives beyond a biomedical view of the damage done to their internal and external sexual organs (White, Faithfull, & Allan, 2013).

Cervical cancer

Women diagnosed with cervical cancer may experience symptoms related to sexual activity before diagnosis. Post-coital bleeding is often the first sign that something is wrong, but women also report dyspareunia and vaginal dryness (Grion et al., 2016). Most women will be treated with a total hysterectomy and bilateral salpingo-oophorectomy causing immediate menopause and associated symptoms (Bae & Park, 2016). Adjuvant radiation is usually required, and this causes multiple physical changes to the vagina and adjacent tissues. Vaginal stenosis and shortening is common and this results in significant problems with being able to have penetrative intercourse (Correa et al., 2016) as well as pelvic examination as part of well-woman care. Younger women are more likely to be distressed by these sexual changes but asking for help remains a problem with just 35% of women in one study talking to a health care provider about this (Vermeer et al., 2015).

For women who still want to have children after a diagnosis of cervical cancer, radical trachelectomy may be a surgical option. Compared to hysterectomy, this surgery appears to cause less sexual distress (Brotto, Smith, Breckon, & Plante, 2013). Sexual intercourse after trachelectomy appears to feel normal to women (Lloyd, Briggs, Kane, Jeyarajah, & Shepherd, 2014) but women may experience other sexual problems that persist for many months (Froeding et al., 2014). These include loss of libido, dryness and dyspareunia, bleeding during intercourse, vaginal shortening, and sexual dissatisfaction.

Endometrial cancer

Endometrial cancer is treated by surgical removal of the uterus but some women may need adjuvant radiation therapy as well. Younger women may experience greater distress associated with loss of fertility after treatment; older women tend to adjust to this loss better, especially if they are post-menopausal and have already made accommodations in sexual activity to estrogen loss (Rowlands et al., 2014). Adjuvant brachytherapy does not appear to add additional sexual problems (Becker et al., 2011; Quick, Seamon, Abdel-Rasoul, Salani, & Martin, 2012).

Ovarian cancer

Ovarian cancer is often called the 'silent cancer' because symptoms are vague and appear late in the disease. Diagnostic tests are invasive and add to the distress that many women experience (Tan, Sharpe, & Russell, 2020). Treatment involves total hysterectomy and bilateral salpingo-oophorectomy followed by chemotherapy causing immediate menopause; both the physical and psychological side effects impact on sexuality (Wilmoth, Hatmaker-Flanigan, LaLoggia, & Nixon, 2011).

Women describe loss of desire associated with dyspareunia; this is accompanied by avoidance of sexual touch, fearing that it would lead to intercourse. Changes to sensations of orgasm can result in sadness and feelings of loss and grief. Women may also feel guilty about the changes in their sexual relationship and the effects on their partner (Fischer, Marguerie, & Brotto, 2019). Even though the anatomical changes are internal, some women describe alterations in body image (Whicker et al., 2017). This includes loss of hair, especially pubic hair that makes women feel like they are pre-pubescent and not like an adult woman (Jayde, Boughton, & Blomfield, 2013).

Vulvar cancer

While improvements have been made in surgical management, treatment of vulvar cancer is disfiguring and carries with it psychological distress and significant sexual problems. In the past this was seen predominately in older women but more recently, the human papilloma virus (HPV) is seen as the cause of genital warts and vulvar cancer in younger women (Jeffries & Clifford, 2011).

Sexual changes may occur before the cancer is diagnosed with vulvar itching and dryness (Aerts et al., 2012). The invasiveness of surgery is dependent on the stage and grade of the cancer with a trend towards more conservative tissue-sparing surgery in recent years. This has resulted in less severe impacts on sexual functioning and body image; more radical surgery, lymph node dissection causing lymphedema, and multiple surgical excisions are responsible for greater sexual dysfunction (Barlow, Hacker, Hussain, & Parmenter, 2014). More advanced vulvar cancer requires multi-modality treatment including chemo-radiation or radiation alone; this adds morbidity and additional impact on body image, sexuality, and quality of life (Froeding et al., 2018).

Surgery that does not remove the clitoris is theorized to have less impact on sexual functioning, but loss of sensation is seen even after this less radical surgery (Forner, Dakhil, & Lampe, 2013). Vulvectomy results in sexual problems including pain on penetration and with thrusting, abdominal pain during sexual intercourse, and difficulty having orgasms (Aerts, Enzlin, Verhaeghe, Vergote, & Amant, 2014). When women describe their experience of this cancer, their isolation and loneliness are highlighted. Women report significant sexual changes including not being able to tolerate penetration, loss of sensation, loss of libido, incontinence, and the fear of the end of their relationship (Jeffries & Clifford, 2011). Because of the location of the cancer, it is invisible and for some women, this means that it is difficult to talk about and the lack of peer support means that women often have to deal with this on their own, further increasing their sense of isolation and invisibility (Jeffries & Clifford, 2012). This is particularly cogent for women in smaller cities and towns because of the rarity of the cancer.

Effect on couple/partner

As with all cancers, the partner of the woman with gynecologic cancer experiences changes in their own quality of life, including sexuality. Changes to the sexual relationship are important for male partners of women with cervical cancer (Abbott-Anderson, Young, & Eggenberger, 2020; Oldertrøen Solli, de Boer, Nyheim Solbraekke, & Thoresen, 2019; Vermeer, Bakker, Kenter, Stiggelbout, & Ter Kuile, 2016) and other gynecologic cancers (Abbott-Anderson et al., 2020). Men may be particularly vulnerable when their partner is diagnosed and treated (Oldertrøen Solli et al., 2019). The physical side effects of radiation and associated pain and stenosis may make intercourse impossible and this affects men. The man may lose interest in not only the sexual relationship but also the relationship itself or he may pressure the woman to be sexually active despite the limitations caused by treatment (Vermeer et al., 2016). However, if the partner of the woman is supportive, sexuality may not be negatively affected and there is even hope for improvement in sexual function over time (Lindau, Abramsohn, & Matthews, 2015). The couple's relationship may grow closer and communication is key to mutual understanding and developing a new way of being sexual in the aftermath of treatment (Abbott-Anderson et al., 2020).

Communication with health care providers

Information about sexuality and changes to sexual functioning has been identified as an unmet need in many studies (Beesley, Alemayehu, & Webb, 2018). Communication between women with gynecologic cancer and their health care providers shows the same reluctance on the part of professionals to open the conversation with patients as seen in other cancers (Jeffries & Clifford, 2011). Women may not be provided with any anticipatory guidance about what to expect after treatment, verbally or in writing. The gender of the health care provider, in many cases male, was cited as one potential reason for this by a woman with vulvar cancer (Jeffries & Clifford, 2012). The responsibility for a discussion does not lie solely with the physician; oncology nurses should be able to provide education and support for these women (Stilos, Doyle, & Daines, 2008). Nurses are products of society and carry the same values and perceptions of what is acceptable to talk about. This may result in a lack of enquiry into the experiences of women dealing with the side effects of treatment (Williams, Hauck, & Bosco, 2017). Health care providers cite a number of barriers to discussing sexuality with patients including personal embarrassment, lack of time, when in the treatment trajectory this is important to women, as well as lack of education and training about sexuality (Vermeer et al., 2015). Lack of resources and specialists is also cited; however, sex therapists are rarely consulted even if available.

The reluctance of women to raise the topic with health care providers is a barrier to a discussion. This reluctance may be based in embarrassment; however, if the health care provider raises the subject, this provides an opening for the woman to disclose. If the health care provider does not initiate the discussion, the woman may interpret this as something shameful and she remains isolated with her needs unmet. Not being provided with anticipatory guidance about the changes to expect and normalization of these may result in anger and lack of trust (Sekse, Raheim, & Gjengedal, 2015).

When women are presented with an opportunity to talk about their sexual problems, they are often shocked that someone has asked them about this and state that they have no problems. But they are then more likely to ask for help in the future if they know that something can be done. Presenting questions about sexual function in an intake form may negate the perception that sexuality is a taboo topic but this does not guarantee that the health care provider will address the problems identified (Kennedy et al., 2015). Some health care providers think that the patient should guide the timing. While some may prefer this to happen at the end of treatment (Hay et al., 2018), others may want information earlier, including at the time of treatment decision-making. A simple question such as "When would you prefer to talk about sexual changes?" will provide guidance for the health care provider.

Information can be provided in different ways; some women and their partner prefer internet-based information (Vermeer et al., 2015) while others are happy with printed material (Lubotzky et al., 2016). Still others would prefer to have a face-to-face discussion with their health care provider (McCallum, Lefebvre, Jolicoeur, Maheu, & Lebel, 2012). Finally, populations such as adolescents and young adults and sexual minorities may have unique needs related to information about sexuality that need to be addressed (Harris, 2019). Care should be taken to not make assumptions about sexual orientation and partner status; gender neutral language should be used with all patients if and until they disclose with terms they want to be used.

Interventions

The most frequently recommended intervention in the literature is the use of dilators for women who have had radiation or surgery. The rationale for dilator use is to mitigate the vaginal shortening, tightening, and stenosis seen after radiation therapy in particular. Dilators are usually made of plastic or silicone and come in various sizes (Liu, Juravic, Mazza, & Krychman, 2020). The radiation oncologist may suggest a specific size; if using a graduated set, women should move to the larger size once they can insert the dilator comfortably. Women are advised to use the dilator 2–3 times a week with lubricant beginning 4 weeks after the end of radiation therapy. Earlier initiation when inflammation is present should be avoided because if the woman experiences pain or bleeding she is unlikely to continue long-term use. The dilator should remain in place for 5–10 minutes and should be used for an indefinite amount of time, depending on clinical assessment (Matos et al., 2019).

Acceptance and consistent use of the dilator is challenging for many women. Some view this as a sex toy and are not willing to use it. Others find the dilator to be intrusive and a reminder of the invasiveness of treatment (Cullen et al., 2012). Resistance to use may be presented as being too tired, lacking privacy, or simply forgetting (Bakker et al., 2015). Supporting women in the use of dilators is vitally important. This can be achieved by clear and straightforward instructions and the rationale for use including the need for monitoring of their disease and well-woman pelvic examinations. It is also important to understand the woman's values and beliefs about sexuality and to be empathetic in response to her emotional reaction (Cullen et al., 2013). Information should also be provided about the need for lubricants and how to access them. Anticipatory guidance about the possibility of bleeding and pain with use may help to prevent cessation of use. A nurse-led group intervention for women using dilators showed promise in promoting adherence to use (Bakker et al., 2017); this may be more helpful than one-on-one counseling due to the consistent nature of the information presented.

Other interventions include the use of local estrogen for vulvo-vaginal atrophy that has been shown to be safe for women with gynecologic cancers. The only contraindication to the use of local estrogen is hormone-dependent cancer and most gynecologic cancers are not (Guidozzi, 2013). Estrogen cream can be used with the dilator instead of a lubricant. Mindfulness-based cognitive behavioral therapy has been shown to improve sexual function across all domains and may also decrease distress (Brotto et al., 2012). Web-based peer support has been shown to improve body image and sexual concerns and openness to discussion of sexuality among participants (Wiljer et al., 2011).

Box 9.2 Case study

Pat R. is a 59-year old woman who was diagnosed with endometrial cancer six months ago. She counts herself fortunate that it was caught early, but she still had to have surgery and internal radiation that was completed three weeks ago. She regards herself as very healthy and has always exercised every day so why this happened to her is something that confuses her. But she knows she has to let go of that and focus on getting back to her normal life. She is married to Joe, her husband of 35 years but they have not been sexually active for almost 10 years. She started experiencing pain during intercourse, likely due to peri-menopause, and sex fell by the wayside. She says that they still kiss and cuddle, but sex was something she didn't really enjoy anyway, so she doesn't miss it. Joe is understanding, she says, and has been very supportive during her treatment. He has even started cooking a couple of nights a week and this is something she never thought she would see.

She was told by the nurse at her last appointment that it is now time for her to start using a dilator. She is terrified at the prospect and afraid that it is going to hurt and that she is going to cause damage to her body. She tells the nurse all of this in a teary phone call where she can hardly get the word out. She has never even used tampons and the thought of the dilator makes her panic. The nurse reassures her that she will be able to do this, and that it is important for her ongoing care that she keeps her vagina open so that she can have pelvic exams. This does not seem to help; she hates those examinations and finds herself not sleeping for a week before she sees the gyne-oncologist in anticipation of this.

The nurse talks to her about doing some deep breathing to relax before she uses the dilator and Pat laughs to herself; relax indeed! Her husband had bought a water-based lubricant just as the pamphlet said, and she was grateful that he had gone to the drugstore instead of her. The nurse gave her some tips; she needed to insert the dilator towards her tail bone and she should not force it. She was told that it would feel strange the first few times, and that she may only be able to insert it a little bit at the beginning. She wrote all of this down in her neat handwriting but her hands were shaking a little. She wasn't sure she was going to be able to do this.

> *The next day she woke an hour before she needed to. Her hands were shaking as she took the dilator out of the bag. Joe was still asleep so she went into the den, thinking that she would do it before he woke up. She read the notes she had made again and also the instructions in the pamphlet the nurse had given her. She lay down on the couch, took a deep breath and then realized that she hadn't used the lubricant! Back to the bathroom she went, her courage fading fast. But to her credit, she managed to insert the dilator, just a little bit. As the nurse had warned her, it felt weird but at least she had managed to get that far. Tomorrow was another day, she said to herself, and maybe it'll be better ...*

A detailed description of lubricants and moisturizers and other interventions is provided in Chapter 14.

Colorectal cancer

Treatment for colorectal cancer usually involves surgery, radiation, and chemotherapy and has significant effects on sexual functioning for women. Abdominoperineal resection appears to have the worst sexual outcomes (Milbury, Cohen, Jenkins, Skibber, & Schover, 2013) associated with internal scarring and nerve damage (Schmidt, Bestmann, Kuchler, & Kremer, 2005). For women who engage in anal penetration, surgical removal of the rectum or occlusion of the anal sphincter may make this impossible. The presence of a stoma results in sexual dysfunction and the reduced likelihood of being sexually active. The addition of radiation therapy to the treatment regimen for women with rectal cancer increases dyspareunia (Thyø, Elfeki, Laurberg, & Emmertsen, 2019).

Vaginal dryness and dyspareunia are common and as a result, libido decreases. Sexual satisfaction is also impacted and lack of communication further compromises relationship satisfaction (Stulz, Lamore, Montalescot, Favez, & Flahault, 2020). Some women will continue to have sexual intercourse; however, they may not enjoy it as much as they did previously (Leon-Carlyle et al., 2015). Women may have to experiment with alternative positions for penetrative intercourse; if this is not possible or desirable, they may have to consider non-penetrative activities such as outercourse- or oral/manual sex (Katz, 2018. p. 119).

Those diagnosed with rectal cancer experience more sexual problems than individuals with colon cancer (Almont et al., 2019) and having an ostomy is associated with worse problems persisting for years after treatment (Sun et al., 2016). Pain during sex and body image issues are described as reasons for lack of sexual activity. Fecal incontinence in those who do not have an ostomy is distressing as is the noise, odor, and sight of feces in the ostomy bag (Tripaldi, 2019) that can impact on the partner's willingness to be sexual with the woman. Ultimately, having an ostomy alters the person's sense of self (Smith, Spiers, Simpson, & Nicholls, 2017).

As with other cancers, discussion with a health care provider is limited with just 11% of women in one study recalling a conversation (Almont et al., 2019). Women also felt that having their partner present for the discussion was important and that if the health care provider did not initiate the discussion, they would be too embarrassed to do it themselves (Leon-Carlyle et al., 2015).

Hematologic cancer

Hematologic cancers including leukemia and lymphomas occur across the lifespan including in young adults. A detailed description of the challenges to sexuality in young adults with cancer and other chronic diseases is presented in Chapter 11. These cancers have global effects on sexuality and sexual functioning in women that are long lasting and are associated with the kind of treatment the woman has. Bone marrow- or stem cell transplants have the most impact on sexual functioning due to the radiation and high-dose chemotherapy given prior to transplant (Thygesen, Schjodt, & Jarden, 2012). Sexual changes include loss of libido, vaginal and vulvar dryness causing dyspareunia, as well as body image changes (Tierney, Palesh, & Johnston, 2015). Women may worry about the effects of their sexual problems on their relationship (Astarita et al., 2016). Graft versus host disease is not uncommon after transplant and this syndrome may affect vaginal and vulvar tissues, eventually leading to stenosis and occlusion of the vagina (Nørskov, Schmidt, & Jarden, 2015).

Loss of libido affects not just the person with cancer but also their partner and for some is associated with sadness. Some relationships may become non-sexual due to treatment side effects or because the partner is concerned about exposing the woman to infection and this may be echoed by the person with cancer (Booker, Walker, & Raffin Bouchal, 2019). Couples do not communicate openly about this, much like with other cancers (Yoo et al., 2018).

Interventions include the importance of anticipatory guidance before treatment to allow individuals and couples to be forewarned about the potential for sexual problems and encouragement to seek help if they occur. Regular assessment of the vulva and vagina is not part of routine post-transplant care and so symptoms of graft versus host disease may not be noticed until at an advanced stage (Booker et al., 2019). Local estrogen can be used to alleviate vulvo-vaginal atrophy and dyspareunia (Sadovsky et al., 2010). Dilators and/or steroid cream applied to the vulva and/or vagina can help to alleviate tissue damage or stenosis associated with graft versus host disease (Spinelli et al., 2003).

Conclusions

Cancer profoundly affects a woman's sexual function and sexual self-image. After the chaos of diagnosis, many women go through treatment without thinking about sex and its role in their relationship. When sexual problems do arise, and especially in cancers affecting the sexual organs, women and their partners may be surprised at the changes they experience both individually and as a couple. It is not always easy for them to find help as communication with health care providers may not be as forthcoming as needed. Women may feel shame and embarrassment asking for help, further complicating their sex life and relationship.

References

Abbott-Anderson, K., Young, P.K., & Eggenberger, S.K. (2020). Adjusting to sex and intimacy: Gynecological cancer survivors share about their partner relationships. *Journal of Women and Aging, 32*(3), 329–348. doi: 10.1080/08952841.2019.1591888

Aerts, L., Enzlin, P., Vergote, I., Verhaeghe, J., Poppe, W., & Amant, F. (2012). Sexual, psychological, and relational functioning in women after surgical treatment for vulvar malignancy: A literature review. *Journal of Sexual Medicine, 9*(2), 361–371. doi: 10.1111/j.1743-6109.2011.02520.x

Aerts, L.M.D., Enzlin, P.P., Verhaeghe, J.M.D.P., Vergote, I.M.D.P., & Amant, F.M.D.P. (2014). Psychologic, relational, and sexual functioning in women after surgical treatment of vulvar malignancy: A prospective controlled study. *International Journal of Gynecological Cancer*, *24*(2), 372–380.

Alcorso, J., & Sherman, K.A. (2016). Factors associated with psychological distress in women with breast cancer-related lymphoedema. *Psycho-Oncology*, *25*(7), 865–872. doi: 10.1002/pon.4021

Almont, T., Bouhnik, A.D., Ben Charif, A., Bendiane, M.K., Couteau, C., Manceau, C., Mancini, J., & Huyghe, É. (2019). Sexual health problems and discussion in colorectal cancer patients two years after diagnosis: A national cross-sectional study. *Journal of Sexual Medicine*, *16*(1), 96–110. doi: 10.1016/j.jsxm.2018.11.008

Archangelo, S.C.V., Sabino Neto, M., Veiga, D.F., Garcia, E.B., & Ferreira, L.M. (2019). Sexuality, depression and body image after breast reconstruction. *Clinics (Sao Paulo)*, *74*, e883. doi: 10.6061/clinics/2019/e883

Astarita, S., Caruso, L., Barron, A.M., & Rissmiller, P. (2016). Experiences in sexual health among women after hematopoietic cell transplantation. *Oncology Nursing Forum*, *43*(6), 754–759. doi: 10.1188/16.ONF.754-759

Bae, H., & Park, H. (2016). Sexual function, depression, and quality of life in patients with cervical cancer. *Supportive Care in Cancer*, *24*(3), 1277–1283. doi: 10.1007/s00520-015-2918-z

Bakker, R.M., Mens, J.W.M., de Groot, H.E., Tuijnman-Raasveld, C.C., Braat, C., Hompus, W.C.P., … ter Kuile, M.M. (2017). A nurse-led sexual rehabilitation intervention after radiotherapy for gynecological cancer. *Supportive Care in Cancer*, *25*(3), 729–737. doi: 10.1007/s00520-016-3453-2

Bakker, R.M., Vermeer, W.M., Creutzberg, C.L., Mens, J.W.M., Nout, R.A., & ter Kuile, M.M. (2015). Qualitative accounts of patients' determinants of vaginal dilator use after pelvic radiotherapy. *Journal of Sexual Medicine*, *12*(3), 764–773. doi: 10.1111/jsm.12776

Barlow, E.L., Hacker, N.., Hussain, R., & Parmenter, G. (2014). Sexuality and body image following treatment for early-stage vulvar cancer: A qualitative study. *Journal of Advanced Nursing*, *70*(8), 1856–1866. doi: 10.1111/jan.12346

Baumgart, J., Nilsson, K., Evers, A.S., Kallak, T.K., & Poromaa, I.S. (2013). Sexual dysfunction in women on adjuvant endocrine therapy after breast cancer. *Menopause*, *20*(2), 162–168. doi: 10.1097/GME.0b013e31826560da

Becker, M., Malafy, T., Bossart, M., Henne, K., Gitsch, G., & Denschlag, D. (2011). Quality of life and sexual functioning in endometrial cancer survivors. *Gynecologic Oncology*, *121*(1), 169–173. doi: 10.1016/j.ygyno.2010.11.024

Beesley, V.L., Alemayehu, C., & Webb, P.M. (2018). A systematic literature review of the prevalence of and risk factors for supportive care needs among women with gynaecological cancer and their caregivers. *Supportive Care in Cancer*, *26*(3), 701–710. doi: 10.1007/s00520-017-3971-6

Benoot, C., Saelaert, M., Hannes, K., & Bilsen, J. (2017). The sexual adjustment process of cancer patients and their partners: A qualitative evidence synthesis. *Archives of Sexual Behavior*, *46*(7), 2059–2083. doi: 10.1007/s10508-016-0868-2

Biglia, N., Bounous, V.E., D'Alonzo, M., Ottino, L., Tuninetti, V., Robba, E., & Perrone, T. (2017). Vaginal atrophy in breast cancer survivors: Attitude and approaches among oncologists. *Clinical Breast Cancer*, *17*(8), 611–617. doi: 10.1016/j.clbc.2017.05.008

Blouet, A., Zinger, M., Capitain, O., Landry, S., Bourgeois, H., Seegers, V.T., & Pointreau, Y. (2019). Sexual quality of life evaluation after treatment among women with breast cancer under 35 years old. *Supportive Care in Cancer*, *27*(3), 879–885. doi: 10.1007/s00520-018-4374-z

Boehmer, U., Ozonoff, A., Timm, A., Winter, M., & Potter, J. (2014). After breast cancer: Sexual functioning of sexual minority survivors. *Journal of Sex Research*, *51*(6), 681–689. doi: 10.1080/00224499.2013.772087

Booker, R., Walker, L., & Raffin Bouchal, S. (2019). Sexuality after hematopoietic stem cell transplantation: A mixed methods study. *European Journal of Oncology Nursing*, *39*, 10–20. doi: 10.1016/j.ejon.2019.01.001

Borstelmann, N.A., Rosenberg, S.M., Ruddy, K.J., Tamimi, R.M., Gelber, S., Schapira, L., … Partridge, A.H. (2015). Partner support and anxiety in young women with breast cancer. *Psycho-Oncology*, *24*(12), 1679–1685. doi: 10.1002/pon.3780

Brotto, L., Erskine, Y., Carey, M., Ehlen, T., Finlayson, S., Heywood, M., ... Miller, D. (2012). A brief mindulness-based cognitive behavioral intervention improves sexual functioning versus wait-list control in women treated for gynecologic cancer. *Gynecologic Oncology*, *125*(2), 320–325. doi: 10.1016/j.ygyno.2012.01.035

Brotto, L.A., Smith, K.B., Breckon, E., & Plante, M. (2013). Pilot study of radical hysterectomy versus radical trachelectomy on sexual distress. *Journal of Sex and Marital Therapy*, *39*(6), 510–525. doi: 10.1080/0092623x.2012.667054

Brown, M.T., & McElroy, J.A. (2018). Unmet support needs of sexual and gender minority breast cancer survivors. *Supportive Care in Cancer*, *26*(4), 1189–1196. doi: 10.1007/s00520-017-3941-z

Buki, L.P., Reich, M., & Lehardy, E.N. (2016). "Our organs have a purpose": Body image acceptance in Latina breast cancer survivors. *Psycho-Oncology*, *25*(11), 1337–1342. doi: 10.1002/pon.4270

Burstein, H.J., Lacchetti, C., Anderson, H., Buchholz, T.A., Davidson, N.E., Gelmon, K.E., ... Griggs, J.J. (2016). Adjuvant endocrine therapy for women with hormone receptor-positive breast cancer: American Society of Clinical Oncology clinical practice guideline update on ovarian suppression. *Journal of Clinical Oncology*, *34*(14), 1689–1701. doi: 10.1200/jco.2015.65.9573

Canzona, M.R., Fisher, C.L., & Ledford, C.J.W. (2019). Perpetuating the cycle of silence: The intersection of uncertainty and sexual health communication among couples after breast cancer treatment. *Supportive Care in Cancer*, *27*(2), 659–668. doi: 10.1007/s00520-018-4369-9

Carroll, A.J., Baron, S.R., & Carroll, R.A. (2016). Couple-based treatment for sexual problems following breast cancer: A review and synthesis of the literature.(Review Article). *Supportive Care in Cancer*, *24*(8), 3651. doi: 10.1007/s00520-016-3218-y

Cathcart-Rake, E.J. (2018). Cancer in sexual and gender minority patients: Are we addressing their needs? *Current Oncology Reports*, *20*(11), 85. doi: 10.1007/s11912-018-0737-3

Colleoni, M., & Munzone, E. (2015). Navigating the challenges of endocrine treatments in premenopausal women with ER-positive early breast cancer. *Drugs*, *75*(12), 1311–1321. doi: 10.1007/s40265-015-0433-7

Committee opinion no. 659: The use of vaginal estrogen in women with a history of estrogen-dependent breast cancer. (2016). *Obstetrics and Gynecology*, *127*(3), e93–e96. doi: 10.1002/cam4.1016

Congard, A., Christophe, V., Duprez, C., Baudry, A.S., Antoine, P., Lesur, A., ... Vanlemmens, L. (2019). The self-reported perceptions of the repercussions of the disease and its treatments on daily life for young women with breast cancer and their partners. *Journal of Psychosocial Oncology*, *37*(1), 50–68. doi: 10.1080/07347332.2018.1479326

Cornell, L.F., Mussallem, D.M., Gibson, T.C., Diehl, N.N., Bagaria, S.P., & McLaughlin, S.A. (2017). Trends in sexual function after breast cancer surgery. *Annals of Surgical Oncology*, *24*(9), 2526–2538. doi: 10.1245/s10434-017-5894-3

Correa, C.S., Leite, I.C., Andrade, A.P., de Souza Sérgio Ferreira, A., Carvalho, S.M., & Guerra, M.R. (2016). Sexual function of women surviving cervical cancer. *Archives of Gynecology and Obstetrics*, *293*(5), 1053–1063. doi: 10.1007/s00404-015-3857-0

Cullen, K., Fergus, K., Dasgupta, T., Fitch, M., Doyle, C., & Adams, L. (2012). From "sex toy" to intrusive imposition: A qualitative examination of women's experiences with vaginal dilator use following treatment for gynecological cancer. *Journal of Sexual Medicine*, *9*(4), 1162–1173. doi: 10.1111/j.1743-6109.2011.02639.x

Cullen, K., Fergus, K., DasGupta, T., Kong, I., Fitch, M., Doyle, C., & Adams, L. (2013). Toward clinical care guidelines for supporting rehabilitative vaginal dilator use with women recovering from cervical cancer. *Supportive Care in Cancer*, *21*(7), 1911–1917. doi: 10.1007/s00520-013-1726-6

Dahl, C.A.F., Reinertsen, K.V., Nesvold, I.-L., Fosså, S.D., & Dahl, A.A. (2010). A study of body image in long-term breast cancer survivors. *Cancer*, *116*(15), 3549–3557. doi: 10.1002/cncr.25251

Daldoul, A., Ben Ahmed, K., Tlili, G., Krir, M.W., Gharbi, O., & Ben Ahmed, S. (2017). Female sexuality in premenopausal patients with breast cancer on endocrine therapy. *Breast Journal*. doi: 10.1111/tbj.12778

de Boer, M., Zeiler, K., & Slatman, J. (2019). Sharing lives, sharing bodies: Partners negotiating breast cancer experiences. *Medicine, Health Care, and Philosophy*, *22*(2), 253–265. doi: 10.1007/s11019-018-9866-6

Den Ouden, M.E.M., Pelgrum-Keurhorst, M.N., Uitdehaag, M.J., & De Vocht, H.M. (2019). Intimacy and sexuality in women with breast cancer: Professional guidance needed. *Breast Cancer (Tokyo, Japan)*, *26*(3), 326–332. doi: 10.1007/s12282-018-0927-8

Donders, G., Neven, P., Moegele, M., Lintermans, A., Bellen, G., Prasauskas, V., ... Buchholz, S. (2014). Ultra-low-dose estriol and Lactobacillus acidophilus vaginal tablets (Gynoflor®) for vaginal atrophy in postmenopausal breast cancer patients on aromatase inhibitors: Pharmacokinetic, safety, and efficacy phase I clinical study. *Breast Cancer Research and Treatment*, *145*(2), 371–379. doi: 10.1007/s10549-014-2930-x

Donders, G.G.G., Ruban, K., Bellen, G., & Grinceviciene, S. (2019). Pharmacotherapy for the treatment of vaginal atrophy. *Expert Opinion on Pharmacotherapy*, *20*(7), 821–835. doi: 10.1080/14656566.2019.1574752

Dunberger, G.L., Steineck, H., Waldenstrom, G., Nyberg, A., al-Abany, T.M., ... Avall-Lundqvist, E. (2010). Fecal incontinence affecting quality of life and social functioning among long-term gynecological cancer survivors. International Journal *of* Gynecological Cancer, *20*(3), 449–460. doi:10.1111/IGC.0b013e3181d373bf

Eaton, A.A., Baser, R.E., Seidel, B., Stabile, C., Canty, J.P., Goldfrank, D.J., & Carter, J. (2017). Validation of clinical tools for vaginal and vulvar symptom assessment in cancer patients and survivors. *Journal of Sexual Medicine*, *14*(1), 144–151. doi: 10.1016/j.jsxm.2016.11.317

Eden, J. (2016). ENDOCRINE DILEMMA: Managing menopausal symptoms after breast cancer. *European Journal of Endocrinology*, *174*(3), R71–R77. doi: 10.1530/eje-15-0814

Emilee, G., Ussher, J.M., & Perz, J. (2010). Sexuality after breast cancer: A review. *Maturitas*, *66*(4), 397–407. doi: 10.1016/j.maturitas.2010.03.027

Fallbjörk, U., Rasmussen, B.H., Karlsson, S., & Salander, P. (2013). Aspects of body image after mastectomy due to breast cancer—A two-year follow-up study. *European Journal of Oncology Nursing*, *17*(3), 340–345. doi: 10.1016/j.ejon.2012.09.002

Fallbjork, U., Salander, P., & Rasmussen, B.H. (2012). From "no big deal" to "losing oneself": Different meanings of mastectomy. *Cancer Nursing*, *35*(5), E41–E48. doi: 10.1097/NCC.0b013e31823528fb

Faubion, S.S., Larkin, L., Stuenkel, C.A., Bachmann, G.A., Chism, L.A., Kagan, R., ... Kingsberg, S.A. (2018). Management of genitourinary syndrome of menopause in women with or at high risk for breast cancer: Consensus recommendations from the North American Menopause Society and the International Society for the Study of Women's Sexual Health. *Menopause*, *25*(6), 596–608. doi: 10.1097/GME.0000000000001121

Fergus, K.D., & Gray, R.E. (2009). Relationship vulnerabilities during breast cancer: Patient and partner perspectives. *Psycho-Oncology*, *18*(12), 1311–1322. doi: 10.1002/pon.1555

Fischer, O.J., Marguerie, M., & Brotto, L.A. (2019). Sexual function, quality of life, and experiences of women with ovarian cancer: A mixed-methods study. *Sexual Medicine*. doi: 10.1016/j.esxm.2019.07.005

Forner, D.M., Dakhil, R., & Lampe, B. (2013). Can clitoris-conserving surgery for early vulvar cancer improve the outcome in terms of quality of life and sexual sensation? *European Journal of Obstetrics and Gynecology and Reproductive Biology*, *171*(1), 150–153. doi: 10.1016/j.ejogrb.2013.08.028

Froeding, L.P., Greimel, E., Lanceley, A., Oberguggenberger, A., Schmalz, C., Radisic, V.B., ... Jensen, P.T. (2018). Assessing patient-reported quality of life outcomes in vulva cancer patients: A systematic literature review. *International Journal of Gynecological Cancer*, *28*(4), 808–817. doi: 10.1097/igc.0000000000001211

Froeding, L.P., Ottosen, C., Rung-Hansen, H., Svane, D., Mosgaard, B.J., & Jensen, P.T. (2014). Sexual functioning and vaginal changes after radical vaginal trachelectomy in early stage cervical cancer patients: A longitudinal study. *Journal of Sexual Medicine*, *11*(2), 595–604. doi: 10.1111/jsm.12399

Gandhi, C., Butler, E., Pesek, S., Kwait, R., Edmonson, D., Raker, C., ... Gass, J. (2019). Sexual dysfunction in breast cancer survivors: Is it surgical modality or adjuvant therapy? *American Journal of Clinical Oncology*, *42*(6), 500–506. doi: 10.1097/coc.0000000000000552

Gass, J., Mitchell, S., & Hanna, M. (2019). How do breast cancer surgery scars impact survivorship? Findings from a nationwide survey in the United States. *BMC Cancer*, *19*(1), 342. doi: 10.1186/s12885-019-5553-0

Gass, J.S., Onstad, M., Pesek, S., Rojas, K., Fogarty, S., Stuckey, A., … Dizon, D.S. (2017). Breast-specific sensuality and sexual function in cancer survivorship: Does surgical modality matter? *Annals of Surgical Oncology*, *24*(11), 3133–3140. doi: 10.1245/s10434-017-5905-4

Ghizzani, A., Bruni, S., & Luisi, S. (2018). The sex life of women surviving breast cancer. *Gynecological Endocrinology: The Official Journal of the International Society of Gynecological Endocrinology*, *34*(10), 821–825. doi: 10.1080/09513590.2018.1467401

Grimm, D., Hasenburg, A., Eulenburg, C., Steinsiek, L., Mayer, S., Eltrop, S., … Woelber, L. (2015). Sexual activity and function in patients with gynecological malignancies after completed treatment. *International Journal of Gynecological Cancer*, *25*(6), 1134–1141. doi: 10.1097/igc.0000000000000468

Grion, R.C., Baccaro, L.F., Vaz, A.F., Costa-Paiva, L., Conde, D.M., & Pinto-Neto, A.M. (2016). Sexual function and quality of life in women with cervical cancer before radiotherapy: A pilot study. *Archives of Gynecology and Obstetrics*, *293*(4), 879–886. doi: 10.1007/s00404-015-3874-z

Guidozzi, F. (2013). Estrogen therapy in gynecological cancer survivors. *Climacteric*, *16*(6), 611–617. doi: 10.3109/13697137.2013.806471

Harris, M.G. (2019). Sexuality and menopause: Unique issues in gynecologic cancer. *Seminars in Oncology Nursing*, *35*(2), 211–216. doi: 10.1016/j.soncn.2019.02.008

Hart, A.M., Pinell-White, X., Egro, F.M., & Losken, A. (2015). The psychosexual impact of partial and total breast reconstruction: A prospective one-year longitudinal study. *Annals of Plastic Surgery*, *75*(3), 281–286. doi: 10.1097/sap.0000000000000152

Hart, A.M., Pinell-White, X., & Losken, A. (2016). The psychosexual impact of postmastectomy breast reconstruction. *Annals of Plastic Surgery*, *77*(5), 517–522. doi: 10.1097/sap.0000000000000665

Hay, C.M., Donovan, H.S., Hartnett, E.G., Carter, J., Roberge, M.C., Campbell, G.B., … Taylor, S.E. (2018). Sexual health as part of gynecologic cancer care: What do patients want? *International Journal of Gynecological Cancer*, *28*(9), 1737–1742. doi: 10.1097/igc.0000000000001376

Herring, B., Paraskeva, N., Tollow, P., & Harcourt, D. (2019). Women's initial experiences of their appearance after mastectomy and/or breast reconstruction: A qualitative study. *Psycho-Oncology*, *28*(10), 2076–2082. doi: 10.1002/pon.5196

Iavazzo, C., Johnson, K., Savage, H., Gallagher, S., Datta, M., & Winter-Roach, B.A. (2015). Sexuality issues in gynaecological oncology patients: Post treatment symptoms and therapeutic options. *Archives of Gynecology and Obstetrics*, *291*(3), 653–656. doi: 10.1007/s00404-014-3491-2

Jayde, V., Boughton, M., & Blomfield, P. (2013). The experience of chemotherapy-induced alopecia for Australian women with ovarian cancer. *European Journal of Cancer Care*, *22*(4), 503–512. doi: 10.1111/ecc.12056

Jeffries, H.C.C., & Clifford, C. (2011). Aloneness: The lived experience of women with cancer of the vulva. *European Journal of Cancer Care*, *20*(6), 738–746. doi: 10.1111/j.1365-2354.2011.01246.x

Jeffries, H.C.C., & Clifford, C. (2012). Invisibility: The lived experience of women with cancer of the vulva. *Cancer Nursing*, *35*(5), 382–389. doi: 10.1097/NCC.0b013e31823335a1

Jha, S., Wyld, L., & Krishnaswamy, P.H. (2019). The impact of vaginal laser treatment for genitourinary syndrome of menopause in breast cancer survivors: A systematic review and meta-analysis. *Clinical Breast Cancer*, *19*(4), e556–e562. doi: 10.1016/j.clbc.2019.04.007

Jonsdottir, J.I., Jonsdottir, H., & Klinke, M.E. (2018). A systematic review of characteristics of couple-based intervention studies addressing sexuality following cancer. *Journal of Advanced Nursing*, *74*(4), 760–773. doi: 10.1111/jan.13470

Katz, A. (2018). Colorectal cancer. *Breaking the silence on cancer and sexuality: A handbook for health care providers*. (2nd ed., pp. 115–122). Pittsburgh, PA: Oncology Nursing Society.

Kennedy, V., Abramsohn, E., Makelarski, J., Barber, R., Wroblewski, K., Tenney, M., … Lindau, S.T. (2015). Can you ask? We just did! Assessing sexual function and concerns in patients presenting for initial gynecologic oncology consultation. *Gynecologic Oncology*, *137*(1), 119–124. doi: 10.1016/j.ygyno.2015.01.451

Kingsberg, S.A., Larkin, L., Krychman, M., Parish, S.J., Bernick, B., & Mirkin, S. (2019). WISDOM survey: Attitudes and behaviors of physicians toward vulvar and vaginal atrophy (VVA) treatment in women including those with breast cancer history. *Menopause, 26*(2), 124–131. doi: 10.1097/gme.0000000000001194

Krychman, M., & Millheiser, L.S. (2013). Sexual health issues in women with cancer. *Journal of Sexual Medicine, 10*(Suppl. 1), 5–15. doi: 10.1111/jsm.12034

Landi, S.N., Doll, K.M., Bensen, J.T., Hendrix, L., Anders, C.K., Wu, J.M., & Nichols, H.B. (2016). Endocrine therapy and urogenital outcomes among women with a breast cancer diagnosis. *Cancer Causes and Control, 27*(11), 1325–1332. doi: 10.1007/s10552-016-0810-x

Lemke, E., Madsen, L., & Dains, J. (2017). Vaginal testosterone for management of aromatase inhibitor related sexual dysfunction: An integrative review. *Oncology Nursing Forum, 44*(3), 296–301. doi: 10.1188/1

Leon-Carlyle, M., Schmocker, S., Victor, J.C., Maier, B.A., O'Connor, B.I., Baxter, N.N., ... Kennedy, E.D. (2015). Prevalence of physiologic sexual dysfunction is high following treatment for rectal cancer: But is it the only thing that matters? *Diseases of the Colon and Rectum, 58*(8), 736–742. doi: 10.1097/dcr.0000000000000409

Lester, J., Pahouja, G., Andersen, B., & Lustberg, M. (2015). Atrophic vaginitis in breast cancer survivors: A difficult survivorship issue. *Journal of Personalized Medicine, 5*(2), 50–66. doi: 10.3390/jpm5020050

Levin, R.J. (2006). The breast/nipple/areola complex and human sexuality. *Sexual and Relationship Therapy, 21*(2), 237–249. doi: 10.1080/14681990600674674

Levin, R.J., & Meston, C. (2006). Nipple/breast stimulation and sexual arousal in young men and women. *Journal of Sexual Medicine, 3*(3), 450–454. doi: 10.1111/j.1743-6109.2006.00230.x

Lewis, F.M., Cochrane, B.B., Fletcher, K.A., Zahlis, E.H., Shands, M.E., Gralow, J.R., ... Schmitz, K. (2008). Helping Her Heal: A pilot study of an educational counseling intervention for spouses of women with breast cancer. *Psycho-Oncology, 17*(2), 131–137. doi: 10.1002/pon.1203

Lind, H., Waldenstrom, A.C., Dunberger, G., al-Abany, M., Alevronta, E., Johansson, K.A., ... Avall-Lundqvist, E. (2011). Late symptoms in long-term gynaecological cancer survivors after radiation therapy: A population-based cohort study. *British Journal of Cancer, 105*(6), 737–745. doi: 10.1038/bjc.2011.315

Lindau, S.T., Abramsohn, E.M., & Matthews, A.C. (2015). A manifesto on the preservation of sexual function in women and girls with cancer. *American Journal of Obstetrics and Gynecology, 213*(2), 166–174. doi: 10.1016/j.ajog.2015.03.039

Lisy, K., Peters, M.D.J., Schofield, P., & Jefford, M. (2018). Experiences and unmet needs of lesbian, gay, and bisexual people with cancer care: A systematic review and meta-synthesis. *Psychooncology, 27*(6), 1480–1489. doi: 10.1002/pon.4674

Liu, M., Juravic, M., Mazza, G., & Krychman, M.L. (2020). Vaginal dilators: Issues and answers. *Sexual Medicine Reviews.* doi: 10.1016/j.sxmr.2019.11.005

Ljungman, L., Ahlgren, J., Petersson, L.M., Flynn, K.E., Weinfurt, K., Gorman, J.R., ... Lampic, C. (2018). Sexual dysfunction and reproductive concerns in young women with breast cancer: Type, prevalence, and predictors of problems. *Psychooncology, 27*(12), 2770–2777. doi: 10.1002/pon.4886

Lloyd, P.A., Briggs, E.V., Kane, N., Jeyarajah, A.R., & Shepherd, J.H. (2014). Women's experiences after a radical vaginal trachelectomy for early stage cervical cancer. A descriptive phenomenological study. *European Journal of Oncology Nursing, 18*(4), 362–371. doi: 10.1016/j.ejon.2014.03.014

Lovelace, D.L., McDaniel, L.R., & Golden, D. (2019). Long-term effects of breast cancer surgery, treatment, and survivor care. *Journal of Midwifery and Women's Health, 64*(6), 713–724. doi: 10.1111/jmwh.13012

Lubotzky, F., Butow, P., Nattress, K., Hunt, C., Carroll, S., Comensoli, A., ... Juraskova, I. (2016). Facilitating psychosexual adjustment for women undergoing pelvic radiotherapy: Pilot of a novel patient psycho-educational resource. *Health Expectations, 19*(6), 1290–1301. doi: 10.1111/hex.12424

Marino, J.L., Saunders, C.M., & Hickey, M. (2017). Sexual inactivity in partnered female cancer survivors. *Maturitas, 105,* 89–94. doi: 10.1016/j.maturitas.2017.04.020

Matos, S.R.L., Lucas Rocha Cunha, M., Podgaec, S., Weltman, E., Yamazaki Centrone, A.F., & Cintra Nunes Mafra, A.C. (2019). Consensus for vaginal stenosis prevention in patients submitted to pelvic radiotherapy. *PLOS ONE, 14*(8), e0221054. doi: 10.1371/journal.pone.0221054

McCallum, M., Lefebvre, M., Jolicoeur, L., Maheu, C., & Lebel, S. (2012). Sexual health and gynecological cancer: Conceptualizing patient needs and overcoming barriers to seeking and accessing services. *Journal of Psychosomatic Obstetrics and Gynaecology, 33*(3), 135–142. doi:10 .3109/0167482X.2012.709291, doi: 10.3109/0167482X.2012.709291

Miaja, M., Platas, A., & Martinez-Cannon, B.A. (2017). Psychological impact of alterations in sexuality, fertility, and body image in young breast cancer patients and their partners. *Revista de Investigacion Clinica, 69*(4), 204–209. doi: 10.24875/ric.17002279

Milbury, K., Cohen, L., Jenkins, R., Skibber, J.M., & Schover, L.R. (2013). The association between psychosocial and medical factors with long-term sexual dysfunction after treatment for colorectal cancer. *Supportive Care in Cancer, 21*(3), 793–802.

Millman, R., Jacox, N., Sears, C., Robinson, J.W., Turner, J., & Walker, L.M. (2020). Patient interest in the lowdown on down there: Attendance at a vulvovaginal and sexual health workshop post-cancer treatment. *Supportive Care in Cancer, 28*(8), 3889–3896. doi: 10.1007/ s00520-019-05162-9

Moreira, H., & Canavarro, M.C. (2010). A longitudinal study about the body image and psychosocial adjustment of breast cancer patients during the course of the disease. *European Journal of Oncology Nursing, 14*(4), 263–270. doi: 10.1016/j.ejon.2010.04.001

Moreira, H., & Canavarro, M.C. (2013). Psychosocial adjustment and marital intimacy among partners of patients with breast cancer: A comparison study with partners of healthy women. *Journal of Psychosocial Oncology, 31*(3), 282–304. doi: 10.1080/07347332.2013.778934

Nørskov, K.H., Schmidt, M., & Jarden, M. (2015). Patients' experience of sexuality 1-year after allogeneic haematopoietic Stem Cell Transplantation. *European Journal of Oncology Nursing, 19*(4), 419–426. doi: 10.1016/j.ejon.2014.12.005

Oldertrøen Solli, K., de Boer, M., Nyheim Solbraekke, K., & Thoresen, L. (2019). Male partners' experiences of caregiving for women with cervical cancer-a qualitative study. *Journal of Clinical Nursing, 28*(5–6), 987–996. doi: 10.1111/jocn.14688

Paterson, C.L., Lengacher, C.A., Donovan, K.A., Kip, K.E., & Tofthagen, C.S. (2016). Body image in younger breast cancer survivors: A systematic review. *Cancer Nursing, 39*(1), E39–E58. doi: 10.1097/ncc.0000000000000251

Pavlović, R.T., Janković, S.M., Milovanović, J.R., Stefanović, S.M., Folić, M.M., Milovanović, O.Z., ... Milosavljević, M.N. (2019). The safety of local hormonal treatment for vulvovaginal atrophy in women with estrogen receptor-positive breast cancer who are on adjuvant aromatase inhibitor therapy: Meta-analysis. *Clinical Breast Cancer, 19*(6), e731–e740. doi: 10.1016/j. clbc.2019.07.007

Pearson, A., Booker, A., Tio, M., & Marx, G. (2019). Vaginal CO(2) laser for the treatment of vulvovaginal atrophy in women with breast cancer: LAAVA pilot study. *Breast Cancer Research and Treatment, 178*(1), 135–140. doi: 10.1007/s10549-019-05384-9

Perndorfer, C., Soriano, E.C., Siegel, S.D., & Laurenceau, J.P. (2019). Everyday protective buffering predicts intimacy and fear of cancer recurrence in couples coping with early-stage breast cancer. *Psycho-Oncology, 28*(2), 317–323. doi: 10.1002/pon.4942

Pieterse, Q.D., Kenter, G.G., Maas, C.P., de Kroon, C.D., Creutzberg, C.L., Trimbos, J.B., & Ter Kuile, M.M. (2013). Self-reported sexual, bowel and bladder function in cervical cancer patients following different treatment modalities: Longitudinal prospective cohort study. *International Journal of Gynecological Cancer, 23*(9), 1717–1725. doi: 10.1097/IGC.0b013e3182a80a65

Pitsouni, E., Grigoriadis, T., Falagas, M.E., Salvatore, S., & Athanasiou, S. (2017). Laser therapy for the genitourinary syndrome of menopause: A systematic review and meta-analysis. *Maturitas, 103*, 78–88. doi: 10.1016/j.maturitas.2017.06.029

Quick, A.M., Seamon, L.G., Abdel-Rasoul, M., Salani, R., & Martin, D. (2012). Sexual function after intracavitary vaginal brachytherapy for early-stage endometrial carcinoma. *International Journal of Gynecological Cancer, 22*(4), 703–708. doi: 10.1097/IGC.0b013e3182481611

Radina, M.E., Fu, M.R., Horstman, L., & Kang, Y. (2015). Breast cancer-related lymphedema and sexual experiences: A mixed-method comparison study. *Psycho-Oncology, 24*(12), 1655–1662. doi: 10.1002/pon.3778

Recio-Saucedo, A., Gerty, S., Foster, C., Eccles, D., & Cutress, R.I. (2016). Information requirements of young women with breast cancer treated with mastectomy or breast conserving surgery: A systematic review. *Breast, 25*, 1–13. doi: 10.1016/j.breast.2015.11.001

Reese, J.B., Porter, L.S., Casale, K.E., Bantug, E.T., Bober, S.L., Schwartz, S.C., & Smith, K.C. (2016). Adapting a couple-based intimacy enhancement intervention to breast cancer: A developmental study. *Health Psychology, 35*(10), 1085–1096. doi: 10.1037/hea0000413

Reese, J.B., Sorice, K.A., Pollard, W., Zimmaro, L.A., Beach, M.C., Handorf, E., & Lepore, S.J. (2020). Understanding sexual help-seeking for women with breast cancer: What distinguishes women who seek help from those who do not? *Journal of Sexual Medicine, 17*(9), 1729–1739. doi: 10.1016/j.jsxm.2020.06.004

Regan, T.W., Lambert, S.D., Girgis, A., Kelly, B., Kayser, K., & Turner, J. (2012). Do couple-based interventions make a difference for couples affected by cancer? A systematic review. *BMC Cancer, 12*, 279. doi: 10.1186/1471-2407-12-279

Rezaei, M., Elyasi, F., Janbabai, G., Moosazadeh, M., & Hamzehgardeshi, Z. (2016). Factors influencing body image in women with breast cancer: A comprehensive literature review. *Iranian Red Crescent Medical Journal, 18*(10), 1–9. doi: 10.5812/ircmj.39465

Richter, L.A., Han, J., Bradley, S., Lynce, F.C., Willey, S.C., Tefera, E., & Pollack, C.E. (2019). Topical estrogen prescribing patterns for urogenital atrophy among women with breast cancer: Results of a national provider survey. *Menopause, 26*(7), 714–719. doi: 10.1097/gme.0000000000001311

Robinson, P.J., Bell, R.J., Christakis, M.K., Ivezic, S.R., & Davis, S.R. (2017). Aromatase inhibitors are associated with low sexual desire causing distress and fecal incontinence in women: An observational study. *Journal of Sexual Medicine, 14*(12), 1566–1574. doi: 10.1016/j.jsxm.2017.09.018

Rodrigues, A.C., Teixeira, R., Teixeira, T., Conde, S., Soares, P., & Torgal, I. (2012). Impact of pelvic radiotherapy on female sexuality. *Archives of Gynecology and Obstetrics, 285*(2), 505–514. doi: 10.1007/s00404-011-1988-5

Rosenberg, S.M., Tamimi, R.M., Gelber, S., Ruddy, K.J., Kereakoglow, S., Borges, V.F., … Partridge, A.H. (2013). Body image in recently diagnosed young women with early breast cancer. *Psycho-Oncology, 22*(8), 1849–1855. doi: 10.1002/pon.3221

Rottmann, N., Gilså Hansen, D., dePont Christensen, R., Hagedoorn, M., Frisch, M., Nicolaisen, A., … Johansen, C. (2017). Satisfaction with sex life in sexually active heterosexual couples dealing with breast cancer: A nationwide longitudinal study. *Acta Oncologica, 56*(2), 212–219. doi: 10.1080/0284186x.2016.1266086

Rowlands, I.J., Lee, C., Beesley, V.L., Webb, P.M., & Australian National Endometrial Cancer Study Group (2014). Predictors of sexual well-being after endometrial cancer: Results of a national self-report survey. *Supportive Care in Cancer, 22*(10), 2715–2723. doi: 10.1007/s00520-014-2263-7

Rubin, L.R., Chavez, J., Alderman, A., & Pusic, A.L. (2013). 'Use what God has given me': Difference and disparity in breast reconstruction. *Psychology and Health, 28*(10), 1099–1120. doi: 10.1080/08870446.2013.782404

Sadovsky, R., Basson, R., Krychman, M., Morales, A.M., Schover, L., Wang, R., & Incrocci, L. (2010). Cancer and sexual problems. *Journal of Sexual Medicine, 7*(1 Pt 2), 349–373. doi: 10.1111/j.1743-6109.2009.01620.x

Saha, P., Regan, M.M., Pagani, O., Francis, P.A., Walley, B.A., Ribi, K., … International Breast Cancer Study, G. (2017). Treatment efficacy, adherence, and quality of life among women younger than 35 years in the International Breast Cancer Study Group TEXT and SOFT adjuvant endocrine therapy trials. *Journal of Clinical Oncology: Official Journal of the American Society of Clinical Oncology, 35*(27), 3113–3122. doi: 10.1200/JCO.2016.72.0946

Santen, R.J., Stuenkel, C.A., Davis, S.R., Pinkerton, J.V., Gompel, A., & Lumsden, M.A. (2017). Managing menopausal symptoms and associated clinical issues in breast cancer survivors. *Journal of Clinical Endocrinology and Metabolism, 102*(10), 3647–3661. doi: 10.1210/jc.2017-01138

Sassarini, J., Perera, M., Spowart, K., McAllister, K., Fraser, J., Glasspool, R., … Lumsden, M.A. (2018). Managing vulvovaginal atrophy after breast cancer. *Post Reproductive Health*, 2053369118805344, doi: 10.1177/2053369118805344

Schmidt, C.E., Bestmann, B., Kuchler, T., & Kremer, B. (2005). Factors influencing sexual function in patients with rectal cancer. *International Journal of Impotence Research : Official Journal of the International Society for Impotence Research*, *17*(3), 231–238.

Schmidt, J.L., Wetzel, C.M., Lange, K.W., Heine, N., & Ortmann, O. (2017). Patients' experience of breast reconstruction after mastectomy and its influence on postoperative satisfaction. *Archives of Gynecology and Obstetrics*, *296*(4), 827–834. doi: 10.1007/s00404-017-4495-5

Schover, L.R., Baum, G.P., Fuson, L.A., Brewster, A., & Melhem-Bertrandt, A. (2014). Sexual problems during the first 2 years of adjuvant treatment with aromatase inhibitors. *Journal of Sexual Medicine*, *11*(12), 3102–3111. doi: 10.1111/jsm.12684

Sekse, R.J., Gjengedal, E., & Raheim, M. (2013). Living in a changed female body after gynecological cancer. *Health Care for Women International*, *34*(1), 14–33. doi: 10.1080/07399332.2011.645965

Sekse, R.J., Hufthammer, K.O., & Vika, M.E. (2017). Sexual activity and functioning in women treated for gynaecological cancers. *Journal of Clinical Nursing*, *26*(3–4), 400–410. doi: 10.1111/jocn.13407

Sekse, R.J., Raheim, M., & Gjengedal, E. (2015). Shyness and openness—Common ground for dialogue between health personnel and women about sexual and intimate issues after gynecological cancer. *Health Care for Women International*, *36*(11), 1255–1269. doi: 10.1080/07399332.2014.989436

Smith, J.A., Spiers, J., Simpson, P., & Nicholls, A.R. (2017). The psychological challenges of living with an ileostomy: An interpretative phenomenological analysis. *Health Psychology*, *36*(2), 143–151. doi: 10.1037/hea0000427

Soldera, S.V., Ennis, M., Lohmann, A.E., & Goodwin, P.J. (2018). Sexual health in long-term breast cancer survivors. *Breast Cancer Research and Treatment*, *172*(1), 159–166. doi: 10.1007/s10549-018-4894-8

Sousa, M., Peate, M., Lewis, C., Jarvis, S., Willis, A., Hickey, M., & Friedlander, M. (2018). Exploring knowledge, attitudes and experience of genitourinary symptoms in women with early breast cancer on adjuvant endocrine therapy. *European Journal of Cancer Care (Engl)*, *27*(2), e12820. doi: 10.1111/ecc.12820

Spinelli, S., Chiodi, S., Costantini, S., Van Lint, M.T., Raiola, A.M., Ravera, G.B., & Bacigalupo, A. (2003). Female genital tract graft-versus-host disease following allogeneic bone marrow transplantation. *Haematologica*, *88*(10), 1163–1168.

Stilos, K., Doyle, C., & Daines, P. (2008). Addressing the sexual health needs of patients with gynecologic cancers. *Clinical Journal of Oncology Nursing*, *12*(3), 457–463. doi: 10.1188/08.cjon.457-463

Stulz, A., Lamore, K., Montalescot, L., Favez, N., & Flahault, C. (2020). Sexual health in colon cancer patients: A systematic review. *Psycho-Oncology*, *29*(7), 1095–1104. doi: 10.1002/pon.5391

Sun, V., Grant, M., Wendel, C.S., McMullen, C.K., Bulkley, J.E., Herrinton, L.J., … Krouse, R.S. (2016). Sexual function and health-related quality of life in long-term rectal cancer survivors. *Journal of Sexual Medicine*, *13*(7), 1071–1079. doi: 10.1016/j.jsxm.2016.05.005

Tan, J.H., Sharpe, L., & Russell, H. (2020). The impact of ovarian cancer on individuals and their caregivers: A qualitative analysis. *Psycho-Oncology*, n/a. doi: 10.1002/pon.5551

Tat, S., Doan, T., Yoo, G.J., & Levine, E.G. (2018). Qualitative exploration of sexual health among diverse breast cancer survivors. *Journal of Cancer Education*, *33*(2), 477–484. doi: 10.1007/s13187-016-1090-6

Thygesen, K.H., Schjodt, I., & Jarden, M. (2012). The impact of hematopoietic stem cell transplantation on sexuality: A systematic review of the literature. *Bone Marrow Transplantation*, *47*(5), 716–724. doi: 10.1038/bmt.2011.169

Thyø, A., Elfeki, H., Laurberg, S., & Emmertsen, K.J. (2019). Female sexual problems after treatment for colorectal cancer—A population-based study. *Colorectal Disease*, *21*(10), 1130–1139. doi: 10.1111/codi.14710

Tierney, D.K., Palesh, O., & Johnston, L. (2015). Sexuality, menopausal symptoms, and quality of life in premenopausal women in the first year following hematopoietic cell transplantation. *Oncology Nursing Forum*, *42*(5), 488–497. doi: 10.1188/15.onf.488-497

Tripaldi, C. (2019). Sexual function after stoma formation in women with colorectal cancer. *British Journal of Nursing*, 28(16), S4–S15. doi: 10.12968/bjon.2019.28.16.S4

Ussher, J.W., & Perz, J. (2010). A qualitative analysis of changes in relationship dynamics and roles between people with cancer and their primary informal carer. *Health*, 15(6), 650–667. doi: 10.1177.1363459310367440

Ussher, J.M., Perz, J., & Gilbert, E. (2012). Changes to sexual well-being and intimacy after breast cancer. *Cancer Nursing*, 35(6), 456–465. doi: 10.1097/NCC.0b013e3182395401

Vermeer, W.M., Bakker, R.M., Kenter, G.G., de Kroon, C.D., Stiggelbout, A.M., & ter Kuile, M.M. (2015). Sexual issues among cervical cancer survivors: How can we help women seek help? *Psycho-Oncology*, 24(4), 458–464. doi: 10.1002/pon.3663

Vermeer, W.M., Bakker, R.M., Kenter, G.G., Stiggelbout, A.M., & Ter Kuile, M.M. (2016). Cervical cancer survivors' and partners' experiences with sexual dysfunction and psychosexual support. *Supportive Care in Cancer*, 24(4), 1679–1687. doi: 10.1007/s00520-015-2925-0

Whicker, M., Black, J., Altwerger, G., Menderes, G., Feinberg, J., & Ratner, E. (2017). Management of sexuality, intimacy, and menopause symptoms in patients with ovarian cancer. *American Journal of Obstetrics and Gynecology*, 217(4), 395–403. doi: 10.1016/j.ajog.2017.04.012

White, I.D., Faithfull, S., & Allan, H. (2013). The re-construction of women's sexual lives after pelvic radiotherapy: A critique of social constructionist and biomedical perspectives on the study of female sexuality after cancer treatment. *Social Science and Medicine*, 76(1), 188–196. doi: 10.1016/j.socscimed.2012.10.025

Wiljer, D., Urowitz, S., Barbera, L., Chivers, M.L., Quartey, N.K., Ferguson, S.E., … Classen, C.C. (2011). A qualitative study of an internet-based support group for women with sexual distress due to gynecologic cancer. *Journal of Cancer Education*, 26(3), 451–458. doi: 10.1007/s13187-011-0215-1

Williams, N.F., Hauck, Y.L., & Bosco, A.M. (2017). Nurses' perceptions of providing psychosexual care for women experiencing gynaecological cancer. *European Journal of Oncology Nursing*, 30(Suppl. C), 35–42. doi: 10.1016/j.ejon.2017.07.006

Wilmoth, M.C., Hatmaker-Flanigan, E., LaLoggia, V., & Nixon, T. (2011). Ovarian cancer survivors: Qualitative analysis of the symptom of sexuality. *Oncology Nursing Forum*, 38(6), 699–708. doi: 10.1188/11.onf.699-708

Winch, C.J., Sherman, K.A., Koelmeyer, L.A., Smith, K.M., Mackie, H., & Boyages, J. (2015). Sexual concerns of women diagnosed with breast cancer-related lymphedema. *Supportive Care in Cancer*, 23(12), 3481–3491. doi: 10.1007/s00520-015-2709-6

Yoo, K.H., Kang, D., Kim, I.R., Choi, E.K., Kim, J.S., Yoon, S.S., … Cho, J. (2018). Satisfaction with sexual activity and sexual dysfunction in hematopoietic stem cell transplantation survivors and their partners: A couple study. *Bone Marrow Transplantation*, 53(8), 967–976. doi: 10.1038/s41409-018-0097-5

Yu, Y., & Sherman, K.A. (2015). Communication avoidance, coping and psychological distress of women with breast cancer. *Journal of Behavioral Medicine*, 38(3), 565–577. doi: 10.1007/s10865-015-9636-3

Zhu, Y., Cohen, S.M., Rosenzweig, M.Q., & Bender, C.M. (2019). Symptom map of endocrine therapy for breast cancer: A scoping review. *Cancer Nursing*, 42(5), E19–E30. doi: 10.1097/ncc.0000000000000632

Zimmermann, T., Scott, J.L., & Heinrichs, N. (2010). Individual and dyadic predictors of body image in women with breast cancer. *Psycho-Oncology*, 19(10), 1061–1068. doi: 10.1002/pon.1660

RESOURCES

Fight Colorectal Cancer (http://www.fightcolorectalcancer.org)
Leukemia and Lymphoma Society (http://www.lls.org/)
LIVESTRONG (http://www.livestrong.org)
Living Beyond Breast Cancer (http://www.lbbc.org)
Look Good … Feel Better® (http://www.lookgoodfeelbetter.org/)
National Breast Cancer Coalition (http://www.stopbreastcancer.org)

National Cervical Cancer Coalition (http://www.nccc-online.org/)
National Coalition for Cancer Survivorship (http://www.canceradvocacy.org)
National Ovarian Cancer Coalition (http://www.ovarian.org)
Ovarian Cancer National Alliance (http://ocrahope.org/)
Sharsheret (http://www.sharsheret.org)
Sisters Network®, Inc. (http://www.sistersnetworkinc.org)
Susan G. Komen for the Cure® (http://www.komen.org)
Triple Negative Breast Cancer Helpline (http://tnbcfoundation.org/)

10 Cancer in men

Prostate cancer is the most common solid tumor in men and the second leading cause of death in men in the United States. Most men with this cancer do not die from it; there are an estimate 3 million men in the US living after a diagnosis of prostate cancer. The 5-year survival rate for men with localized prostate cancer is almost 100% (https://www.cancer.org/cancer/prostate-cancer/detection-diagnosis-staging/survival-rates.html). Other cancers commonly affecting men include colorectal cancer and testicular cancer.

Prostate cancer

Men who are diagnosed with localized prostate cancer generally have the ability to choose what treatment they want to have. Their choices include active surveillance where the growth of the cancer is monitored regularly in an attempt to delay or defer treatment, thus preserving quality of life for as long as possible. Radical prostatectomy is accepted by many men who think that removing the prostate, the source of the cancer, they do not have to worry about recurrence and can lead a normal life. This however is not completely accurate and they may be left dealing with long-term side effects including urinary incontinence and sexual dysfunction. External beam radiation is usually reserved for older men who often already have sexual dysfunction but other forms of radiation, including brachytherapy and stereotactic body radiation therapy, are used for men of all ages, and also have potential side effects.

1. Effects of radical prostatectomy on sexual function

Surgery has significant and long-lasting effects on erectile functioning with 14–90% of men reporting problems (DeFade et al., 2011); 73% report the inability to have an erection 12 months after surgery when improvements should be seen (Capogrosso et al., 2019). While some men will see some degree of improvement (Donovan et al., 2016), erections remain difficult to both achieve and maintain. Younger men tend to opt for surgery and just 43% see a return to baseline erectile functioning and these men are often bothered by this (Barocas et al., 2017). Sexual satisfaction may remain low, even for men who are able to achieve erections rigid enough for penetration or who see a return to baseline erectile function (Terrier, Masterson, Mulhall, & Nelson, 2018). This information is important for men to know before surgery as it presents a realistic prediction of what may lie ahead.

Men report that erectile function and self-esteem are closely related and sexuality is important for a variety of reasons (Hilger et al., 2019). Some men report that their physician painted an unrealistic picture of their future sexual functioning resulting in disappointment when their predictions were not fulfilled (Pietilä, Jurva, Ojala, & Tammela, 2018). Other

DOI: 10.4324/9781003145745-10

men mourn the loss of spontaneity that once characterized their sexual function and now find themselves unable to express themselves sexually (Laursen, 2017). Their sexual difficulties extend in their friendships with other men; they felt diminished and ashamed and could not talk about what they were experiencing.

Men may need to find a way to redefine what their sexuality meant to them with some explaining that since they no longer wanted more children, the importance of sexuality was no longer of importance (Pietilä, Jurva, Ojala, & Tammela, 2018). Even men who retain erectile function sufficient for penetration may be distressed because their erections are not as good as they were before (Nelson, Deveci, Stasi, Scardino, & Mulhall, 2010). Men who are distressed about their sexual function tend to be depressed, regard sex as less important and are less satisfied with their adaptation to their new sexual reality as well as being less likely to have found a solution to their sexual problems (Walker & Santos-Iglesias, 2020).

Other impacts on sexuality and sexual function include penile shrinkage in both length and girth with an average loss of 1 cm/1/2 inch (Vasconcelos, Figueiredo, Nascimento, Damiao, & da Silva, 2012). This is traumatic for some men (Laursen, 2017) and impacts on self-esteem and quality of life (Carlsson et al., 2012). It is suggested that men be made aware of this as a potential side effect of surgery to reduce distress (Eylert, Bahl, & Persad, 2012). Men can still have orgasms without erections (Hollenbeck, Dunn, Wei, Montie, & Sanda, 2003) but will also experience dry orgasms due to the removal of the seminal vesicles. They will still experience orgasms but they may feel different, either weaker or stronger, perhaps to the point of pain (Messaoudi, Menard, Ripert, Parquet, & Staerman, 2011).

Urinary incontinence, especially during arousal and/or orgasm, termed climacturia, (Nilsson et al., 2011), is described as embarrassing and infantalizing (Palmer et al., 2003). This phenomenon has been reported to occur in as many as 45% of men (Lee, Hersey, Lee, & Fleshner, 2006). Urethral sling surgery may improve climacturia for some men (Nolan et al., 2020). Men also report pain with orgasm (Matsushita, Tal, & Mulhall, 2012; Mogorovich et al., 2013) and about 10% may develop curvature of the penis or Peyronie's disease (Frey et al., 2014). Men are extremely bothered by the sight of the curvature, but their partners are more accepting. This deformity of the erect penis makes vaginal intercourse difficult for both men and women with pain as the most commonly reported symptom (Farrell, Ziegelmann, Bajic, & Levine, 2020).

Reactive loss of libido in response to the inability to have erections is common (Namiki et al., 2012) and this will impact on the partner who may blame his/her self for his lack of initiation. A circular pattern may emerge with the partner reluctant to hug or kiss the man in case he interprets this as wanting sex that he cannot provide and the man avoids anything that could be perceived by his partner as an overture for sex (Laursen, 2017). But some men find that in the absence of the desire for sexual intercourse they are able to appreciate non-penetrative activities with their partner that are surprising but satisfying (Klaeson, Sandell, & Bertero, 2012).

Men who do not have a partner experience increased distress related to sexual dysfunction (Chambers et al., 2017; Matheson et al., 2017) and find it difficult to date, assuming that they have 'nothing to offer' a potential partner if they cannot have erections. Men in their 60s who are single may either by looking for a younger partner but in reality, women who would be involved with an older man are post-menopausal themselves and may not see sexual dysfunction as a deal breaker.

The support of a partner is important but the assumption of the partner about the man's sexual recovery may lead to difficulties in the relationship. Men may be more realistic than their partner in anticipating erectile dysfunction and changes in sexual activity after surgery (Paich et al., 2016). Sexual problems lead to a loss of perceived masculinity for African American and African Caribbean men (Bamidele et al., 2018); loss of erections is associated with the fear of losing their partner(s). In turn, the female partners of these men report significant changes in the relationship (Bamidele, Lagan, McGarvey, Wittmann, & McCaughan, 2019). Younger men with prostate cancer, a product of the wide acceptance of prostate specific antigen (PSA) screening, experience perhaps a greater loss of sexuality because the disease and treatment happen before they experience a decline in sexual function (Matheson et al., 2017).

2. Effects of radiation therapy on sexual function

External radiation therapy tends to impact negatively on erectile function at 6 months after treatment and then improvement is seen (Donovan et al., 2016). Men who have radiation therapy are often older and with poorer baseline erectile function and yet sexual outcomes are better three years after treatment than in men who had surgery (Barocas et al., 2017). Damage to blood vessels and nerves are responsible for these changes (Incrocci & Jensen, 2013). Men who have brachytherapy as treatment tend to fare better and are satisfied with their functioning (Crook, 2011) but they too see a gradual decline in the quality of erections over years (Roeloffzen et al., 2010). Stereotactic body radiation (CyberKnife) has similar outcomes (Bhattasali et al., 2014; Loi, Wortel, Francolini, & Incrocci, 2019). Cryotherapy has poor erectile outcomes (Shah et al., 2014; Tay et al., 2016) and may be reserved for men who are no longer sexually active.

3. Androgen deprivation therapy

Androgen deprivation therapy (ADT), commonly (and inaccurately) termed 'hormone therapy,' has the most profound effect on men's sexual functioning. Androgen deprivation causes global sexual side effects including profound erectile dysfunction and loss of genital sensitivity (Higano, 2012) as well as genital shrinkage (Park, Lee, & Chung, 2011). Body image changes and loss of masculine self-image are common and these all impact on the couple's relationship and loss of sexual thoughts and libido are common (Navon & Morag, 2003; Walker & Robinson, 2012).

Men are distressed about not being able to be sexual in the way they were before but the partner(s) often feels distressed about the man's lack of attention and desire for them While it may seem logical that the man who is not able to have erections will suffer less if his libido is absent, this is not necessarily what happens to men, especially those who are younger, as they may experience significant distress at this change (Hamilton, Van Dam, & Wassersug, 2016). In fact, as sexual function worsens over time, bother about this increases too (Donovan et al., 2018). Intermittent therapy, where men are given a 'holiday' off androgen deprivation and then resume treatment when their prostate specific antigen (PSA) rises, allows for relief from these sexual symptoms (Abrahamsson, 2017).

Many men are interested to know when their testosterone levels, and as a result their sexual function, may return to normal. Older age (above 65 years) and duration on androgen deprivation therapy longer than 6 months is associated with a slower recovery (Nascimento et al., 2019). Twenty-four months after the end of ADT, about half of men (51%) saw a return to their baseline level of testosterone but 8% of men remained at castrate levels. About a quarter of men did not return to a normal level of testosterone after 24 months.

It is important to remember that many female partners are not distressed at the loss of sexual potential as they may be post-menopausal and experiencing their own loss of libido and sexual dysfunction. The quality of the sexual relationship declines for both members of the couple over time, starting within 3–6 months of androgen deprivation (Walker, Santos-Iglesias, & Robinson, 2018). Other factors may help or hinder the man's sexual performance including sleep quality, co-morbidities, depression and its treatment, physical activity, and access to psycho-sexual education and support (Duthie, Calich, Rapsey, & Wibowo, 2020).

Sexual minority men

Sexual minority men, i.e. men who have sex with men or gay men in some instances, experience the same sexual side effects from prostate cancer treatment; however, these occur in the context of a specific culture and social environment that differs from heterosexual men. It has been shown that sexual minority men are more distressed with sexual changes (Hart et al., 2014). Erectile dysfunction causes changes in spontaneity, loss of sexual confidence and performance anxiety, and fear of rejection from a new or casual partner (Thomas, Wootten, & Robinson, 2013). These men may place great importance on erections and ejaculation that are hallmarks of sexual attraction and satisfaction (Lee et al., 2015). The prostate gland is a source of sexual pleasure for some men and the absence of the organ results in a loss of an elemental sexual experience (Jägervall, Brüggemann, & Johnson, 2019). Pain may be experienced for those who are the receptive partner in anal intercourse (Rosser et al., 2020; Ussher et al., 2017).

Many sexual minority men have sexual preferences that are cemented in their sexual identity and may not be amenable to change. Men who are 'tops' or the insertive partner may experience challenges if they have erectile dysfunction; men need a more rigid erection for anal penetration compared to vaginal penetration (Goldstone, 2005). Men who are 'bottoms,' the receptive partner, may be less concerned about their ability to achieve and maintain an erection. Some same-sex couples cope by either changing their roles, the insertive partner becoming receptive and vice versa (Lee, Breau, & Eapen, 2013). Others open their relationship so that the unaffected partner can find sexual experiences with other men (Hartman et al., 2014). Still others see this as an opportunity to deepen their emotional connection (Jägervall et al., 2019).

For sexual minority men who are single or in an open relationship, sexual problems after treatment pose challenges in engaging in sex or finding a new partner. Men report feeling sexually inferior and incapable of attracting other men for sex (Lee et al., 2015; Ussher et al., 2017). This can lead to isolation from their community, marginalization and loss of identity (Matheson et al., 2017).

Interacting with health care providers can be fraught with misunderstanding and missed opportunities to provide support and education for these men. Heteronormativity, assuming that everyone is heterosexual, continues to dominate health care facilities and individual providers (Rose, Ussher, & Perz, 2016). Assumptions about the patient's sexual identity may result in advice and education that does not apply to a sexual minority man and his relationship and/or sexual practices. This assumption may prevent the man from disclosing his sexual identity as he may feel unseen or unwelcome and vulnerable to homophobia or hurtful comments and care. Sexual minority men are frequently dissatisfied with the information they receive from health care providers about their sexual functioning (McInnis & Pukall, 2020).

It is important for health care providers to ask about sexual identity in a non-judgmental manner ("do you have sex with men, women or both") and tailor their communication accordingly (Kelly, Sakellariou, Fry, & Vougioukalou, 2018). Sexual minority men may be impacted by a purely medical approach to treatments for sexual problems that do not take into account their psycho-sexual identity and efforts to address their unique concerns (Katz, 2018, p. 213). Support groups for heterosexual men may not provide appropriate resources or help for sexual minority men who may also fear homophobia from the older men who often attend these meetings and may not be comfortable with this population.

Effects on the partner

The couple relationship is profoundly affected by treatment and the loss of sexual performance and agency. The female partner may feel isolated and unable to reach the man on an emotional level; at the same time, the man may be feeling diminished and a failure. Mutual loss of emotional connection leads to avoidance and withdrawal. A focus on physical effects of sexual dysfunction limits the understanding of the depth and breadth of the impact on the couple. It is for this reason that erectile aids in the form of medication or devices often fail. These interventions cannot replace the spontaneity and playfulness that once was a part of the couple's sexual relationship (Tucker, Speer, & Peters, 2016). While interventions for men may be useful if they target options for erectile functioning, female partners need attention to relational factors (Nelson, Emanu, & Avildsen, 2015). It may take months for the couple to adjust to the changes in their sexual relationship (Kelly, Forbat, Marshall-Lucette, & White, 2015).

Women report feeling burdened by the role of caretaker and feel responsible for supporting the man's emotional response that is often one of depression and anxiety (Pinks, Davis, & Pinks, 2018). Not knowing what to expect after treatment, whether from health care providers not including them in pre-treatment discussion or by the man excluding them from attending medical appointments, leads to an impact on their own quality of life and coping. Women report constant grief but being unable to express this to the man or others. In an attempt to protect and avoid making things worse for the man, they do not give voice to their own suffering. In this way they feel like invisible victims of the disease, ignored by the medical team, and their needs ignored. For older couples, the loss of sex was not that important but younger women actively mourned the loss of sexual activity and were distressed by the impact of this on their relationship. But instead of talking about this, they ignored this loss in an attempt to not distress their partner.

Some women describe a loss of self-esteem on their part when their partner no longer approaches them or initiates sex (Collaço et al., 2018). Despite knowing the cause of their partner's withdrawal, women can experience self-doubt about their own attractiveness and the strength of the partner bond. Failure of sexual aids to aid the man in being able to perform sexually may lead to frustration on the part of the woman, especially if her partner persists in trying to find something that will work. The use of these aids detracts from the spontaneity of their pre-treatment sexual relationship and are ultimately not satisfactory.

While men may avoid non-sexual activity, women feel loved and valued when the couple tries to maintain physical closeness by alternative means (Lyons, Winters-Stone, Bennett, & Beer, 2016). Verbal assurances of caring and acceptance of communication about feelings in a bi-directional manner can help in promoting emotional intimacy (Manne et al., 2018). Couples who are able to talk effectively about sexual function find that the man's self-esteem is preserved but those who cannot experience a decrease in masculine self-esteem and lack of partner support (Seidler, Lawsin, Hoyt, & Dobinson, 2016).

Some couples may be able to find a new and alternative way to explore both sexuality and sensuality (Collaço et al., 2018). Being able to accept the changes in their sex life is key to adapting and moving forward with a new way of being sexual. Replacing penetrative sex with mutual genital touch, kissing, caressing, and oral sex can lead to mutual satisfaction. A focus on emotional connectedness can detract in part from the loss of sexual intercourse, but this does not work for all couples who may persist in pursuing solutions within a biomedical model.

Box 10.1 5As model to address side effects of androgen deprivation

Ask: "Dr Biggs said that you had some questions about your husband's treatment, Ms. Lassiter. How can I help you today?"

Mrs Lassiter: "I'm not sure anyone can help me … I think that Bill's having an affair. In fact, I'm pretty certain about that. Why would he do this after 45 years of marriage? It's not right!"

Assess: "What makes you think that your husband is having an affair? What has changed in his behavior to suggest this?"

Mrs Lassiter: "Well, he doesn't touch me anymore. We used to hold hands and all that … and well, we'd do more than that, you know … And now, nothing! So he must be having an affair!"

Advise: "So you think that since he no longer approaches you for sex that he is having an affair? What did Dr Biggs tell you about the side effects of the medication he is taking?"

Mrs Lassiter: "I wasn't there when he put Bill on those injections and Bill doesn't say much after he comes back from his appointments …"

Assist: "The medication your husband is on, the injections, they stop his body from producing the male hormone called testosterone. This will take away his desire for sex and often men just stop touching their partner completely. It's really upsetting for women but if he doesn't show desire for you, he in all likelihood doesn't desire anyone else either!"

Mrs Lassiter: "Well, that's interesting. The other week when I accused Bill of having an affair he got really upset. Maybe it's not his fault, now that you tell me this about the medication … now I feel really awful about accusing him … oh, dear …"

Arrange: "You're not the first woman to think like this, Mrs Lassiter. Perhaps both of you can come and see me next week and we can talk about the side effects of the medication. I also have some suggestions for how you two can remain connected under these circumstances. How does that sound?"

Mrs Lassiter: "Well, that's very kind of you. I'd have to talk to Bill of course, but I bet he'll do anything if it stops me from accusing him of something he's not done."

Interventions

A detailed discussion about the after-effects of prostate cancer treatment on sexual function is important for these men and their partner but the timing of this is not well established. Anticipatory guidance may be ignored as it may be provided at a time when the man has just heard that he has cancer, or he may engage in magical thinking that nothing bad will happen to him. Immediately after treatment may be too soon, because the man is likely to be experiencing the most acute side effects and may not be concerned about sexual activity when he is dealing with radiation side effects or incontinence after surgery. Repeated discussions both before and after surgery may be necessary for the man to understand the impact of radical prostatectomy on his sexual function (Faris, Montague, & Gill, 2019). It is suggested that a discussion with a knowledgeable health care provider 3 months after treatment is optimal and the man's partner should be present (Palacios et al., 2018). Information from the man's partner is important as the man may minimize how he is feeling and not ask for help; the partner may more accurately report his struggles (Garos, Kluck, & Aronoff, 2007; O'Shaughnessy, Ireland, Pelentsov, Thomas, & Esterman, 2013). Partner involvement in establishing a return to sexual functioning is seen as important; this may occur through a process of acceptance of the need for erectile aids and the partner's interest in sex (Wittmann et al., 2015).

Pelvic floor physiotherapy has been shown to be effective in managing urinary incontinence after surgery, including for men who experience leakage with orgasm (Geraerts et al., 2016; Wong, Louie, & Beach, 2020). It may also be of benefit for men who experience pelvic pain, including painful orgasms (Cohen, Gonzalez, & Goldstein, 2016).

Communication needs to take into account the individual and unique attributes of the man's psycho-sexual needs, including partner status, sexual identity, motivation and values (Speer, Tucker, McPhillips, & Peters, 2017). A biopsychosocial model of male sexuality after cancer (Katz & Dizon, 2016) proposes that male sexuality is influenced by societal messages about how sexuality is expressed with a focus on lifelong sex drive. Body image and treatment side effects impact on sexual performance that relies on communication with his partner for individual or mutual satisfaction.

The approach to erectile dysfunction in these men usually takes a step-wise approach with a trial of phosphodiesterase-5 inhibitors (PDE5-*i*) and then moving on to more mechanical or invasive interventions such as penile pumps, alprostadil suppositories, and penile self-injections. A detailed description of these is presented in Chapter 13. The intervention of last resort is usually a penile prosthesis that while requiring surgery, is generally well accepted by men (Pillay et al., 2017).

The sole focus on erectile function after treatment does not address the more existential issues of loss and grief; interventions that support the man in accepting the reality of his situation and paying attention to sensation in a mindful manner may improve sexual satisfaction if not erectile function (Bossio, Miller, O'Loughlin, & Brotto, 2019). Erectile aids do not help couples with restoring or maintaining an emotional bond (Tucker et al., 2016). Interventions that promote communication, mutual understanding of values, and goal setting within the couple's approach to problem solving are effective for increasing relationship satisfaction but not sexual problems (Walker, King, Kwasny, & Robinson, 2017). Increasing recognition of the complex nature of men's sexuality has led to the use of multi-disciplinary clinical approaches to help men after treatment (Matthew, 2016) that includes active participation of his partner (Matthew et al., 2018).

Penile rehabilitation

Beginning in the late 1990s, the concept of penile rehabilitation was proposed, primarily as a way of decreasing the incidence of erectile dysfunction after radical prostatectomy (Montorsi et al., 1997). The theory behind the concept is to prevent tissue fibrosis in the penile tissues by maintaining blood flow by the use of PDE-5*i*s. Some success was seen initially in small studies with the use of sildenafil 50mg or 100mg at night (Padma-Nathan et al., 2008). Other protocols have been used including other PDE-5*i*s (Montorsi et al., 2008), including the penile pump for stretching (Qian, 2016; Raina et al., 2006), and intercavernosal injections (Gandaglia et al., 2015) alone or in combination. A study intended to answer the question about which protocol is the most effective was stopped after failure to recruit an adequate sample (Miranda, Benfante, Kunzel, Nelson, & Mulhall, 2020). A meta-analysis of studies has shown that while any of these interventions may help a man achieve an erection, spontaneous erections are not improved by penile rehabilitation (Liu, Lopez, Chen, & Wang, 2017). Recommendations from the Fourth International Consultation for Sexual Medicine (ICSM 5) state that the data does not support any one particular regimen for penile rehabilitation and also that there is not enough significant data to support the use of the oral medications in the return of spontaneous erections (Salonia et al., 2017). Pre-operative use of PDE-5*i*s may improve erectile function after surgery but additional evidence is needed before this can be recommended (Hisasue et al., 2018).

Adherence to daily dosing of oral medications and the use of a penile pump on a regular basis is poor (Albaugh, Kirwen, & Chang, 2019).The costs of medication are significant and are usually not covered by insurance (Patel et al., 2019); this may add to the attrition from protocols for penile rehabilitation.

Colorectal cancer

Treatment for colorectal cancer (cancer of the colon, rectum or anus) usually involves surgery, radiation and chemotherapy in various combinations. Treatment for rectal cancer appears to have worse sexual outcomes compared to colon cancer (Almont et al., 2019). Sexual problems are more common in men than women (42.8% vs. 23.5%) (Downing et al., 2019) and evidence to date has focused on erectile difficulties in men (Almont et al., 2019). Abdominoperineal resection (APR) has the worst sexual outcomes for men with erectile dysfunction the most common symptom (Costa et al., 2018). Other sexual problems also occur including loss of libido (Zhu et al., 2017) and anorgasmia (Haney, Alzweri, & Hellstrom, 2018).

The presence of an ostomy increases sexual problems and these may persist when the ostomy is reversed (Downing et al., 2019). Visible changes to the body in addition to the stoma such as weight gain, scars and muscle loss contribute to altered body image (Stuhlfauth, Melby, & Hellesø, 2018). Fear of leakage, odor, gas, or noises from the stoma during sexual activity are common (Neuman et al., 2011). In addition, fear of the response from a sexual partner may be at the forefront of the person's mind, especially if with a new partner who may react with disgust or fear at the sight of the stoma and/or ostomy bag. But even for those without a stoma, sexual function is impacted negatively (Näsvall et al., 2017).

Overall, treatment for these cancers impacts not only sexual functioning but also body image and distress as well as health-related quality of life (Reese, Handorf, & Haythornthwaite, 2018). Masculine self-image may also be disturbed (Traa, De Vries, Roukema, Rutten, &

Den Oudsten, 2014) but men do tend to adjust to these changes over time while their female partner may continue to experience greater levels of distress (Kayser et al., 2018).

Sexual minority men experience the same sexual consequences but for those who engage in receptive anal intercourse, rectal cancer causes some specific issues. They may need to find alternative methods of sexual expression (Katz, 2018, p. 213). Anal cancer is caused by certain strains of the human papilloma virus and is found more often in HIV-infected individuals who are often men who have sex with men (Wang, Sparano, & Palefsky, 2017). Treatment for these cancers is associated with decreased sexual satisfaction (Sodergren et al., 2015) as well as erectile dysfunction (Frick et al., 2017). Fecal incontinence is common after treatment and this has a deleterious impact on sexual activity (Knowles, Haigh, McLean, & Phillips, 2015).

Testicular cancer

Testicular cancer is the most common cancer in young men, aged between 15 and 40 years (Chia et al., 2010). While most will be cured after definitive treatment, the location of the cancer and the symbolic meaning of the testicles affects these men and can have far-reaching psychosocial and psychosexual impacts (Hoyt, McCann, Savone, Saigal, & Stanton, 2015). Treatment is usually multi-modal with orchiectomy and chemotherapy as the gold standard; retroperitoneal lymph node dissection is performed to identify any lymph node involvement that can lead to death (Dimitropoulos et al., 2016). The latter causes retrograde ejaculation that impacts on fertility but may also complicate sexual functioning.

The most common sexual side effects of treatment in addition to ejaculatory dysfunction are erectile difficulties (Kim et al., 2012), decreased libido and sexual enjoyment (Rossen, Pedersen, Zachariae, & Maase, 2012). Two years after treatment, 43% of young men report ongoing issues with sexual functioning, mainly in the areas of dissatisfaction with sex life, not having a partner and experiencing poor body image (Ljungman et al., 2019). Erectile dysfunction is associated with radiation therapy but not with chemotherapy or retroperitoneal lymph node dissection (Capogrosso et al., 2016).

Orchiectomy alone with ongoing surveillance has the least side effects (Bandak et al., 2018) suggesting that the cause of sexual problems is related to chemotherapy and/or radiation. However, body image may be compromised by the loss of a testicle (Cappuccio et al., 2018) and cultural values related to the role of the testicle in male identity also play a role. Men who are partnered and have children are seen to adjust better after treatment (Alexis, Adeleye, & Worsley, 2020).

Men are offered a testicular prothesis after orchiectomy and acceptance of this is linked to improved cosmetic appearance of the scrotum and increased self-confidence in some men (Srivatsav et al., 2019). Men may not be satisfied with the prosthesis however, for reasons including the placement in the scrotal sac, the size discrepancy between their natural testicle and the prosthesis or how the prosthesis felt, generally too firm as compared to their other testicle (Catanzariti, Polito, & Polito, 2016).

As with other cancers, communication about the disease and sexual side effects by health care providers is limited with nurses reporting discomfort talking about these issues with men (Moore, Higgins, & Sharek, 2013) and not all surgeons discussing testicular prostheses with their patients (Ashwin Srivatsav et al., 2019).

Conclusion

Cancer in men presents challenges to sexual function and masculine self-image. Men are often regarded as stoic with little emotional response to physical challenges, but this is not accurate. The consequences of treatment for cancer and the location of the cancer itself affect men and their partner deeply. Interventions to address sexual problems tend to be biomedical and often do not address the psycho-sexual impact of these cancers.

References

Abrahamsson, P.-A. (2017). Intermittent androgen deprivation therapy in patients with prostate cancer: Connecting the dots. *Asian Journal of Urology*, *4*(4), 208–222. doi: 10.1016/j.ajur.2017.04.001

Albaugh, J., Kirwen, N., & Chang, C. (2019). 163 adherence and outcomes with penile rehabilitation over a 2 year period. *Journal of Sexual Medicine*, *16*(4), S82–S83. doi: 10.1016/j.jsxm.2019.01.172

Alexis, O., Adeleye, A.O., & Worsley, A.J. (2020). Men's experiences of surviving testicular cancer: An integrated literature review. *Journal of Cancer Survivorship*, *14*(3), 284–293. doi: 10.1007/s11764-019-00841-2

Almont, T., Bouhnik, A.D., Ben Charif, A., Bendiane, M.K., Couteau, C., Manceau, C., Mancini, J., & Huyghe, E. (2019). Sexual health problems and discussion in colorectal cancer patients two years after diagnosis: A national cross-sectional study. *Journal of Sexual Medicine*, *16*(1), 96–110. doi: 10.1016/j.jsxm.2018.11.008

Bamidele, O., Lagan, B.M., McGarvey, H., Wittmann, D., & McCaughan, E. (2019). "...It might not have occurred to my husband that this woman, his wife who is taking care of him has some emotional needs as well...": The unheard voices of partners of Black African and Black Caribbean men with prostate cancer. *Supportive Care in Cancer*, *27*(3), 1089–1097. doi: 10.1007/s00520-018-4398-4

Bamidele, O., McGarvey, H., Lagan, B.M., Ali, N., Chinegwundoh Mbe, F., Parahoo, K., & McCaughan, E. (2018). Life after prostate cancer: A systematic literature review and thematic synthesis of the post-treatment experiences of Black African and Black Caribbean men. *European Journal of Cancer Care (Engl)*, *27*(1). doi: 10.1111/ecc.12784

Bandak, M., Lauritsen, J., Johansen, C., Kreiberg, M., Skøtt, J.W., Agerbaek, M., ... Daugaard, G. (2018). Sexual function in a nationwide cohort of 2,260 survivors of testicular cancer after 17 years of followup. *Journal of Urology*, *200*(4), 794–800. doi: 10.1016/j.juro.2018.04.077

Barocas, D.A., Alvarez, J., Resnick, M.J., Koyama, T., Hoffman, K.E., Tyson, M.D., ... Penson, D.F. (2017). Association between radiation therapy, surgery, or observation for localized prostate cancer and patient-reported outcomes after 3 years. *JAMA*, *317*(11), 1126–1140. doi: 10.1001/jama.2017.1704

Bhattasali, O., Chen, L.N., Woo, J., Park, J.-W., Kim, J.S., Moures, R., ... Collins, S.P. (2014). Patient-reported outcomes following stereotactic body radiation therapy for clinically localized prostate cancer. *Radiation Oncology*, *9*(1), 52. doi: 10.1186/1748-717x-9-52

Bossio, J.A., Miller, F., O'Loughlin, J.I., & Brotto, L.A. (2019). Sexual health recovery for prostate cancer survivors: The proposed role of acceptance and mindfulness-based interventions. *Sexual Medicine Reviews*. doi: 10.1016/j.sxmr.2019.03.001

Capogrosso, P., Boeri, L., Ferrari, M., Ventimiglia, E., La Croce, G., Capitanio, U., ... Salonia, A. (2016). Long-term recovery of normal sexual function in testicular cancer survivors. *Asian Journal of Andrology*, *18*(1), 85–89. doi: 10.4103/1008-682x.149180

Capogrosso, P., Vertosick, E.A., Benfante, N.E., Eastham, J.A., Scardino, P.J., Vickers, A.J., & Mulhall, J.P. (2019). Are we improving erectile function recovery after radical prostatectomy? Analysis of patients treated over the last decade. *European Urology*, *75*(2), 221–228. doi: 10.1016/j.eururo.2018.08.039

Cappuccio, F., Rossetti, S., Cavaliere, C., Iovane, G., Taibi, R., D'Aniello, C., ... Facchini, G. (2018). Health-related quality of life and psychosocial implications in testicular cancer survivors: A literature review. *European Review for Medical and Pharmacological Sciences*, *22*(3), 645–661. doi: 10.26355/eurrev_201802_14290

Carlsson, S., Nilsson, A.E., Johansson, E., Nyberg, T., Akre, O., & Steineck, G. (2012). Self-perceived penile shortening after radical prostatectomy. *International Journal of Impotence Research*, *24*, 179.

Catanzariti, F., Polito, B., & Polito, M. (2016). Testicular prosthesis: Patient satisfaction and sexual dysfunctions in testis cancer survivors. *Archivio Italiano di Urologia e Andrologia*, *88*(3), 186–188. doi: 10.4081/aiua.2016.3.186

Chambers, S.K., Ng, S.K., Baade, P., Aitken, J.F., Hyde, M.K., Wittert, G., … Dunn, J. (2017). Trajectories of quality of life, life satisfaction, and psychological adjustment after prostate cancer. *Psychooncology*, *26*(10), 1576–1585. doi: 10.1002/pon.4342

Chia, V.M., Quraishi, S.M., Devesa, S.S., Purdue, M.P., Cook, M.B., & McGlynn, K.A. (2010). International trends in the incidence of testicular cancer, 1973–2002. *Cancer Epidemiology Biomarkers & Prevention*, *19*(5), 1151–1159. doi: 10.1158/1055-9965.epi-10-0031

Cohen, D., Gonzalez, J., & Goldstein, I. (2016). The role of pelvic floor muscles in male sexual dysfunction and pelvic pain. *Sexual Medicine Reviews*, *4*(1), 53–62. doi: 10.1016/j.sxmr.2015.10.001

Collaço, N., Rivas, C., Matheson, L., Nayoan, J., Wagland, R., Alexis, O., … Watson, E. (2018). Prostate cancer and the impact on couples: A qualitative metasynthesis. *Supportive Care in Cancer*, *26*(6), 1703–1713. doi: 10.1007/s00520-018-4134-0

Costa, P., Cardoso, J.M., Louro, H., Dias, J., Costa, L., Rodrigues, R., … Ferraz, L. (2018). Impact on sexual function of surgical treatment in rectal cancer. *International Brazilian Journal of Urology*, *44*(1), 141–149. doi: 10.1590/s1677-5538.ibju.2017.0318

Crook, J. (2011). The role of brachytherapy in the definitive management of prostate cancer. *Cancer Radiotherapie: Journal de la Societe Francaise de Radiotherapie Oncologique*, *15*(3), 230–237. doi: 10.1016/j.canrad.2011.01.004

Danemalm Jägervall, C., Brüggemann, J., & Johnson, E. (2019). Gay men's experiences of sexual changes after prostate cancer treatment-a qualitative study in Sweden. *Scandinavian Journal of Urology*, *53*(1), 40–44. doi: 10.1080/21681805.2018.1563627

DeFade, B.P., Carson, C.C., & Kennelly, M.J. (2011). Postprostatectomy erectile dysfunction: The role of penile rehabilitation. *Reviews in Urology*, *13*(1), 6–13. doi: 1-.3909/riu0501

Dimitropoulos, K., Karatzas, A., Papandreou, C., Daliani, D., Zachos, I., Pisters, L.L., & Tzortzis, V. (2016). Sexual dysfunction in testicular cancer patients subjected to post-chemotherapy retroperitoneal lymph node dissection: A focus beyond ejaculation disorders. *Andrologia*, *48*(4), 425–430. doi: 10.1111/and.12462

Donovan, J.L., Hamdy, F.C., Lane, J.A., Mason, M., Metcalfe, C., Walsh, E., … Neal, D.E. (2016). Patient-reported outcomes after monitoring, surgery, or radiotherapy for prostate cancer. *New England Journal of Medicine*, *375*(15), 1425–1437. doi: 10.1056/NEJMoa1606221

Donovan, K.A., Gonzalez, B.D., Nelson, A.M., Fishman, M.N., Zachariah, B., & Jacobsen, P.B. (2018). Effect of androgen deprivation therapy on sexual function and bother in men with prostate cancer: A controlled comparison. *Psychooncology*, *27*(1), 316–324. doi: 10.1002/pon.4463

Downing, A., Glaser, A.W., Finan, P.J., Wright, P., Thomas, J.D., Gilbert, A., … Sebag-Montefiore, D. (2019). Functional outcomes and health-related quality of life after curative treatment for rectal cancer: A population-level study in England. *International Journal of Radiation Oncology Biology Physics*, *103*(5), 1132–1142. doi: 10.1016/j.ijrobp.2018.12.005

Duthie, C.J., Calich, H.J., Rapsey, C.M., & Wibowo, E. (2020). Maintenance of sexual activity following androgen deprivation in males. *Critical Reviews in Oncology/Hematology*, *153*, 103064, doi: 10.1016/j.critrevonc.2020.103064

Eylert, M.F., Bahl, A., & Persad, R. (2012). Do we need to obtain consent for penile shortening as a complication of treatment for organ-confined prostate cancer? *BJU International*, *110*(10), 1491–1500. doi: 10.1111/j.1464-410X.2012.11102.x

Faris, A.E.R., Montague, D.K., & Gill, B.C. (2019). Perioperative educational interventions and contemporary sexual function outcomes of radical prostatectomy. *Sexual Medicine Reviews*, *7*(2), 293–305. doi: 10.1016/j.sxmr.2018.05.003

Farrell, M.R., Ziegelmann, M.J., Bajic, P., & Levine, L.A. (2020). Peyronie's disease and the female sexual partner: A comparison of the male and female experience. *Journal of Sexual Medicine*, *17*(12), 2456–2461. doi: 10.1016/j.jsxm.2020.08.010

Frey, A., Sønksen, J., Jakobsen, H., & Fode, M. (2014). Prevalence and predicting factors for commonly neglected sexual side effects to radical prostatectomies: Results from a cross-sectional questionnaire-based study. *Journal of Sexual Medicine*, *11*(9), 2318–2326. doi: 10.1111/jsm.12624

Frick, M.A., Vachani, C.C., Hampshire, M.K., Bach, C., Arnold-Korzeniowski, K., Metz, J.M., & Hill-Kayser, C.E. (2017). Survivorship after lower gastrointestinal cancer: Patient-reported outcomes and planning for care. *Cancer*. doi: 10.1002/cncr.30527

Gandaglia, G., Suardi, N., Cucchiara, V., Bianchi, M., Shariat, S.F., Roupret, M., ... Briganti, A. (2015). Penile rehabilitation after radical prostatectomy: Does it work? *Translational Andrology and Urology*, *4*(2), 110–123. doi: 10.3978/j.issn.2223-4683.2015.02.01

Garos, S., Kluck, A., & Aronoff, D. (2007). Prostate cancer patients and their partners: Differences in satisfaction indices and psychological variables. *Journal of Sexual Medicine*, *4*(5), 1394–1403. doi: 10.1111/j.1743-6109.2007.00545.x

Geraerts, I., Van Poppel, H., Devoogdt, N., De Groef, A., Fieuws, S., & Van Kampen, M. (2016). Pelvic floor muscle training for erectile dysfunction and climacturia 1 year after nerve sparing radical prostatectomy: A randomized controlled trial. *International Journal of Impotence Research*, *28*(1), 9–13. doi: 10.1038/ijir.2015.24

Goldstone, S.E. (2005). The ups and downs of gay sex after prostate cancer treatment. *Journal of Gay and Lesbian Psychotherapy*, *9*(1–2), 43–55. doi: 10.1300/J236v09n01_04

Grondhuis Palacios, L.A., Krouwel, E.M., den Oudsten, B.L., den Ouden, M.E.M., Kloens, G.J., van Duijn, G., ... Elzevier, H.W. (2018). Suitable sexual health care according to men with prostate cancer and their partners. *Supportive Care in Cancer*, *26*(12), 4169–4176. doi: 10.1007/s00520-018-4290-2

Hamilton, L.D., Van Dam, D., & Wassersug, R.J. (2016). The perspective of prostate cancer patients and patients' partners on the psychological burden of androgen deprivation and the dyadic adjustment of prostate cancer couples. *Psycho-Oncology*, *25*(7), 823–831. doi: 10.1002/pon.3930

Haney, N.M., Alzweri, L.M., & Hellstrom, W.J.G. (2018). Male orgasmic dysfunction post-radical pelvic surgery. *Sexual Medicine Reviews*, *6*(3), 429–437. doi: 10.1016/j.sxmr.2017.12.003

Hart, T.L., Coon, D.W., Kowalkowski, M.A., Zhang, K., Hersom, J.I., Goltz, H.H., ... Latini, D.M. (2014). Changes in sexual roles and quality of life for gay men after prostate cancer: Challenges for sexual health providers. *Journal of Sexual Medicine*, *11*(9), 2308–2317. doi: 10.1111/jsm.12598

Hartman, M.E., Irvine, J., Currie, K.L., Ritvo, P., Trachtenberg, L., Louis, A., ... Matthew, A.G. (2014). Exploring gay couples' experience with sexual dysfunction after radical prostatectomy: A qualitative study. *Journal of Sex and Marital Therapy*, *40*(3), 233–253. doi: 10.1080/0092623x.2012.726697

Higano, C.S. (2012). Sexuality and intimacy after definitive treatment and subsequent androgen deprivation therapy for prostate cancer. *Journal of Clinical Oncology*, *30*(30), 3720–3725. doi: 10.1200/jco.2012.41.8509

Hilger, C., Schostak, M., Neubauer, S., Magheli, A., Fydrich, T., Burkert, S., & Kendel, F. (2019). The importance of sexuality, changes in erectile functioning and its association with self-esteem in men with localized prostate cancer: Data from an observational study. *BMC Urology*, *19*(1), 9. doi: 10.1186/s12894-019-0436-x

Hisasue, S., Takeuchi, H., Ota, S., Natsuyama, T., Shiozawa, S., Matsumoto, S., & Mitsui, Y. (2018). 423 The impact of preoperative daily PDE5 inhibitors on the early recovery of erectile function following robot-assisted radical prostatectomy. *Journal of Sexual Medicine*, *15*(7), S274. doi: 10.1016/j.jsxm.2018.04.329

Hollenbeck, B.K., Dunn, R.L., Wei, J.T., Montie, J.E., & Sanda, M.G. (2003). Determinants of long-term sexual health outcome after radical prostatectomy measured by a validated instrument. *Journal d'urologie*, *169*(4), 1453–1457.

Hoyt, M.A., McCann, C., Savone, M., Saigal, C.S., & Stanton, A.L. (2015). Interpersonal sensitivity and sexual functioning in young men with testicular cancer: The moderating role of coping. *International Journal of Behavioral Medicine*, *22*(6), 709–716. doi: 10.1007/s12529-015-9472-4

Incrocci, L., & Jensen, P.T. (2013). Pelvic radiotherapy and sexual function in men and women. *Journal of Sexual Medicine*, *10*(Suppl. 1), 53–64. doi: 10.1111/jsm.12010

Katz, A. (2018). Sexual minority patients. *Breaking the silence on cancer and sexuality: A handbook for health care providers*. (pp. 207–218.). Pittsburgh, PA: Oncology Nursing Society.

Katz, A., & Dizon, D.S. (2016). Sexuality after cancer: A model for male survivors. *Journal of Sexual Medicine*, *13*(1), 70–78. doi: 10.1016/j.jsxm.2015.11.006

Kayser, K., Acquati, C., Reese, J.B., Mark, K., Wittmann, D., & Karam, E. (2018). A systematic review of dyadic studies examining relationship quality in couples facing colorectal cancer together. *Psychooncology*, *27*(1), 13–21. doi: 10.1002/pon.4339

Kelly, D., Forbat, L., Marshall-Lucette, S., & White, I. (2015). Co-constructing sexual recovery after prostate cancer: A qualitative study with couples. *Translational Andrology and Urology*, *4*(2), 131–138. doi: 10.3978/j.issn.2223-4683.2015.04.05

Kelly, D., Sakellariou, D., Fry, S., & Vougioukalou, S. (2018). Heteronormativity and prostate cancer: A discursive paper. *Journal of Clinical Nursing*, *27*(1–2), 461–467. doi: 10.1111/jocn.13844

Kim, C., McGlynn, K.A., McCorkle, R., Li, Y., Erickson, R.L., Ma, S., ... Zhang, Y. (2012). Sexual functioning among testicular cancer survivors: A case-control study in the U.S. *Journal of Psychosomatic Research*, *73*(1), 68–73. doi: 10.1016/j.jpsychores.2012.02.011

Klaeson, K., Sandell, K., & Bertero, C.M. (2012). Sexuality in the context of prostate cancer narratives. *Qualitative Health Research*, *22*(9), 1184–1194. doi: 10.1177/1049732312449208

Knowles, G., Haigh, R., McLean, C., & Phillips, H. (2015). Late effects and quality of life after chemo-radiation for the treatment of anal cancer. *European Journal of Oncology Nursing*, *19*(5), 479–485. doi: 10.1016/j.ejon.2015.02.007

Lee, J., Hersey, K., Lee, C.T., & Fleshner, N. (2006). Climacturia following radical prostatectomy: Prevalence and risk factors. *Journal of Urology*, *176*(6), 2562–2565. doi: 10.1016/j.juro.2006.07.158

Lee, T., Breau, R., & Eapen, L. (2013). Pilot study on quality of life and sexual function in men-who-have-sex-with-men treated for prostate cancer. *Journal of Sexual Medicine*, *10*(8), 2094–2100. doi: 10.1111/jsm.12208

Lee, T.K., Handy, A.B., Kwan, W., Oliffe, J.L., Brotto, L.A., Wassersug, R.J., & Dowsett, G.W. (2015). Impact of prostate cancer treatment on the sexual quality of life for men-who-have-sex-with-men. *Journal of Sexual Medicine*, *12*(12), 2378–2386. doi: 10.1111/jsm.13030

Liu, C., Lopez, D.S., Chen, M., & Wang, R. (2017). Penile rehabilitation therapy following radical prostatectomy: A meta-analysis. *Journal of Sexual Medicine*. doi: 10.1016/j.jsxm.2017.09.020

Ljungman, L., Eriksson, L.E., Flynn, K.E., Gorman, J.R., Ståhl, O., Weinfurt, K., ... Wettergren, L. (2019). Sexual dysfunction and reproductive concerns in young men diagnosed with testicular cancer: An observational study. *Journal of Sexual Medicine*, *16*(7), 1049–1059. doi: 10.1016/j.jsxm.2019.05.005

Loi, M., Wortel, R.C., Francolini, G., & Incrocci, L. (2019). Sexual function in patients treated with stereotactic radiotherapy for prostate cancer: A systematic review of the current evidence. *Journal of Sexual Medicine*, *16*(9), 1409–1420. doi: 10.1016/j.jsxm.2019.05.019

Lyons, K.S., Winters-Stone, K.M., Bennett, J.A., & Beer, T.M. (2016). The effects of partnered exercise on physical intimacy in couples coping with prostate cancer. *Health Psychology*, *35*(5), 509–513. doi: 10.1037/hea0000287

Manne, S., Kashy, D.A., Zaider, T., Lee, D., Kim, I.Y., Heckman, C., ... Virtue, S.M. (2018). Interpersonal processes and intimacy among men with localized prostate cancer and their partners. *Journal of Family Psychology*, *32*(5), 664–675. doi: 10.1037/fam0000404

Matheson, L., Watson, E.K., Nayoan, J., Wagland, R., Glaser, A., Gavin, A., ... Rivas, C. (2017). A qualitative metasynthesis exploring the impact of prostate cancer and its management on younger, unpartnered and gay men. *European Journal of Cancer Care (Engl)*, *26*(6). doi: 10.1111/ecc.12676

Matsushita, K., Tal, R., & Mulhall, J. (2012). The evolution of orgasmic pain (dysorgasmia) following radical prostatectomy. *Journal of Sexual Medicine*, *9*(5), 1454–1458. doi: 10.1111/j.1743-6109.2012.02699.x

Matthew, A. (2016). Core principles of sexual health treatments in cancer for men. *Current Opinion in Supportive and Palliative Care*, *10*(1), 38–43. doi: 10.1097/spc.0000000000000183

Matthew, A., Lutzky-Cohen, N., Jamnicky, L., Currie, K., Gentile, A., Mina, D.S., ... Elterman, D. (2018). The prostate cancer rehabilitation clinic: A biopsychosocial clinic for sexual dysfunction after radical prostatectomy. *Current Oncology*, *25*(6), 393–402. doi: 10.3747/co.25.4111

McInnis, M.K., & Pukall, C.F. (2020). Sex after prostate cancer in gay and bisexual men: A review of the literature. *Sexual Medicine Reviews*, *8*(3), 466–472. doi: 10.1016/j.sxmr.2020.01.004

Messaoudi, R., Menard, J., Ripert, T., Parquet, H., & Staerman, F. (2011). Erectile dysfunction and sexual health after radical prostatectomy: Impact of sexual motivation. *International Journal of Impotence Research*, *23*(2), 81–86. Retrieved from http://www.nature.com/ijir/journal/v23/n2/sup pinfo/ijir20118s1.html

Miranda, E.P., Benfante, N., Kunzel, B., Nelson, C.J., & Mulhall, J.P. (2020). A randomized, controlled, 3-arm trial of pharmacological penile rehabilitation in the preservation of erectile function after radical prostatectomy. *Journal of Sexual Medicine*. doi: 10.1016/j.jsxm.2020.10.022

Mogorovich, A., Nilsson, A.E., Tyritzis, S.I., Carlsson, S., Jonsson, M., Haendler, L., … Wiklund, N.P. (2013). Radical prostatectomy, sparing of the seminal vesicles, and painful orgasm. *Journal of Sexual Medicine*, *10*(5), 1417–1423. doi: 10.1111/jsm.12086

Montorsi, F., Brock, G., Lee, J., Shapiro, J., Van Poppel, H., Graefen, M., & Stief, C. (2008). Effect of nightly versus on-demand vardenafil on recovery of erectile function in men following bilateral nerve-sparing radical prostatectomy. *European Urology*, *54*(4), 924–931. doi: 10.1016/j. eururo.2008.06.083

Montorsi, F., Guazzoni, G., Strambi, L.F., Da Pozzo, L.F., Nava, L., Barbieri, L., … Miani, A. (1997). Recovery of spontaneous erectile function after nerve-sparing radical retropubic prostatectomy with and without early intracavernous injections of alprostadil: Results of a prospective, randomized trial. *Journal d'urologie*, *158*(4), 1408–1410.

Moore, A., Higgins, A., & Sharek, D. (2013). Barriers and facilitators for oncology nurses discussing sexual issues with men diagnosed with testicular cancer. *European Journal of Oncology Nursing*, *17*(4), 416–422. doi: 10.1016/j.ejon.2012.11.008

Namiki, S., Ishidoya, S., Nakagawa, H., Ito, A., Kaiho, Y., Tochigi, T., … Arai, Y. (2012). The relationships between preoperative sexual desire and quality of life following radical prostatectomy: A 5-year follow-up study. *Journal of Sexual Medicine*, *9*(9), 2448–2456. doi: 10.1111/j.1743-6109.2012.02788.x

Nascimento, B., Miranda, E.P., Jenkins, L.C., Benfante, N., Schofield, E.A., & Mulhall, J.P. (2019). Testosterone recovery profiles after cessation of androgen deprivation therapy for prostate cancer. *Journal of Sexual Medicine*, *16*(6), 872–879. doi: 10.1016/j.jsxm.2019.03.273

Näsvall, P., Dahlstrand, U., Löwenmark, T., Rutegård, J., Gunnarsson, U., & Strigård, K. (2017). Quality of life in patients with a permanent stoma after rectal cancer surgery. *Quality of Life Research*, *26*(1), 55–64. doi: 10.1007/s11136-016-1367-6

Navon, L., & Morag, A. (2003). Advanced prostate cancer patients' ways of coping with the hormonal therapy's effect on body, sexuality, and spousal ties. *Qualitative Health Research*, *13*(10), 1378–1392.

Nelson, C.J., Deveci, S., Stasi, J., Scardino, P.T., & Mulhall, J.P. (2010). Sexual bother following radical prostatectomy. *Journal of Sexual Medicine*, *7*(1), 129–135. doi: 10.1111/j.1743-6109.2009.01546.x

Nelson, C.J., Emanu, J.C., & Avildsen, I. (2015). Couples-based interventions following prostate cancer treatment: A narrative review. *Translational Andrology and Urology*, *4*(2), 232–242. doi: 10.3978/j.issn.2223-4683.2015.04.04

Neuman, H.B., Patil, S., Fuzesi, S., Wong, W.D., Weiser, M.R., Guillem, J.G., … Temple, L.K. (2011). Impact of a temporary stoma on the quality of life of rectal cancer patients undergoing treatment. *Annals of Surgical Oncology*, *18*(5), 1397–1403. doi: 10.1245/s10434-010-1446-9

Nilsson, A.E., Carlsson, S., Johansson, E., Jonsson, M.N., Adding, C., Nyberg, T., … Wiklund, N.P. (2011). Orgasm-associated urinary incontinence and sexual life after radical prostatectomy. *Journal of Sexual Medicine*, *8*(9), 2632–2639. doi: 10.1111/j.1743-6109.2011.02347.x

Nolan, J., Kershen, R., Staff, I., McLaughlin, T., Tortora, J., Gangakhedkar, A., … Wagner, J. (2020). Use of the urethral sling to treat symptoms of climacturia in men after radical prostatectomy. *Journal of Sexual Medicine*, *17*(6), 1203–1206. doi: 10.1016/j.jsxm.2020.03.001

O'Shaughnessy, P.K., Ireland, C., Pelentsov, L., Thomas, L.A., & Esterman, A.J. (2013). Impaired sexual function and prostate cancer: A mixed method investigation into the experiences of men and their partners. *Journal of Clinical Nursing*, *22*(23–24), 3492–3502. doi: 10.1111/jocn.12190

Padma-Nathan, H., McCullough, A.R., Levine, L.A., Lipshultz, L.I., Siegel, R., Montorsi, F., ... on behalf of the Study, G. (2008). Randomized, double-blind, placebo-controlled study of postoperative nightly sildenafil citrate for the prevention of erectile dysfunction after bilateral nerve-sparing radical prostatectomy. *International Journal of Impotence Research, 20*(5), 479–486. doi: 10.1038/ijir.2008.33

Paich, K., Dunn, R., Skolarus, T., Montie, J., Hollenbeck, B., Palapattu, G., ... Wittmann, D. (2016). Preparing patients and partners for recovery from the side effects of prostate cancer surgery: A group approach. *Urology, 88*, 36–42. doi: 10.1016/j.urology.2015.07.064

Palmer, M.H., Fogarty, L.A., Somerfiled, M.R., & Powell, L,L. (2003). Incontinence after prostate cancer surgery. *Oncology Nursing Forum, 30*(2), 229–238.

Park, K.K., Lee, S.H., & Chung, B.H. (2011). The effects of long-term androgen deprivation therapy on penile length in patients with prostate cancer: A single-center, prospective, open-label, observational study. *Journal of Sexual Medicine, 8*(11), 3214–3219. doi: 10.1111/j.1743-6109.2011.02364.x

Patel, M., Hudnall, M., Cooley, L., Fitzgerald, M.K., Pham, M., Wren, J., ... Bennett, N. (2019). 159 Two year cost analysis of penile rehabilitation post-prostatectomy for various regimens at a single institution. *Journal of Sexual Medicine, 16*(4), S81. doi: 10.1016/j.jsxm.2019.01.168

Pietilä, I., Jurva, R., Ojala, H., & Tammela, T. (2018). Seeking certainty through narrative closure: Men's stories of prostate cancer treatments in a state of liminality. *Sociology of Health and Illness, 40*(4), 639–653. doi: 10.1111/1467-9566.12671

Pillay, B., Moon, D., Love, C., Meyer, D., Ferguson, E., Crowe, H., ... Wootten, A. (2017). Quality of life, psychological functioning, and treatment satisfaction of men who have undergone penile prosthesis surgery following robot-assisted radical prostatectomy. *Journal of Sexual Medicine, 14*(12), 1612–1620. doi: 10.1016/j.jsxm.2017.10.001

Pinks, D., Davis, C., & Pinks, C. (2018). Experiences of partners of prostate cancer survivors: A qualitative study. *Journal of Psychosocial Oncology, 36*(1), 49–63. doi: 10.1080/07347332.2017.1329769

Qian, S.Q., Gao, L., Wei, Q., & Yuan, J. (2016). Vacuum therapy in penile rehabilitation after radical prostatectomy: Review of hemodynamic and antihypoxic evidence. *Asian Journal of Andrology, 18*(3), 446–451. doi: 10.4103/1008-682X.159716.

Raina, R., Agarwal, A., Ausmundson, S., Lakin, M.M., Nandipati, K., Montague, D.K., ... Zippe, C. (2006). Early use of vacuum constriction device following radical prostatectomy facilitates early sexual activity and potential early return of erectile function. *International Journal of Impotence Research: Official Journal of the International Society for Impotence Research, 18*, 77–81.

Reese, J.B., Handorf, E., & Haythornthwaite, J.A. (2018). Sexual quality of life, body image distress, and psychosocial outcomes in colorectal cancer: A longitudinal study. *Supportive Care in Cancer, 26*(10), 3431–3440. doi: 10.1007/s00520-018-4204-3

Roeloffzen, E.M.A., Lips, I.M., van Gellekom, M.P.R., van Roermund, J., Frank, S.J., Battermann, J.J., & van Vulpen, M. (2010). Health-related quality of life up to six years after 125I brachytherapy for early-stage prostate cancer. *International Journal of Radiation Oncology Biology Physics, 76*(4), 1054–1060. doi: 10.1016/j.ijrobp.2009.03.045

Rose, D., Ussher, J.M., & Perz, J. (2016). Let's talk about gay sex: Gay and bisexual men's sexual communication with healthcare professionals after prostate cancer. *European Journal of Cancer Care (Engl)*. doi: 10.1111/ecc.12469

Rossen, P., Pedersen, A.F., Zachariae, R., & Maase, H. (2012). Sexuality and body image in long-term survivors of testicular cancer. *European Journal of Cancer, 48*(4), 571–578.

Rosser, B.R.S., Kohli, N., Polter, E.J., Lesher, L., Capistrant, B.D., Konety, B.R., ... Kilian, G. (2020). The sexual functioning of gay and bisexual men following prostate cancer treatment: Results from the restore study. *Archives of Sexual Behavior, 49*(5), 1589–1600. doi: 10.1007/s10508-018-1360-y

Salonia, A., Adaikan, G., Buvat, J., Carrier, S., El-Meliegy, A., Hatzimouratidis, K., ... Khera, M. (2017). Sexual rehabilitation after treatment for prostate cancer-part 2: Recommendations from the fourth international consultation for sexual medicine (ICSM 2015). *Journal of Sexual Medicine, 14*(3), 297–315. doi: 10.1016/j.jsxm.2016.11.324

Schantz Laursen, B. (2017). Sexuality in men after prostate cancer surgery: A qualitative interview study. *Scandinavian Journal of Caring Sciences, 31*(1), 120–127. doi: 10.1111/scs.12328

Seidler, Z.E., Lawsin, C.R., Hoyt, M.A., & Dobinson, K.A. (2016). Let's talk about sex after cancer: Exploring barriers and facilitators to sexual communication in male cancer survivors. *Psycho-Oncology*, *25*(6), 670–676. doi: 10.1002/pon.3994

Shah, T.T., Ahmed, H., Kanthabalan, A., Lau, B., Ghei, M., Maraj, B., & Arya, M. (2014). Focal cryotherapy of localized prostate cancer: A systematic review of the literature. *Expert Review of Anticancer Therapy*, *14*(11), 1337–1347. doi: 10.1586/14737140.2014.965687

Sodergren, S.C., Vassiliou, V., Dennis, K., Tomaszewski, K.A., Gilbert, A., Glynne-Jones, R., ... Johnson, C.D. (2015). Systematic review of the quality of life issues associated with anal cancer and its treatment with radiochemotherapy. *Supportive Care in Cancer*, *23*(12), 3613–3623. doi: 10.1007/s00520-015-2879-2

Speer, S.A., Tucker, S.R., McPhillips, R., & Peters, S. (2017). The clinical communication and information challenges associated with the psychosexual aspects of prostate cancer treatment. *Social Science and Medicine*, *185*, 17–26. doi: 10.1016/j.socscimed.2017.05.011

Srivatsav, A., Balasubramanian, A., Butaney, M., Thirumavalavan, N., McBride, J.A., Gondokusumo, J., ... Lipshultz, L. (2019). Patient attitudes toward testicular prosthesis placement after orchiectomy. *American Journal of Men's Health*, *13*(4), 1557988319861019. doi: 10.1177/1557988319861019

Stuhlfauth, S., Melby, L., & Hellesø, R. (2018). Everyday life after colon cancer: The visible and invisible challenges. *Cancer Nursing*, *41*(6), E48–E57. doi: 10.1097/ncc.0000000000000506

Tay, K.J., Polascik, T.J., Elshafei, A., Cher, M.L., Given, R.W., Mouraviev, V., ... Jones, J.S. (2016). Primary cryotherapy for high-grade clinically localized prostate cancer: Oncologic and functional outcomes from the COLD registry. *Journal of Endourology*, *30*(1), 43–48. doi: 10.1089/end.2015.0403

Terrier, J.E., Masterson, M., Mulhall, J.P., & Nelson, C.J. (2018). Decrease in intercourse satisfaction in men who recover erections after radical prostatectomy. *Journal of Sexual Medicine*, *15*(8), 1133–1139. doi: 10.1016/j.jsxm.2018.05.020

Thomas, C., Wootten, A., & Robinson, P. (2013). The experiences of gay and bisexual men diagnosed with prostate cancer: Results from an online focus group. *European Journal of Cancer Care (Engl)*, *22*(4), 522–529. doi: 10.1111/ecc.12058

Traa, M.J., De Vries, J., Roukema, J.A., Rutten, H.J., & Den Oudsten, B.L. (2014). The sexual health care needs after colorectal cancer: The view of patients, partners, and health care professionals. *Supportive Care in Cancer*, *22*(3), 763–772. doi: 10.1007/s00520-013-2032-z

Tucker, S.R., Speer, S.A., & Peters, S. (2016). Development of an explanatory model of sexual intimacy following treatment for localised prostate cancer: A systematic review and meta-synthesis of qualitative evidence. *Social Science and Medicine*, *163*, 80–88. doi: 10.1016/j.socscimed.2016.07.001

Ussher, J.M., Perz, J., Rose, D., Dowsett, G.W., Chambers, S., Williams, S., ... Latini, D. (2017). Threat of sexual disqualification: The consequences of erectile dysfunction and other sexual changes for gay and bisexual men with prostate cancer. *Archives of Sexual Behavior*, *46*(7), 2043–2057. doi: 10.1007/s10508-016-0728-0

Vasconcelos, J.S., Figueiredo, R.T., Nascimento, F.L., Damiao, R., & da Silva, E.A. (2012). The natural history of penile length after radical prostatectomy: A long-term prospective study. *Urology*, *80*(6), 1293–1296. doi: 10.1016/j.urology.2012.07.060

Walker, L.M., King, N., Kwasny, Z., & Robinson, J.W. (2017). Intimacy after prostate cancer: A brief couples' workshop is associated with improvements in relationship satisfaction. *Psychooncology*, *26*(9), 1336–1346. doi: 10.1002/pon.4147

Walker, L.M., & Robinson, J.W. (2012). Sexual adjustment to androgen deprivation therapy: Struggles and strategies. *Qualitative Health Research*, *22*(4), 452–465. doi: 10.1177/1049732311422706

Walker, L.M., & Santos-Iglesias, P. (2020). On the relationship between erectile function and sexual distress in men with prostate cancer. *Archives of Sexual Behavior*, *49*(5), 1575–1588. doi: 10.1007/s10508-019-01603-y

Walker, L.M., Santos-Iglesias, P., & Robinson, J. (2018). Mood, sexuality, and relational intimacy after starting androgen deprivation therapy: Implications for couples. *Supportive Care in Cancer*, *26*(11), 3835–3842. doi: 10.1007/s00520-018-4251-9

Wang, C.J., Sparano, J., & Palefsky, J.M. (2017). Human immunodeficiency virus/AIDS, human papillomavirus, and anal cancer. *Surgical Oncology Clinics of North America, 26*(1), 17–31. doi: 10.1016/j.soc.2016.07.010

Wittmann, D., Northouse, L., Crossley, H., Miller, D., Dunn, R., Nidetz, J., … Montie, J.E. (2015). A pilot study of potential pre-operative barriers to couples' sexual recovery after radical prostatectomy for prostate cancer. *Journal of Sex and Marital Therapy, 41*(2), 155–168. doi: 10.1080/0092623x.2013.842194

Wong, C., Louie, D.R., & Beach, C. (2020). A systematic review of pelvic floor muscle training for erectile dysfunction after prostatectomy and recommendations to guide further research. *Journal of Sexual Medicine, 17*(4), 737–748. doi: 10.1016/j.jsxm.2020.01.008

Zhu, X., Chen, Y., Tang, X., Chen, Y., Liu, Y., Guo, W., & Liu, A. (2017). Sexual experiences of Chinese patients living with an ostomy. *Journal of Wound, Ostomy, and Continence Nursing, 44*(5), 469–474. doi: 10.1097/won.0000000000000357

RESOURCES

USToo

https://www.ustoo.org

Prostate Cancer Foundation

https://www.pcf.org/patient-resources/patient-navigation/support-groups/

Cancer Care

https://www.cancercare.org/support_groups/126-prostate_cancer_patient_support_group

BOOKS

Saving Your Sex Life: A Guide for Men with Prostate Cancer by John Mulhall (2011) CIACT, Inc. Publishing.

Prostate Cancer and the Man You Love: Supporting and Caring for Your Partner by Anne Katz (2012) Rowman & Littlefield.

What Every Gay Man Needs to Know about Prostate Cancer: The Essential Guide to Diagnosis, Treatment, and Recovery by Gerald Perlman (2012) Magnus Books.

Gay and Bisexual Men Living with Prostate Cancer: From Diagnosis. Edited by J. Ussher, J. Perz and S. Rosser (2018) Harrington Park Press.

11 Adolescents and young adults with cancer

Adolescent and young adulthood, occurring between the ages of 15 and 39 years of age, are critical phases when multiple developmental milestones should be achieved. These are discussed in detail in Chapter 2. Briefly, these include the development of sexual and gender identity, establishment of romantic and sexual relationships, making decisions about long-term relationship commitments as well as having children. Cancer during this time interrupts the achievement of these milestones to a lesser or greater extent.

The most common cancers affecting adolescents and young adults include leukemia, Hodgkin's lymphoma, bone sarcoma, brain, thyroid, breast, cervical, and testicular (Soanes & White, 2018). Treatments may include surgery, radiation, chemotherapy, and usually some combination of all three; bone marrow- and stem cell transplants are commonly used to treat hematologic cancers. Global sexual side effects are seen accompanied by psychosocial effects such as low self-esteem, anxiety, and changes in body image.

Box 11.1 Case study

Crystal is a 17-year-old young woman who was diagnosed and treated for a sarcoma in her left femur. She had an above-knee amputation and while she has recovered well from the surgery, she has become very quiet and withdrawn. Her mother slept in her room while she was in hospital and both her parents attend out-patient visits with her. Her parents, Rick and Stacey, appear baffled by the change in her personality.

When she was admitted to hospital before her surgery, the nurses noted that she was anxious but still seemed outgoing and upbeat. She had a lot of visitors and was upbeat when they were there. She appeared to be coping well and seemed fine when she was transferred to the rehabilitation facility. She progressed well according to the physio- and occupational therapists there. She adapted rapidly to her prosthesis and never complained about anything. Now at follow-up visits, the nurse practitioner responsible for care has noticed that her demeanor has changed. She rarely makes eye contact and shrugs her shoulders when asked how she is doing. She is almost never alone and her parents often answer questions posed to her; she doesn't seem bothered by this.

Nancy, the nurse practitioner, calls the social worker who is responsible for the adolescent- and young adult program at the cancer center. There is just something

---

DOI: 10.4324/9781003145745-11

that is bothering Nancy although she can't quite articulate what it is. The social worker suggests that Nancy tell Crystal's parents that she wants to see her without them. Nancy is not sure they will agree but she decides that she will try and find a way to talk to Crystal without them.

At her next visit, Nancy tells Crystal that she needs to get a urine sample. Stacey, Crystal's mother, starts to get out of her chair to go with her daughter to the restroom but Nancy stops her.

"I'll take it from here," she says firmly, and stands in front of Stacey as Crystal stands up.

"But ... ." Stacey starts to protest, but Nancy has moved behind Crystal and they leave the room together.

Nancy and Crystal walk slowly down the hallway. Nancy has found a way to get the young woman alone and she feels quite proud of herself.

"Hey, Crystal," she starts, "How are you doing, like really doing?"

Crystal shrugs, her usual response to any question about her coping.

"You know you can tell me anything, right?" Nancy stops at the restroom door, "I can feel that something is just not right with you, and I want to help in any way I can."

Crystal pushes her way past Nancy and enters the restroom. She puts out her hand to take the specimen jar from Nancy, but the nurse practitioner doesn't have anything to give her.

"Okay, so I got you here under false pretences ... But I think that maybe you don't want to talk in front of your parents ... ."

Crystal's response is more emotional than Nancy expected. In between sobs and gulps of air, Crystal tells her everything. Her friends don't seem to care about her and they don't include her in their social activities after school. She can see from the way they look at her that they pity her and she can't stand that. She's lonely and isolated and this was supposed to be such a great year, her senior year, and it's just a mess.

Nancy has put a hand on Crystal's shoulder as she talks but the young woman seems not to have noticed.

"What else, Crystal?" she says softly.

Crystal looks at Nancy and hesitates.

"I can't believe I'm telling you this but ..." She starts to cry again and Nancy moves closer and hugs her. Crystal starts to talk, her head buried in Nancy's shoulder.

"It's Jared ... . We started seeing each other before I was diagnosed and well, please don't tell my parents, but I, we ... . well we had sex and now he won't talk to me and he ignores me and I know it's because of how I look! But it's not fair! I didn't ask for this and I'm deformed and no one is ever going to want to date me never mind have sex with me and my life may as well be over!"

Her whole body is shaking now and Nancy has to brace herself to support Crystal's weight. She wonders if Crystal's parents have any idea about what is going on and how distressed their daughter is. This young woman needs help, and she needs it now. She wonders if the social worker is free to talk with Crystal and after that with her parents. If only Crystal would stop crying … .

Cancer in adolescence

Given the developmental stage of adolescents, cancer in this age group provides significant challenges. In a study of adolescents aged 15 to 19 years, a number of side effects of cancer and its treatment were identified (Veneroni et al., 2020). These include negative changes to body image in 56% of respondents and how they related to others (53%). Sexual desire was not changed in the majority (69.7%) who participated. Most had not had the opportunity to discuss sexual changes (67%) with health care providers despite 79% stating that this was important. When they did talk about it, it was generally with friends and/or their partner; they were mostly told to avoid sex or ask permission from their doctor. Given that many in this age group are exploring their sexuality alone or with partner(s), avoiding sex may not be something they are willing to do, or they have sex with anxiety. Speaking to a doctor may be fraught with embarrassment and not something they will do.

The contextual factors of adolescent life are important. Cancer interrupts the development of sexual identity with an existential crisis, where death is never far away. Many adolescents have not experienced the death of friends or family members, so dealing with the threat to their own life may be overwhelming. While their friends and peer group are exploring and experimenting with their sexuality, for adolescents with cancer, their nascent sexuality takes a much lower priority in their identity compared to the pressing nature of cancer treatment (Estefan, Moules, & Laing, 2019). Despite the normal experiences of adolescence with sexuality as a driving force physically and emotionally, these young people are forced to mature quickly.

Physical changes after treatment impact on their sense of physical attractiveness and self-esteem. They may have lost weight, have a puffy face from steroids, stretch marks from rapid weight gain, and alopecia from chemotherapy. Adolescents have described how cancer changed the image of their physical appearance both for themselves and in how others saw them. Cancer also took away some of the focus on their own sexuality and replaced it with uncertainty about the possibility of establishing loving relationships. During treatment, sexuality was secondary to the desire to survive and be cured of the cancer but at the same time they worried about side effects such as infertility and how that would affect their future (Moules et al., 2017).

Discussing sexuality with adolescents is not necessarily easy. This can be anxiety provoking for the adolescent not only because it is potentially embarrassing but also because they don't want to be punished by adults who may perceive their behaviors or ideas as unacceptable (Ashcraft & Murray, 2017). In turn, health care providers may be unsure about talking to a young person and concerned that parents and others may deem this as unnecessary or inappropriate (Halpern, 2010). Sexuality in adolescence is often seen as problematic and a risk for unplanned pregnancy or sexually transmitted infections. Discussions about sexual side effects of treatment are seen in the context of danger rather than a healthy aspect of development (Estefan et al., 2019). However, opening the discussion is itself an intervention in that it gives the adolescent permission to ask questions and alerts them to the willingness of a health care provider to talk about it at another time (Moules et al., 2017).

Young adults with cancer

As many as one-third of young adult cancer survivors report sexual problems and this is seen in both reproductive cancers as well as those not involving the reproductive organs (Mütsch et al., 2019). Changes in appearance are common, including weight gain, scars, and hair loss (Brierley, Sansom-Daly, Baenziger, McGill, & Wakefield, 2019). Feeling unattractive as a result of these changes has an effect on their willingness to flirt and/or establish a romantic relationship; low or absent libido is also experienced, perhaps as a result of these feelings or because of sexual problems that make sexual activity problematic (Graugaard, Sperling, Hølge-Hazelton, Boisen, & Petersen, 2018). Young women appear to be more affected than young men; however, the latter may experience more distress related to sexual changes (Soanes & White, 2018).

Young adult females reported decreased orgasm frequency compared to matched controls and young men reported lower desire than controls (Olsson, Steineck, Enskär, Wilderäng, & Jarfelt, 2018). Another study found that young women reported decreased desire and young men poor erectile, ejaculatory, and orgasmic function (Stanton, Handy, & Meston, 2017). Dyspareunia and decreased arousal to sexual stimuli have also been reported (Robinson, Miedema, & Easley, 2014).

Changes in romantic relationships for young adults with cancer are common. Seventy two percent of women with cancer reported having less intercourse than men (45%) but despite this, their relationship satisfaction was high. Effects on relationships included remaining in an unsatisfactory relationship longer than they would have without their cancer diagnosis, or getting married sooner than they would have under normal circumstances. In addition, some individuals with cancer avoid relationships to avoid burdening a potential partner. Cancer affects partners too with some describing playing a secondary or excluded role when the parents of the person with cancer take over (Moules, Laing, Estefan, Schulte, & Guilcher, 2018). But one study found that the partners of individuals with cancer report fewer negative effects (19%) than individuals with cancer themselves (13%) (Geue, Schmidt, Sender, Sauter, & Friedrich, 2015).

The supportive care- and sexual support-needs of young adults are high (Sender, Friedrich, Schmidt, & Geue, 2020) but may not be adequately met by health care providers. In one study, 61% of young adults reported that they had not had a discussion or only had a limited discussion with their health care provider about sex (Graugaard et al., 2018). A bio-psycho-social approach should be taken with attention to physical, mental, social, and cultural aspects of life (Condorelli et al., 2019). A brief checklist to identify sexual problems in the clinical setting is presented below.

Box 11.2: Clinical screener for sexual concerns (adapted from Soanes & White, 2018)

In the past 12 months, has there been a period of 3 months or more where you had one or more of the following:

- You wanted to feel more desire for sexual activity
- (Men only) You had problems with erections
- (Women only) Your vagina felt dry
- You had pain during or after sex
- You had problems having an orgasm
- You felt anxious about sex

- You did not enjoy sex
- Other sexual problems or concerns
- No sexual problems or concerns

Communication between health care providers and this population are infrequent. Nurses in a study from Australia reported that they rarely talked about sexuality during survivorship care (Chan, Button, Thomas, Gates, & Yates, 2018). In dedicated adolescent and young adult units a more comprehensive approach to caring for this population identified three key areas that need to be addressed (Ricadat, Schwering, Fradkin, Boissel, & Aujoulat, 2019). These include a focus on separation from parents and self-determination; gender and sexual identity; and social life and connection with peers. Many of the existing guidelines for survivorship care focus on fertility with little about sexuality and sexual functioning (Murphy et al., 2015).

Childhood-cancer survivors

There is a paucity of evidence on the long-term sexual side effects of treatment on survivors of childhood cancer. Most recently, studies have identified risk factors for sexual dysfunction later in life from radiation therapy as well as surgery to the pelvis in women. Twice as many women than men experienced sexual dysfunction later in life after treatment in childhood (Greenberg, Khandwala, Bhambhvani, Simon, & Eisenberg, 2020) but men may be more distressed (Zebrack, Foley, Wittmann, & Leonard, 2010). In another study of female survivors, 19.9% reported sexual dysfunction, primarily related to pelvic surgery, and just 2.9% had received any help in this regard (Bjornard et al., 2020). They may also experience age-related sexual changes at an earlier than unaffected individuals (Haavisto, Henriksson, Heikkinen, Puukko-Viertomies, & Jahnukainen, 2016).

Childhood-cancer survivors may have difficulty disclosing their cancer history to prospective partners (Thompson, Long, & Marsland, 2013); those who were treated as a young child may not know their treatment history and may have little to no memory of what happened to them.

Conclusion

Cancer in the formative adolescent and young adult years presents unique psycho-sexual and psycho-social challenges. These are times of great personal growth with developmental milestones related to sexuality and relationships that should be achieved. Gaps in social engagement because of hospitalization and out-patient treatments result in loss of connection with peer groups with the potential of being left behind the peer group. It is important to recognize these challenges when providing care to this population.

RESOURCES

WEBSITES

LIVESTRONG

https://www.livestrong.org/we-can-help/young-adults

Stupid Cancer

https://stupidcancer.org/

Ulman Foundation

https://ulmanfoundation.org/

Teen Cancer America

https://teencanceramerica.org/

The Samfund

http://www.thesamfund.org/

Lacuna Loft

https://lacunaloft.org/

Young Survivor Coalition

https://www.youngsurvival.org/

Imerman Angels

https://imermanangels.org/

References

Ashcraft, A.M., & Murray, P.J. (2017). Talking to parents about adolescent sexuality. *Pediatric Clinics of North America*, *64*(2), 305–320. doi: 10.1016/j.pcl.2016.11.002

Bjornard, K.L., Howell, C.R., Klosky, J.L., Chemaitilly, W., Srivastava, D.K., Brinkman, T.M., Green, D., Willard, W., Jacola, L., Krasin, M., Hudson, M., Robison, L., & Ness, K.K. (2020). Psychosexual functioning of female childhood cancer survivors: A report from the St. Jude lifetime cohort study. *Journal of Sexual Medicine*, *17*(10), 1981–1994.

Brierley, M.-E.E., Sansom-Daly, U.M., Baenziger, J., McGill, B., & Wakefield, C.E. (2019). Impact of physical appearance changes reported by adolescent and young adult cancer survivors: A qualitative analysis. *European Journal of Cancer Care*, *28*(4), e13052. doi: 10.1111/ecc.13052

Chan, R.J., Button, E., Thomas, A., Gates, P., & Yates, P. (2018). Nurses attitudes and practices towards provision of survivorship care for people with a haematological cancer on completion of treatment. *Supportive Care in Cancer*, *26*(5), 1401–1409. doi: 10.1007/s00520-017-3972-5

Condorelli, M., Lambertini, M., Del Mastro, L., Boccardo, F., Demeestere, I., & Bober, S.L. (2019). Fertility, sexuality and cancer in young adult women. *Current Opinion in Oncology*, *31*(4), 259–267. doi: 10.1097/cco.0000000000000540

Estefan, A., Moules, N.J., & Laing, C.M. (2019). Composing sexuality in the midst of adolescent cancer. *Journal of Pediatric Oncology Nursing*, *36*(3), 191–206. doi: 10.1177/1043454219836961

Geue, K., Schmidt, R., Sender, A., Sauter, S., & Friedrich, M. (2015). Sexuality and romantic relationships in young adult cancer survivors: Satisfaction and supportive care needs. *Psycho-Oncology*, *24*(11), 1368–1376. doi: 10.1002/pon.3805

Graugaard, C., Sperling, C.D., Hølge-Hazelton, B., Boisen, K.A., & Petersen, G.S. (2018). Sexual and romantic challenges among young Danes diagnosed with cancer: Results from a cross-sectional nationwide questionnaire study. *Psychooncology*, *27*(6), 1608–1614. doi: 10.1002/pon.4700

Greenberg, D.R., Khandwala, Y.S., Bhambhvani, H.P., Simon, P.J., & Eisenberg, M.L. (2020). Male and female sexual dysfunction in pediatric cancer survivors. *Journal of Sexual Medicine*, *17*(9), 1715–1722. doi: 10.1016/j.jsxm.2020.05.014

Haavisto, A., Henriksson, M., Heikkinen, R., Puukko-Viertomies, L.-R., & Jahnukainen, K. (2016). Sexual function in male long-term survivors of childhood acute lymphoblastic leukemia. *Cancer*, *122*(14), 2268–2276. doi: 10.1002/cncr.29989

Halpern, C.T. (2010). Reframing research on adolescent sexuality: Healthy sexual development as part of the life course. *Perspectives on Sexual and Reproductive Health*, *42*(1), 6–7. doi: 10.1363/4200610

Moules, N.J., Estefan, A., Laing, C.M., Schulte, F., Guilcher, G.M.T., Field, J.C., & Strother, D. (2017). "A Tribe Apart": Sexuality and cancer in adolescence. *Journal of Pediatric Oncology Nursing*, *34*(4), 295–308. doi: 10.1177/1043454217697669

Moules, N.J., Laing, C.M., Estefan, A., Schulte, F., & Guilcher, G.M.T. (2018). Family is who they say they are(a): Examining the effects of cancer on the romantic partners of adolescents and young adults. *Journal of Family Nursing*, *24*(3), 374–404. doi: 10.1177/1074840718786985

Murphy, D., Klosky, J.L., Reed, D.R., Termuhlen, A.M., Shannon, S.V., & Quinn, G.P. (2015). The importance of assessing priorities of reproductive health concerns among adolescent and young adult patients with cancer. *Cancer*, *121*(15), 2529–2536. doi: 10.1002/cncr.29466

Mütsch, J., Friedrich, M., Leuteritz, K., Sender, A., Geue, K., Hilbert, A., & Stöbel-Richter, Y. (2019). Sexuality and cancer in adolescents and young adults—A comparison between reproductive cancer patients and patients with non-reproductive cancer. *BMC Cancer*, *19*(1), 828. doi: 10.1186/s12885-019-6009-2

Olsson, M., Steineck, G., Enskär, K., Wilderäng, U., & Jarfelt, M. (2018). Sexual function in adolescent and young adult cancer survivors-a population-based study. *Journal of Cancer Survivorship*, *12*(4), 450–459. doi: 10.1007/s11764-018-0684-x

Ricadat, É., Schwering, K.-L., Fradkin, S., Boissel, N., & Aujoulat, I. (2019). Adolescents and young adults with cancer: How multidisciplinary health care teams adapt their practices to better meet their specific needs. *Psycho-Oncology*, *28*(7), 1576–1582. doi: 10.1002/pon.5135

Robinson, L., Miedema, B., & Easley, J. (2014). Young adult cancer survivors and the challenges of intimacy. *Journal of Psychosocial Oncology*, *32*(4), 00–00. doi: 10.1080/07347332.2014.917138

Sender, A., Friedrich, M., Schmidt, R., & Geue, K. (2020). Cancer-specific distress, supportive care needs and satisfaction with psychosocial care in young adult cancer survivors. *European Journal of Oncology Nursing*, *44*, 101708, doi: 10.1016/j.ejon.2019.101708

Soanes, L., & White, I. (2018). Sexuality and cancer: The experience of adolescents and young adults. *Pediatric Blood and Cancer*, *65*(12), e27396. doi: 10.1002/pbc.27396

Stanton, A.M., Handy, A.B., & Meston, C.M. (2017). Sexual function in adolescents and young adults diagnosed with cancer: A systematic review. *Journal of Cancer Survivorship*. doi: 10.1007/s11764-017-0643-y

Thompson, A.L., Long, K.A., & Marsland, A.L. (2013). Impact of childhood cancer on emerging adult survivors' romantic relationships: A qualitative account. *Journal of Sexual Medicine*, *10*(Suppl. 1), 65–73. doi: 10.1111/j.1743-6109.2012.02950.x

Veneroni, L., Bagliacca, E.P., Sironi, G., Silva, M., Casanova, M., Bergamaschi, L. Terenziani, M., Trombatore, J., Clerici, C., Prunas, A., Silvaggi, M., Massimino, M., & Ferrari, A. (2020). Investigating sexuality in adolescents with cancer: Patients talk of their experiences. *Pediatric Hematology and Oncology*, *37*(3), 223–234. doi: 10.1080/08880018.2020.1712502

Zebrack, B.J., Foley, S., Wittmann, D., & Leonard, M. (2010). Sexual functioning in young adult survivors of childhood cancer. *Psycho-Oncology*, *19*(8), 814–822. doi: 10.1002/pon.1641

12 Sexuality and infertility

Infertility presents singular challenges to couples when sexual activity becomes focused on conception rather than pleasure. The primary relationship may become strained and it is not unusual to see conflict and even relationship breakdown in the aftermath of treatment for infertility. The connection between infertility and sexuality or sexual function is clear with infertility and its treatment causing sexual problems for some, while sexual dysfunction can also cause infertility. These associations will be discussed in depth in this chapter.

Infertility may be primary (not able to conceive at all despite at least two or more years without of the use of contraceptives) or secondary (not able to conceive after the birth of one or more babies and not using contraceptives since the last birth). Fifteen percent of couples globally experience infertility; the 35 to 39-year age group has the highest prevalence of infertility (Sun et al., 2019). The cause of infertility may be related to the man or woman, or sometimes both. Sexual dysfunction in couples dealing with infertility is significant with 43–90% of women and 48–58% of men experiencing sexual problems (Starc et al., 2019).

Sexual problems in men with infertility

Male causes of infertility include erectile dysfunction, anejaculation, retrograde ejaculation, premature ejaculation, and altered sperm production including azoospermia (Lotti & Maggi, 2018). Infertility causes decreased self-esteem and loss of confidence in some men (Jamil, Shoaib, Aziz, & Ather, 2020) as well as decreased sexual- and general quality of life (Smith et al., 2009). Specifically, male infertility causes erectile dysfunction or premature ejaculation in one out of six men and orgasmic problems in 10% of men. More prevalent are low desire and poor sexual satisfaction (Lotti & Maggi, 2018). For many men, fertility is a sign of virility (Halcomb, 2018) and this may play a role in the psychological burden that they may carry.

Sexual problems in women with infertility

Female causes of infertility include premature ovarian insufficiency, polycystic ovary syndrome, endometriosis, uterine fibroids, and polyps; fertility also decreases with increasing age (Vander Borght & Wyns, 2018). Women who think or know that the problems with conception are their fault are more likely to experience a negative impact on their sexual function (Winkelman, Katz, Smith, & Rowen, 2016) and in one study, 26% of women met the criteria for female sexual dysfunction (Nelson, Shindel, Naughton, Ohebshalom, & Mulhall, 2008). Commonly reported sexual problems include lack of desire, vaginal dryness and pain, and anorgasmia (Smith, Madeira, & Millard, 2015).

DOI: 10.4324/9781003145745-12

Impact of infertility on couple sexual functioning

Sexual problems in couples experiencing infertility include loss of pleasure and less frequent sexual activity (Süli, Kopa, Benyó, & Vereczkey, 2017) and reactive loss of desire for both (Piva, Lo Monte, Graziano, & Marci, 2014). Fifty percent of couples report changes in their sex life due to childlessness; women are more affected than their male partners (Wischmann, 2010). Men may feel pressured to have sex and develop performance anxiety that affects their erections; this leads to shame and a sense of failure that increases performance anxiety (Wischmann, 2010). Sex becomes less about fun and eroticism and instead revolves around the time of ovulation and positions that maximize the possibility of conception.

Some couples avoid sex during the woman's ovulation period to prevent the negative effects of not conceiving when she gets her next menstrual period (Piva et al., 2014). Some couples do return to their previous level of sexual functioning after treatment for infertility; however, for others sexual problems persist particularly if they are not successfully treated and do not conceive (Wirtberg, Möller, Hogström, Tronstad, & Lalos, 2006). Sex for the sole purpose of getting pregnant is often not pleasurable and causes pain for the woman due to lack of arousal/lubrication; this contributes to the woman's anxiety about sex itself that further causes anticipation of pain (Purcell-Lévesque, Brassard, Carranza-Mamane, & Péloquin, 2019).

The pressure to conceive may lead to coercion to have intercourse; more men (37%) report this than women (12%) (Peterson & Buday, 2020). The coercion is usually verbal and rarely physical and some report that they pressure themselves; women report that they experience pressure from their fertility specialist to have sex when they are told to and this is distressing. When the decision is made to use assisted reproductive technology to conceive, the pressure on the couple decreases and their sexual relationship improves.

Box 12.1 The PLISSIT model to address sexual problems in couples experiencing infertility

Permission: Couples going through infertility treatment often experience changes to their sex life. What information can I give you about this?

Limited Information: Sex is often different when you are trying to conceive. It's as if all the fun has gone from what used to be spontaneous and pleasurable. I have some suggestions that may help.

Specific suggestion: It's helpful to have sex for fun in a different room than sex to get pregnant. That may help to bring some of the joy back!

Intensive Therapy: The pressure to get pregnant can cause couples to stop communicating and conflict can happen. We have a counselor that we can refer you to if you find that you need some support in that area.

Assisted reproductive technology

Assisted reproductive technology (ART) has made pregnancy possible for many couples experiencing infertility; however, this too may have a negative effect on both male and female sexuality. It is important to remember that no matter the cause of the infertility, the woman bears the brunt of the treatments that have significant side effects including mood swings, fluid retention, weight gain, and feelings of unattractiveness (Piva et al., 2014).

The man's contribution to ART is basically the need to produce semen samples by masturbation; this is contradicted by some religious and cultural groups and the man may feel guilty when contravening this prohibition. For men with azoospermia, the use of donor sperm for insemination or ART lessens the impact on sexual functioning but the man may experience guilt and feeling less masculine; these can both impact on sexual functioning (Indekeu et al., 2012).

Many couples have high expectations that ART will be successful and with repeated cycles that are not successful, men may become anxious and distressed. Men of reproductive age are often infrequent users of the health care system and infertility throws them into a highly technical but also intrusive environment where their manhood is questioned (Bechoua, Hamamah, & Scalici, 2016). But men may also use the highly technical nature of ART to reconstruct their masculinity by framing their infertility as a medical condition and not reflective of their identity (Halcomb, 2018).

This medicalization of infertility and the use of ART are suggested to allow men to alleviate any shame or guilt they may feel (Bell, 2016a). The focus of infertility treatment predominately falls on the female partner even if the cause of the infertility is the man's problem. He is thus distanced from the treatments she undergoes and instead is seen as the main source of support for her; this emphasizes his masculinity and prevents him from feeling any guilt. The use of intracytoplasmic sperm injection (ICSE) where a single sperm in injected directly into the woman's egg further removes the man from the act of procreation. Financial considerations may cause additional distress and when the man wants to stop treatment, his partner may react negatively.

For women in same-sex relationships, the desire for pregnancy means that ART is necessary in most instances. Women report that undergoing treatments is challenging as heteronormativity prevails in many fertility practices (Bell, 2016b) and their unique needs are not met. Some women also describe receiving demeaning comments from staff and feeling marginalized. For women who have experienced sexual trauma, the need for repeated invasive investigations such as intravaginal ultrasound to monitor follicle development can be traumatizing.

Interventions for treatment-related sexual dysfunction

For men who experience sexual problems such as erectile dysfunction, the use of oral erectile aids such as sildenafil may be helpful. Other more mechanical aids such as the penile pump or intra-cavernosal injections may be needed and are discussed in greater detail in Chapter 13. Low libido should not be treated with testosterone as this inhibits conception (Berger, Messore, Pastuszak, & Ramasamy, 2016).Treatment of anejaculation by electrostimulation of the prostate or penile vibratory stimulation may produce semen but for some men, surgical sperm extraction from the testicle may be necessary. Lack of lubrication in women can be treated with lubricants; care should be taken to suggest Pre-Seed™ that will not affect sperm negatively as most other lubricants do. Pelvic floor physiotherapy is helpful for women who experience pain with penetration that precludes intercourse. Any pre-existing medical conditions that may impact on fertility should of course be treated before attempting ART. Sexuality counseling or sex therapy using a variety of psychotherapeutic techniques is helpful for these couples.

The close association between infertility and sexual dysfunction may not be recognized by fertility specialists who are focused on technical aspects of assisted reproduction.

Couples may not get any support for the sexual problems they have while trying to conceive and persistent problems may result, perhaps leading to relationship breakdown. While psychological assessment is usually prescribed as part of the work-up for fertility treatment, this may not include anticipatory guidance about sexual problems and how to find help for these.

Referral to a sex therapist or sexuality counselor can help couples to find ways to make sex pleasurable and reduce the pressure to perform. Couples can be helped to connect sensually without intercourse and to focus on the relationship outside of the desire to conceive. Simple strategies such as having sex for pleasure in the bedroom and sex for conception in another room can be helpful. Removing the paraphernalia of ART such as medications, syringes, books about fertility, and ovulation kits can also protect the bedroom as a space for love and sex not connected to conception.

Conclusion

Sexual dysfunction is common during attempts at conception as well as during the process of fertility treatment. Anxiety and depression because of infertility further complicate sexual problems and cause additional distress and stress for couples. Insufficient support for sexual problems is common and is an unmet need for many.

RESOURCES

Fertility IQ
   https://www.fertilityiq.com/

References

Bechoua, S., Hamamah, S., & Scalici, E. (2016). Male infertility: An obstacle to sexuality? *Andrology*, *4*(3), 395–403. doi: 10.1111/andr.12160

Bell, A.V. (2016a). 'I don't consider a cup performance; I consider it a test': Masculinity and the medicalization of infertility. *Sociology of Health and Illness*, *38*(5), 706–720. doi: 10.1111/1467-9566.12395

Bell, A.V. (2016b). The margins of medicalization: Diversity and context through the case of infertility. *Social Science and Medicine*, *156*, 39–46. doi: 10.1016/j.socscimed.2016.03.005

Berger, M.H., Messore, M., Pastuszak, A.W., & Ramasamy, R. (2016). Association between infertility and sexual dysfunction in men and women. *Sexual Medicine Reviews*, *4*(4), 353–365. doi: 10.1016/j.sxmr.2016.05.002

Halcomb, L. (2018). Men and infertility: Insights from the sociology of gender. *Sociology Compass*, *12*(10), e12624. doi: 10.1111/soc4.12624

Indekeu, A., D'Hooghe, T., De Sutter, P., Demyttenaere, K., Vanderschueren, D., Vanderschot, B., Welkenhuysen, M., & Rober, P. (2012). Parenthood motives, well-being and disclosure among men from couples ready to start treatment with intrauterine insemination using their own sperm or donor sperm. *Human Reproduction*, *27*(1), 159–166. doi: 10.1093/humrep/der366

Jamil, S., Shoaib, M., Aziz, W., & Ather, M.H. (2020). Does male factor infertility impact on self-esteem and sexual relationship? *Andrologia*, *52*(2), e13460. doi: 10.1111/and.13460

Lotti, F., & Maggi, M. (2018). Sexual dysfunction and male infertility. *Nature Reviews. Urology*, *15*(5), 287. doi: 10.1038/nrurol.2018.20

Nelson, C.J., Shindel, A.W., Naughton, C.K., Ohebshalom, M., & Mulhall, J.P. (2008). Prevalence and predictors of sexual problems, relationship stress, and depression in female partners of infertile couples. *Journal of Sexual Medicine*, *5*(8), 1907–1914. doi: 10.1111/j.1743-6109.2008.00880.x

Peterson, Z.D., & Buday, S.K. (2020). Sexual coercion in couples with infertility: Prevalence, gender differences, and associations with psychological outcomes. *Sexual and Relationship Therapy*, *35*(1), 30–45. doi: 10.1080/14681994.2018.1435863

Piva, I., Lo Monte, G., Graziano, A., & Marci, R. (2014). A literature review on the relationship between infertility and sexual dysfunction: Does fun end with baby making? *European Journal of Contraception and Reproductive Health Care*, *19*(4), 231–237. doi: 10.3109/13625187.2014.919379

Purcell-Lévesque, C., Brassard, A., Carranza-Mamane, B., & Péloquin, K. (2019). Attachment and sexual functioning in women and men seeking fertility treatment. *Journal of Psychosomatic Obstetrics and Gynecology*, *40*(3), 202–210. doi: 10.1080/0167482x.2018.1471462

Smith, J.F., Walsh, T.J., Shindel, A.W., Turek, P.J., Wing, H., Pasch, L. (2009). Sexual, marital, and social impact of a man's perceived infertility diagnosis. *Journal of Sexual Medicine*, *6*(9), 2505–2515. doi: 10.1111/j.1743-6109.2009.01383.x

Smith, N.K., Madeira, J., & Millard, H.R. (2015). Sexual function and fertility quality of life in women using in vitro fertilization. *Journal of Sexual Medicine*, *12*(4), 985–993. doi: 10.1111/jsm.12824

Starc, A., Trampuš, M., Pavan Jukić, D., Rotim, C., Jukić, T., & Polona Mivšek, A. (2019). Infertility and sexual dysfunctions: A systematic literature review. *Acta Clinica Croatica*, *58*(3), 508–515. doi: 10.20471/acc.2019.58.03.15

Süli, Á., Kopa, Z., Benyó, M., & Vereczkey, A. (2017). Factors affecting sexuality in infertile couples. *Journal of Sexual Medicine*, *14*(5), e260. doi: 10.1016/j.jsxm.2017.04.278

Sun, H., Gong, T.-T., Jiang, Y.-T., Zhang, S., Zhao, Y.-H., & Wu, Q.-J. (2019). Global, regional, and national prevalence and disability-adjusted life-years for infertility in 195 countries and territories, 1990–2017: Results from a global burden of disease study, 2017. *Aging*, *11*(23), 10952–10991. doi: 10.18632/aging.102497

Vander Borght, M., & Wyns, C. (2018). Fertility and infertility: Definition and epidemiology. *Clinical Biochemistry*, *62*, 2–10. doi: 10.1016/j.clinbiochem.2018.03.012

Winkelman, W.D., Katz, P.P., Smith, J.F., Rowen, T.S., & Infertility Outcomes Program Project Group (2016). The sexual impact of infertility among women seeking fertility care. *Sexual Medicine*, *4*(3), e190–e197. doi: 10.1016/j.esxm.2016.04.001

Wirtberg, I., Möller, A., Hogström, L., Tronstad, S.-E., & Lalos, A. (2006). Life 20 years after unsuccessful infertility treatment. *Human Reproduction*, *22*(2), 598–604. doi: 10.1093/humrep/del401

Wischmann, T.H. (2010). Original Research—Couples' sexual dysfunctions: Sexual disorders in infertile couples. *Journal of Sexual Medicine*, *7*(5), 1868–1876. doi: 10.1111/j.1743-6109.2010.01717.x

13 Interventions to treat sexual dysfunction in men

There are a number of medications that are prescribed to treat sexual dysfunction in men. This chapter will provide information about oral medications to treat erectile dysfunction as well as more invasive treatment options such as the penile pump, penile injections, and implants. Hormonal treatments for loss of desire in men are common and available in multiple formats.

Erectile dysfunction

As has been described in previous chapters, erectile dysfunction (ED) is a distressing experience for men who desire penetrative intercourse. Fortunately, there are many different treatments for this; however, their success is limited. There is a large psychological or emotional component to erectile dysfunction and interventions that address this are also important.

Pharmaceutical agents

Since the approval of sildenafil (Viagra™) in 1998, the focus of treatment has been on the use of oral agents in managing ED. The oral agents belong to the class of phosphodiesterase 5 inhibitors (PDE5i) and include sildenafil (Viagra), tadalafil (Cialis™), vardenafil (Levitra™), and avanafil (Stendra™). These medications prolong erections by promoting smooth muscle relaxation and blood flow in the spongy bodies (corpora caversona) of the penis (Huang & Lie, 2013). They are regarded as first line treatment. It is important to note these medications do not cause an erection, but rather work to keep blood in the penis after genital stimulation (Goldstein, Burnett, Rosen, Park, & Stecher, 2019). Sildenafil remains the most commonly prescribed of the oral agents (Mulhall, Chopra, Patel, Hassan, & Tang, 2020). The mechanism of action is similar in all of these; however, the onset of action and length of time that the drug is bioavailable differ. An orodispersable film containing sildenafil is available in Europe (Jannini & Droupy, 2019). Other medications in this group are available outside North America and include udenafil, mirodenafil, and lodenafil (Hatzimouratidis et al., 2016).

Education of the man is important because discontinuation rates are high (approaching 50%) due to cost, ineffectiveness, and adverse events; the latter two factors may be ameliorated or prevented with comprehensive education prior to treatment initiation (Carvalheira, Pereira, Maroco, & Forjaz, 2012). Side effects include headache, dyspepsia, and facial flushing (Cui, Liu, Shi, & Gao, 2016). Men should be warned to avoid purchasing these products on the internet as many of these are counterfeit and pose a safety risk (Hatzimouratidis et al., 2016).

DOI: 10.4324/9781003145745-13

More invasive treatments for ED include intra-cavernosal injections of alprostadil/compound product containing alprostadil, papaverine, and phentolamine (Trimix) (Hatzimouratidis et al., 2016). Quadri-mix does not contain alprostadil and instead atropine is included in this compound product. A small amount of the medication is injected into the side of the shaft of the penis and this promotes a local vasodilation response.

It is essential that men receive comprehensive education about how to draw up the correct dose, where to inject, and how to deal with priapism, the most common side effect. The prescriber is responsible for finding the most appropriate dose in the office, based on a test dose as part of the education of the patient. Discontinuation rates are similar to those of the oral agents and the involvement of the partner in the education session along with couple counseling is suggested to improve outcomes.

Intra-urethral alprostadil (MUSE™) may be prescribed for men who are needle-phobic but efficacy is much less than with intra-corporeal injections (Hatzimouratidis et al., 2016). Pain and burning in the urethra is noted to occur in up to 43% of men using this method. Topical alprostadil (Vitaros™) is available in North America and while not as effective as intra-urethral or intra-cavernosal products, may be appropriate for men who have difficulty with other methods.

Non-pharmaceutical interventions

The penile pump is regarded as second-line intervention for ED (Trost, Munarriz, Wang, Morey, & Levine, 2016). There are multiple commercially available pumps including hand- or battery-operated versions. They all involve a cylinder, a pump, and a constriction band. The penis must be lubricated, and the base of the pump cylinder must form a tight seal with the skin at the base of the penis. Once blood is drawn into the penis by the negative pressure generated by the pump, the constriction ring needs to be released from the cylinder and onto the base of the penis. Side effects are common and include lower temperature of the penis that may be distasteful to the sexual partner, hinging of the penis at the level of the constriction band, and decreased penile sensation. Men who are on blood thinners and who have experienced priapism should not use the penile pump.

The penile implant is a surgical intervention with a long history in the management of ED in men. Semi-rigid prostheses were followed by silicone rods and currently, the inflatable penile prosthesis is the most common device used (Khera, Mulcahy, Wen, & Wilson, 2020). This three-part prosthesis comprises two inflatable cylinders inserted into the spongy bodies of the penis, a reservoir containing fluid in the abdomen, and a small pump inserted into the scrotum. The surgery to place the implant is invasive and some men find that they have difficulty activating the pump; future designs may preclude the need for this. Post-operative pain is significant and some men experience shortening of the penis after surgery, impacting on patient satisfaction (Parker, Bickell, & Carrion, 2017); however overall, men are satisfied with this procedure (Habous et al., 2018). The three-part prosthesis is reported to be more satisfying to both men and their partner than the simpler malleable/semi-rigid devices (Çayan et al., 2019) however, it is also more liable to fail. It is important that men and their partner receive in-depth education before consenting to the procedure (Trost, 2020).

Botanical and 'natural' products

Given the relatively limited success of oral agents in treating ED, the costs involved, and the reluctance of many men to use more invasive interventions, the attraction of 'natural' remedies is understandable. In a review of 718 plants suggested to help men achieve erections, Sin and colleagues (Sin, Anand, & Koh) suggest that additional studies are needed to warrant to address efficacy and safety. They report that the most common plants used to treat ED include *P. yohimbe, P. ginseng* and *L. meyenii* (maca)*;* in most instances the roots of these plants are used. As with many natural products, safety of commercially available products cannot be confirmed; there is potential for contamination, substitution, and interactions with pharmaceuticals and other herbal products.

Other interventions in the management of ED

For some men, dealing with ED means exploring other options that may help, either before they try treatments as described above or when these prove to be unsuccessful. Some men use a constriction band such as the UroStop, a variable tension loop created to help with urine leakage during sexual activity. The use of a constriction band may help to prolong an erection; however, the same risks described above with the penile pump exist (Miranda et al., 2019).

Pelvic floor physiotherapy may be an important adjunct for men, especially for those who have high pelvic floor muscle tone that interferes in arterial blood flow as well as smooth muscle relaxation. Both inflow and relaxation of smooth muscle are vital for erections (Cohen, Gonzalez, & Goldstein, 2016). There is evidence that pelvic floor physiotherapy with biofeedback may improve erectile function after radical prostatectomy for treatment of prostate cancer (Wong, Louie, & Beach, 2020) as well as improvement in the incontinence that occurs almost universally in men following this surgery that may promote early intervention for the return of erectile function (Milios & Green, 2020).

Because of the role that vascular health plays in erectile function, cardiovascular health is a key factor in ED. It is suggested that 160 minutes of supervised exercise training per week for 6 months may improve vascular function and mitigate ED caused by metabolic and/or cardiovascular disease (Gerbild, Larsen, Graugaard, & Areskoug Josefsson, 2018). Rigorous exercise (e.g. 10 hours of cycling per week) has been shown to improve erectile function in men (Fergus et al., 2019). This 'whole body' approach is thought to address the root causes of ED and be more effective than merely treating the condition with PDE5*i* medication (Beecken et al., 2019). The Mediterranean diet has shown some efficacy in improving erectile function and for men who are overweight or obese, weight loss from a low-fat and low-calorie diet is also helpful in improving erections (La, Roberts, & Yafi, 2018).

Cognitive approaches may be useful in conjunction with pharmaceutical treatment for ED. In a small study comparing men who used PDE5*i* alone with those who used medication as well as cognitive behavioral therapy (CBT) (Khan, Amjad, & Rowland, 2019), those who used combined therapy showed improvements in erectile function that persisted at the 18-month mark. A novel group-based mindfulness intervention that included homework exercises showed utility for men with situational ED (Bossio, Basson, Driscoll, Correia, & Brotto, 2018). Mindfulness interventions have shown success in women with sexual problems (See Chapter 14) but have not been widely studied in men.

Experimental treatments for ED

Established treatments for ED are not successful or acceptable for some men and ongoing research has focused on alternative therapies using novel techniques. Shockwave therapy has been used for many years in the treatment of kidney stones and there is interest in this modality as it is non-invasive with minimal reported short-term adverse events (Raheem et al., 2020). There is limited evidence that low intensity extracorporeal shockwave therapy (Li-ESWT) has some efficacy in the treatment of organic ED (Porst, 2021).

Interest in platelet-rich plasma (PRP) and stem cell therapy (SCT) has been growing with direct-to-consumer advertising the benefits of this treatment for multiple conditions. The use of both PRP and SCT in the treatment of ED is not supported by evidence at the present time (Scott, Roberts, & Chung, 2019).

Management of low libido

Testosterone is acknowledged to play a role in the sexual functioning of men; however, other factors play an important role. Chronic disease, relationship functioning, and psychological health have a profound influence on all aspects of sexuality in men (Rastrelli et al., 2019). Testosterone levels decline with age and in response to chronic illness; do low testosterone levels reflect aging or are they a marker of chronic illness that may not be diagnosed? (Rastrelli, Corona, & Maggi, 2018).

Testosterone supplementation is a controversial topic with a divide between those who see a number of risks associated with its use while other who see this as a panacea for male aging. There is evidence that when used in men who are hypogonadal (T < 12 nmoles/L or 300 ng/dL), supplemental testosterone can improve libido and erectile dysfunction without risks to cardiovascular and prostate health (Corona, Torres, & Maggi, 2020). It is also important to monitor men who are taking supplemental testosterone; treatment effectiveness and the presence of adverse events should dictate ongoing therapy (Petering & Brooks, 2017). Testosterone therapy may improve the response to PDE5*i* agents (Gannon & Walsh, 2016) and has been shown to improve libido in hypogonadal men but once testosterone levels rise to within the normal range, no additional improvements are seen with ongoing supplementation (Rizk, Kohn, Pastuszak, & Khera, 2017).

The American Urologic Society guidelines state that testosterone deficiency should only be diagnosed after two total testosterone measurements on separate occasions in the early morning. The man should also have symptoms of low testosterone in order to make the diagnosis. A prostate specific antigen (PSA) test should also be ordered on men over the age of 40 before beginning supplementation (https://www.auanet.org/guidelines/testosterone-deficiency-guideline). Many men are prescribed testosterone supplementation without measuring testosterone levels (Twitchell, Pastuszak, & Khera). This is concerning as side effects may occur including worsening lower urinary tract symptoms, rising PSA levels, polycythemia, and risk of thromboembolism (Petering & Brooks, 2017).

There appears to be some differences in the response depending on the method of providing supplemental testosterone; the gel formulation appears superior to the patch for libido and oral testosterone is inferior to all other formulations (Elliott et al., 2017). So-called 'testosterone boosters' (T-boosters) are available online; however, they have limited evidence to support their use (Balasubramanian et al., 2019). There are significant gaps in men's knowledge about the risks associated with this medication. Men report benefits including improving sexual function (54%), feeling better (51%), and increased energy (53%) but have little knowledge about the risks of stroke (10%), blood clots (8%), or heart attack (16%) (Gilbert, Cimmino, Beebe, & Mehta, 2017).

Conclusion

Since 1998, when sildenafil became the first oral medication approved to treat erectile dysfunction, the focus on treating this condition has moved from psychological methods to biomedical interventions. But attrition is significant and more invasive methods are not acceptable to many men. Lifestyle interventions such as diet, exercise, and mindfulness meditation show promise and may have additional benefits for overall physical and mental health.

References

Balasubramanian, A., Thirumavalavan, N., Srivatsav, A., Yu, J., Lipshultz, L.I., & Pastuszak, A.W. (2019). Testosterone imposters: An analysis of popular online testosterone boosting supplements. *Journal of Sexual Medicine, 16*(2), 203–212. doi: 10.1016/j.jsxm.2018.12.008

Beecken, W.-D., Kersting, M., Kunert, W., Blume, G., Bacharidis, N., Cohen, D.S., Shabeeh, H., & Allen, M.S. (2019). Thinking about pathomechanisms and current treatment of erectile dysfunction—"The Stanley Beamish Problem." review, recommendations, and proposals. *Sexual Medicine Reviews.* doi: 10.1016/j.sxmr.2020.11.004

Bossio, J.A., Basson, R., Driscoll, M., Correia, S., & Brotto, L.A. (2018). Mindfulness-based group therapy for men with situational erectile dysfunction: A mixed-methods feasibility analysis and pilot study. *Journal of Sexual Medicine, 15*(10), 1478–1490. doi: 10.1016/j.jsxm.2018.08.013

Carvalheira, A., Pereira, N., Maroco, J., & Forjaz, V. (2012). Dropout in the treatment of erectile dysfunction with PDE5: A study on predictors and a qualitative analysis of reasons for discontinuation. *Journal of Sexual Medicine, 9*(9), 2361–2369. doi: 10.1111/j.1743-6109.2012.02787.x

Çayan, S., Aşçı, R., Efesoy, O., Bolat, M.S., Akbay, E., & Yaman, Ö. (2019). Comparison of long-term results and couples' satisfaction with penile implant types and brands: Lessons learned from 883 patients with erectile dysfunction who underwent penile prosthesis implantation. *Journal of Sexual Medicine, 16*(7), 1092–1099. doi: 10.1016/j.jsxm.2019.04.013

Cohen, D., Gonzalez, J., & Goldstein, I. (2016). The role of pelvic floor muscles in male sexual dysfunction and pelvic pain. *Sexual Medicine Reviews, 4*(1), 53–62. doi: 10.1016/j.sxmr.2015.10.001

Corona, G., Torres, L.O., & Maggi, M. (2020). Testosterone therapy: What we have learned from trials. *Journal of Sexual Medicine, 17*(3), 447–460. doi: 10.1016/j.jsxm.2019.11.270

Cui, Y., Liu, X., Shi, L., & Gao, Z. (2016). Efficacy and safety of phosphodiesterase type 5 (PDE5) inhibitors in treating erectile dysfunction after bilateral nerve-sparing radical prostatectomy. *Andrologia, 48*(1), 20–28. doi: 10.1111/and.12405

Elliott, J., Kelly, S.E., Millar, A.C., Peterson, J., Chen, L., Johnston, A., … Wells, G.A. (2017). Testosterone therapy in hypogonadal men: A systematic review and network meta-analysis. *BMJ Open, 7*(11), e015284. doi: 10.1136/bmjopen-2016-015284

Fergus, K.B., Gaither, T.W., Baradaran, N., Glidden, D.V., Cohen, A.J., & Breyer, B.N. (2019). Exercise improves self-reported sexual function among physically active adults. *Journal of Sexual Medicine, 16*(8), 1236–1245. doi: 10.1016/j.jsxm.2019.04.020

Gannon, J.R., & Walsh, T.J. (2016). Testosterone and sexual function. *Urologic Clinics of North America, 43*(2), 217–222. doi: 10.1016/j.ucl.2016.01.008

Gerbild, H., Larsen, C.M., Graugaard, C., & Areskoug Josefsson, K. (2018). Physical activity to improve erectile function: A systematic review of intervention studies. *Sexual Medicine, 6*(2), 75–89. doi: 10.1016/j.esxm.2018.02.001

Gilbert, K., Cimmino, C.B., Beebe, L.C., & Mehta, A. (2017). Gaps in patient knowledge about risks and benefits of testosterone replacement therapy. *Urology, 103*, 27–33. doi: 10.1016/j.urology.2016.12.066

Goldstein, I., Burnett, A.L., Rosen, R.C., Park, P.W., & Stecher, V.J. (2019). The serendipitous story of sildenafil: An unexpected oral therapy for erectile dysfunction. *Sexual Medicine Reviews, 7*(1), 115–128. doi: 10.1016/j.sxmr.2018.06.005

Habous, M., Tal, R., Tealab, A., Aziz, M., Sherif, H., Mahmoud, S., ... Mulhall, J.P. (2018). Predictors of satisfaction in men after penile implant surgery. *Journal of Sexual Medicine, 15*(8), 1180–1186. doi: 10.1016/j.jsxm.2018.05.011

Hatzimouratidis, K., Salonia, A., Adaikan, G., Buvat, J., Carrier, S., El-Meliegy, A., ... Khera, M. (2016). Pharmacotherapy for erectile dysfunction: Recommendations from the fourth international consultation for sexual medicine (ICSM 2015). *Journal of Sexual Medicine, 13*(4), 465–488. doi: 10.1016/j.jsxm.2016.01.016

Huang, S.A., & Lie, J.D. (2013). Phosphodiesterase-5 (PDE5) inhibitors in the management of erectile dysfunction, *38*(7), 407–419.

Jannini, E.A., & Droupy, S. (2019). Needs and expectations of patients with erectile dysfunction: An update on pharmacological innovations in phosphodiesterase Type 5 inhibition with focus on sildenafil. *Sexual Medicine, 7*(1), 1–10. doi: 10.1016/j.esxm.2018.10.005

Khan, S., Amjad, A., & Rowland, D. (2019). Potential for long-term benefit of cognitive behavioral therapy as an adjunct treatment for men with erectile dysfunction. *Journal of Sexual Medicine, 16*(2), 300–306. doi: 10.1016/j.jsxm.2018.12.014

Khera, M., Mulcahy, J., Wen, L., & Wilson, S.K. (2020). Is there still a place for malleable penile implants in the United States? Wilson's Workshop #18. *International Journal of Impotence Research.* doi: 10.1038/s41443-020-00376-6

La, J., Roberts, N.H., & Yafi, F.A. (2018). Diet and Men's sexual health. *Sexual Medicine Reviews, 6*(1), 54–68. doi: 10.1016/j.sxmr.2017.07.004

Milios, J.A., Ackland, T.R., & Green, D. (2020). Pelvic floor muscle training and erectile dysfunction in radical prostatectomy: A randomized controlled trial investigating a non-invasive addition to penile rehabilitation. *Journal of Sexual Medicine, 8*(3), 414–421. doi: 10.1016/j.esxm.2020.03.005

Miranda, E.P., Taniguchi, H., Cao, D.L., Hald, G.M., Jannini, E.A., & Mulhall, J.P. (2019). Application of sex Aids in men with sexual dysfunction: A review. *Journal of Sexual Medicine, 16*(6), 767–780. doi: 10.1016/j.jsxm.2019.03.265

Mulhall, J.P., Chopra, I., Patel, D., Hassan, T.A., & Tang, W.Y. (2020). Phosphodiesterase Type-5 inhibitor prescription patterns in the United States among men with erectile dysfunction: An update. *Journal of Sexual Medicine, 17*(5), 941–948. doi: 10.1016/j.jsxm.2020.01.027

Parker, J., Bickell, M., & Carrion, R. (2017). Future of penile implant surgery. *Journal of Sexual Medicine, 14*(4), 486–488. doi: 10.1016/j.jsxm.2016.12.011

Petering, R.C., & Brooks, N.A. (2017). Testosterone therapy: Review of clinical applications. *American Family Physician, 96*(7), 441–449.

Porst, H. (2021). Review of the current status of low intensity extracorporeal shockwave therapy (li-ESWT) in erectile dysfunction (ED), Peyronie's disease (PD), and sexual rehabilitation after radical prostatectomy with special focus on technical aspects of the different marketed ESWT devices including personal experiences in 350 patients. *Sexual Medicine Reviews, 9*(1), 93–122. doi: 10.1016/j.sxmr.2020.01.006

Raheem, O.A., Natale, C., Dick, B., Reddy, A.G., Yousif, A., Khera, M., & Baum, N. (2020). Novel treatments of erectile dysfunction: Review of the current literature. *Sexual Medicine Reviews.* doi: 10.1016/j.sxmr.2020.03.005

Rastrelli, G., Corona, G., & Maggi, M. (2018). Testosterone and sexual function in men. *Maturitas, 112*, 46–52. doi: 10.1016/j.maturitas.2018.04.004

Rastrelli, G., Guaraldi, F., Reismann, Y., Sforza, A., Isidori, A.M., Maggi, M., & Corona, G. (2019). Testosterone replacement therapy for sexual symptoms. *Sexual Medicine Reviews, 7*(3), 464–475. doi: 10.1016/j.sxmr.2018.11.005

Rizk, P.J., Kohn, T.P., Pastuszak, A.W., & Khera, M. (2017). Testosterone therapy improves erectile function and libido in hypogonadal men. *Current Opinion in Urology, 27*(6), 511–515. doi: 10.1097/mou.0000000000000442

Scott, S., Roberts, M., & Chung, E. (2019). Platelet-rich plasma and treatment of erectile dysfunction: Critical review of literature and global trends in platelet-rich plasma clinics. *Sexual Medicine Reviews, 7*(2), 306–312. doi: 10.1016/j.sxmr.2018.12.006

Sin, V.J.-E., Anand, G.S., & Koh, H.-L. Botanical medicine and natural products used for erectile dysfunction. *Sexual Medicine Reviews*. doi: 10.1016/j.sxmr.2020.10.005

Trost, L. (2020). Consenting the patient for penile implant surgery. *Journal of Sexual Medicine*, *17*(1), 4–6. doi: 10.1016/j.jsxm.2019.10.002

Trost, L.W., Munarriz, R., Wang, R., Morey, A., & Levine, L. (2016). External mechanical devices and vascular surgery for erectile dysfunction. *Journal of Sexual Medicine*, *13*(11), 1579–1617. doi: 10.1016/j.jsxm.2016.09.008

Twitchell, D.K., Pastuszak, A.W., & Khera, M. Controversies in testosterone therapy. *Sexual Medicine Reviews*. doi: 10.1016/j.sxmr.2020.09.004

Wong, C., Louie, D.R., & Beach, C. (2020). A systematic review of pelvic floor muscle training for erectile dysfunction after prostatectomy and recommendations to guide further research. *Journal of Sexual Medicine*, *17*(4), 737–748. doi: 10.1016/j.jsxm.2020.01.008

14 Interventions to treat sexual dysfunction in women

Sexual dysfunction in women is complicated by the assumption that problems are 'all in the woman's head' and that female sexuality is complex and mysterious. However, the problems that women face related to illness and treatments for many conditions, while they may have an emotional component, are very real and amenable to intervention. This chapter will highlight evidence-based interventions, both pharmaceutical and non-pharmaceutical.

Pharmaceutical treatments

There are limited pharmaceutical agents approved for use in women with sexual dysfunction despite significant effort by pharmaceutical companies to tap into a potentially lucrative market. There are two FDA-approved medications for women with low desire (flibanserin and bremelanotide) and two hormonal treatments are also available; estrogen is widely used in the treatment of vulvo-vaginal atrophy. Dehydroepiandrosterone (DHEA), a sex hormone precursor is a newer treatment that is FDA approved. Testosterone, while not approved for use in women, is used off-label to treat low libido. Other agents used to treat vulvo-vaginal atrophy are ospemifene and local lidocaine.

1. Estrogen

Local estrogen in pessary (Vagifem or Imvexxy), ring (Estring), or cream form (Premarim), is known to be effective in the treatment of vaginal atrophy resulting in dyspareunia (Lethaby, Ayeleke, & Roberts, 2016). Systemic absorption is minimal with these products (Simon & Maamari, 2013). Systemic estrogen is approved for short-term use only for relief of menopausal symptoms such as hot flashes and not for relief of vulvo-vaginal atrophy (Kohn, Rodriguez, Hotaling, & Pastuszak, 2019). A detailed discussion of the use of local estrogen is presented in Chapter 9 where its use in breast cancer is described.

2. Flibanserin

Flibanserin (Addyi™) is a centrally acting agent, approved in 2015, for the treatment of hypoactive sexual desire disorder (HSDD). Often described in the media as the 'female Viagra,' the medication does not impact arousal like sildenafil (Viagra) but rather is suggested to increase libido (Shapiro, Stevens, & Stahl, 2017). The path to approval of this medication is a long and controversial one beginning in 1996. The FDA voted against approval twice but on the third attempt, the medication was submitted for approval, a concerted effort was made by an advocacy group, called Even the Score, supported by the manufacturer, claiming

DOI: 10.4324/9781003145745-14

that there were 23 approved medications for male sexual dysfunction with none for women (Anderson & Moffatt, 2018). This is not accurate as there are numerous formulations of testosterone for men and three for PDE5-*i*, not 23 individual drugs.

The FDA eventually gave approval but with strict conditions. These included requiring prescribers and pharmacists taking a training course, and patients needing to sign a contract that they will not drink alcohol while taking the medication (Dooley, Miller, & Clayton, 2017). Flibanserin is approved for use in pre-menopausal women; however, off-label use is expected. A study of the medication in naturally post-menopausal women was discontinued early due to lack of efficacy (Portman, Brown, Yuan, Kissling, & Kingsberg, 2017).

Side effects of the medication include hypotension, syncope, dizziness, somnolence, and fatigue. Nausea, insomnia, and dry mouth have also been seen and are worse in women taking anti-depressants in addition to flibanserin (Kingsberg, McElroy, & Clayton, 2019). Efficacy is limited with an additional 0.5 sexually satisfying events in a 4-week period (Jaspers et al., 2016). The medication needs to be taken daily at a cost of $400 per month (the manufacturers state that a monthly supply is $25.00 for insured women and $99.00 for uninsured). Despite the promise suggested by manufacturers and professional advocates, flibanserin appears to work for a limited number of women (Segal 2018) and has not been the best seller it was purported to be.

A significant issue that is not often addressed is the role that desire plays in the life of women and how this affects sexual activity or sexual satisfaction. Low desire may not be distressing for women, is likely culturally bound, and there is no 'normal' level of sexual desire Aftab 2017. If desire is reactive as described by Basson (2015), do women need to feel spontaneous desire? The diagnosis of HSDD is no longer included in the Diagnostic and Statistical Manual of Mental Disorders (DSM-5) and instead a new diagnosis, female sexual interest/arousal disorder (FSAID), is included that links desire and arousal, in keeping with the notion of reactive desire accompanied/preceded by arousal (Basson, 2015).

3. Bremelanotide

In late 2019, the FDA approved another drug to treat low libido in women, this one acting on melanocortin receptors. Bremelanotide (Vyleesi) is injected into the subcutaneous fat in the abdomen or thigh; women should inject the medication 45 minutes before sexual activity. This is confusing; if a drug is purported to increase desire but then needs to be used BEFORE sexual activity, where does desire come into play? A woman with low- or no desire is unlikely to be motivated to inject herself before sex. Side effects include nausea, vomiting, and headache as well as injection site reactions. The medication also raised blood pressure in some women and is not recommended for women with or at high risk for cardiovascular disease. A small number of women in the clinical trials developed hyperpigmentation of the skin on the face, breasts, and gums; this did·not resolve after discontinuation of the medication (Mayer & Lynch, 2020). There was no difference in sexually satisfying sexual events when comparing the drug to placebo in clinical trials. A report of two phase-3 studies of medication (Kingsberg, Clayton, Portman, Williams, Krop, et al., 2019) has been heavily criticized for omitting critical data such as not reporting on protocol-listed outcomes, not disclosing that the drop-out rate was higher for those on bremelanotide, and participants preferred the placebo (Spielmans, 2021). This calls into question the validity of the clinical trials as well as the DFA approval of the medication.

Only one dose can be used in a 24-hour period and no more than eight doses per month should be used. The medication costs $948.00 for 4 doses according to the manufacturer.

4. Testosterone

Testosterone plays a role in vaginal tissue structure as well as in smooth muscle relaxation that is essential for arousal and lubrication (Maseroli & Vignozzi, 2020). It is also suggested to play a role in sexual desire in women; however, this is not strongly supported, so prescribing testosterone may not be useful beyond the placebo effect (Brotto, Bitzer, Laan, Leiblum, & Luria, 2010). There are no approved testosterone products for women in North America, despite interest by pharmaceutical companies and certain groups within the sexual medicine field for this (Simon & Kapner, 2020). Despite the lack of FDA approval, various formulations of testosterone (gels and pellets) are used off-label to treat low desire in women. In a global consensus statement (Davis et al., 2019), the use of testosterone in post-menopausal women only is suggested to be safe when resulting in physiologic levels but the safety of long-term use is not known. Of concern for this statement is that 'normal' levels of testosterone have not been established and laboratory assays are not accurate for women even if the normal range of testosterone for women was known (Simon & Kapner, 2020).

In part because of the lack of an approved product and the expense of doing clinical trials in women with sexual dysfunction due to the placebo effect, not much progress is being made in this area. A small double-blind, randomized controlled study of intravaginal testosterone showed no effects on libido but some improvement in sexual satisfaction and dyspareunia in post-menopausal women taking aromatase inhibitors (Davis et al., 2018). The long-term impact of testosterone on cardiovascular and breast cancer risk is unknown Vegunta 2019, adding to the caution that must be taken when prescribing off-label medication.

5. Dehydroepiandrosterone (DHEA)

DHEA is a precursor of sex hormones and is secreted primarily by the adrenal glands, the major source of sex hormones after menopause (Heo, 2019). A synthetic form of DHEA (Prasterone. Introsa®) is FDA approved for the treatment of dyspareunia after menopause (Portman, Goldstein, & Kagan, 2019). In clinical trials, intravaginal DHEA has been shown to decrease pain and improve vaginal pH as well as improvements in multiple aspects of sexual functioning, including lubrication (Bouchard et al., 2016). Efficacy has been shown in peri- and post-menopausal women (Peixoto et al., 2017) with minimal side effects (Labrie et al., 2018); the most commonly reported side effect is vaginal discharge (Heo, 2019). The impact on cardiovascular and cancer risk has not been established (Sauer, Talaulikar, & Davies, 2018); however, during one year of daily use, serum levels of sex hormone metabolites fell with the normal range for post-menopausal women (Heo, 2019).

6. Ospemifine

Ospemifine is a selective estrogen receptor modulator (SERM) that is taken orally (60 mg daily) and is FDA approved to treat moderate to severe vulvo-vaginal dryness due to menopause. It has been shown in multiple studies to improve dyspareunia and vaginal pH (Donato et al., 2019; Portman, Bachmann, Simon, & Group, 2013; Pup & Sánchez-Borrego, 2020). Improvements in a number of other sexual function domains have been shown; these include desire, arousal, orgasm, and satisfaction (Constantine, Graham, Portman, Rosen, & Kingsberg, 2015). An advantage of an oral treatment for dyspareunia is that it does not have any of the local effects that women find distasteful including difficulty in inserting something into the vagina, interference with sexual spontaneity, and itching or burning (Kingsberg

& Krychman, 2013). Effects of the treatment are seen within the first four weeks and are long lasting (Palacios & Cancelo, 2016). Side effects occurred in below 10% of women and included hot flashes, muscle spasms, headache, and vaginal discharge (Simon, Cort, Jiang, Pinkerton, 2018).

7. Local lidocaine

A novel approach using 4% aqueous lidocaine applied to the lower part of the vaginal introitus has been shown to be effective in reducing pain (Goetsch et al., 2015). Women can learn how to do this before penetration; there is no transfer to the partner, a problem with lidocaine gel.

Plant-based products

Women may choose to manage their sexual symptoms with neutraceuticals or so-called bio-identical hormones. Phytoestrogens have been shown to be effective in reducing vaginal dryness (Franco et al., 2016) but the studies supporting this are methodologically weak. Traditional Chinese medicine has mostly studied interventions for men and the highly individual focus of the treatments makes controlled trials almost impossible (Chubak & Doctor, 2018).

Bio-identical hormones are purported to be as effective as those manufactured by pharmaceutical companies but safer and more 'natural.' Celebrity endorsements and advertising on the internet have added to the uptake of these treatments. Why women would choose to use products that are not FDA approved or regulated is complex (Thompson, Ritenbaugh, & Nichter, 2017). Women may be fearful about the safety of conventional hormone therapy and/or distrustful of Western medicine and its practitioners. They may believe that alternatives are safer, more effective and/or tailored their individual needs when compounded by pharmacists. One other factor may be the attention paid to them by naturopaths as opposed to what they perceive as hurried care from physicians and nurse practitioners. The latter is important; when women feel heard and understood and are treated as respected partners in their care, they may be more amenable to evidence-based treatment.

Non-pharmaceutical treatments

1. Lubricants

Lubricants are used to provide comfort and alleviate pain from vaginal dryness during sexual activity. There are many different products available in drugstores, sex stores, and online.

Lubricants are divided into three categories: water-based, silicone-based, and oil-based. Oil-based formulations are not recommended as they stain fabric, alter the pH of the vagina, and are not compatible with condoms. Water-based lubricants are non-staining, widely available, and generally are non-irritating to genital tissues. But they often contain a range of humectants and preservatives to increase viscosity and these can have an impact on the pH of the vaginal tissues (Edwards & Panay, 2016b). Other additives include parabens, propylene glycol, glucose, and perfumes; these all alter the pH of the vagina and may promote the growth of bacteria (Hung et al., 2020) as well as being potentially cytotoxic to the tissues (Wilkinson, Łaniewski, Herbst-Kralovetz, & Brotman, 2019). Parabens are weakly estrogenic and glycols are known to be associated with bacterial vaginosis (Edwards & Panay, 2016a). Silicone-based lubricants are not absorbed and remain on tissues longer than water-based lubricants but they are more expensive and not as commonly available as water-based products (Hickey, Marino, Braat, & Wong, 2016). Silicone-based lubricants should not be used with silicone dilators or sex toys as they degrade these devices. Lubricants that claim to be warming and/or intensifying contain irritants and should be avoided, especially in women who experience vulvo-vaginal atrophy.

Both water- and silicone-based lubricants are associated with greater sexual pleasure and satisfaction for women, even those who do not experience pain with penetration (Herbenick et al., 2011). Women report using lubricants to make sex more fun and more comfortable (Herbenick, Reece, Schick, Sanders, & Fortenberry, 2014) and are often used as part of sex play with a partner. In this study, 65.5% of women reported using a lubricant during sexual activity.

The World Health Organization suggests that lubricants should not exceed an osmolality of 380 mOsm/kg and should have a pH of about 4.5 (Kagan, Kellogg-Spadt, & Parish, 2019). A commonly recommended lubricant, KY Jelly has a pH of 4.49 and an osmolality of 2007, well above what is regarded as acceptable (380 Osm/kg). It also contains glycerin, hydroxyethylcellulose, chlorhexidine gluconate, gluconolactone, methylparaben, and sodium hydroxide. For a detailed list of lubricant properties, see Edwards and Panay (2016) (Edwards & Panay, 2016).

2. Moisturizers

Vaginal moisturizers contain polymers that adhere to the vaginal tissues and promote hydration of the vaginal walls. They are suggested to provide daily comfort but are not to be confused with lubricants that are used for sexual activity. One such product from Brazil was shown to be as effective as local estrogen in postmenopausal women (Vale, Rezende, Raciclan, Bretas, & Geber, 2019). Hyaluronic acid has also been shown to be as effective as local estrogen and thus can be used in women for whom hormones are not advisable (dos Santos et al., 2021). Moisturizers are available in gel form (Gynetrof™, Hyalo-Gyn) or ovules (Repa-Gyn™, Revaree™). Vitamin E oil can also be used externally but caution should be taken to avoid inserting any oil into the vagina; this includes coconut or other plant oils.

Psychological interventions

Non-pharmaceutical/hormonal interventions have been the mainstay of mitigating and improving sexual problems in women for decades; there is very limited data on the effectiveness of psychological interventions for men. Despite the uptake of pharmaceutical products in recent years, there is much to be gained from considering psychological or educational methods that have been shown to be effective in multiple studies with no negative or systemic side effects.

1. Mindfulness-based meditation

Mindfulness-based interventions have been shown to be effective in helping women with sexual problems. Mindfulness-based meditation focuses on a state of being present, with non-judgmental awareness of negative thoughts and distractions (Arora & Brotto, 2017). It is suggested that this is important for women who have negative body image and sexual self-image. Women who experience sexual problems such as lack of libido or decreased arousal are likely to worry about this during sexual activity, thus distracting themselves from what is happening and any physical sensations. It is suggested that this intervention acts by decreasing the psychological barriers to sexually satisfying encounters through decreasing cognitive distractions, as well as anxiety and depression and awareness of physical sensations (Arora & Brotto, 2017). Two of the key principles of mindfulness, self-acceptance and self-compassion, are also thought to play a role.

Importantly, mindfulness has been shown to reduce the fear and negative thoughts that some women experience when planning or engaging in sexual activity (Jaderek & Lew-Starowicz, 2019). Participating in a structured program of mindfulness-based cognitive therapy improved sexual desire and reduced sexual distress (Gunst et al., 2019; Paterson, Handy, & Brotto, 2017). Improving arousal involves focusing on physical sensations during sexual activity; this has been shown to improve both awareness of arousal and concordance with genital arousal (Brotto, Chivers, Millman, & Albert, 2016; Velten, Margraf, Chivers, & Brotto, 2018). In addition, video-based mindfulness cognitive therapy improved achievement of orgasm as well as decreasing distress (Adam, De Sutter, Day, & Grimm, 2020). A meta-analysis of mindfulness-based interventions suggests that all aspects of female sexual dysfunction improve in addition to subjective sexual well-being (Stephenson & Kerth, 2017). It has also been shown that being sexually mindful, paying specific attention to the sensations in the body during sexual activity, contributes to sexual and relationship satisfaction (Leavitt, Lefkowitz, & Waterman, 2019). This requires practice and focus when often the natural cognitive state is one of anxiety and distraction. Mindfulness interventions for sexual pain have also shown positive results (Brotto, Bergeron, Zdaniuk, & Basson, 2020) including the ability of women to engage in vaginal penetration when they previously could not (Zarski 2017).

A number of studies have examined mindfulness interventions in the context of cancer, mostly in gynecologic cancer. Velten and colleagues (Velten et al., 2018) studied women with endometrial or cervical cancer who participated in group sessions; in addition to improvements in many aspects of sexuality, they also experienced a reduction in distress about the changes resulting from treatment. Dr Lori Brotto has shown that after participating in mindfulness interventions, female cancer survivors report hope that they would return to some level of sexual activity (Brotto et al., 2008). Body image has also been shown to improve after learning mindfulness-based meditation (Villena et al., 2018).

This intervention is relatively simple to learn and requires no formal instruction. However, mindfulness requires patience and discipline; this is not a 'when I feel like it or can fit it into my day' intervention but rather one that requires daily practice and an extended period of time to notice any benefits (Brotto & Goldmeier, 2015).

Many websites are available to help learn and practice this state of being in the moment and allowing distractions to pass. These include Mindspace, Calm, and others. There are also books (see resources) and dedicated courses that are useful.

2. Psycho-educational approaches

Psycho-educational interventions are the cornerstone of non-pharmaceutical interventions for sexual problems in women (Kingsberg et al., 2017). These include bibliotherapy, sexuality counseling and sex therapy, as well as cognitive behavioral therapy. Paying attention to the factors potentially impacting on the woman's sexual functioning is vital. These include:

- Relationship factors such as communication and conflict
- Cultural and religious beliefs

- Stress
- Emotional well-being including the presence of depression and/or anxiety
- Knowledge of anatomy and sexual functioning

Cognitive behavioral therapy has been used in the treatment of sexual problems that relate to maladaptive thoughts, unrealistic expectations, and relationships issues such as lack of trust or conflict (Wheeler & Guntupalli, 2020) An internet-based program of cognitive behavioral therapy was acceptable and showed improvement in desire, arousal, and satisfaction (Zippan, Stephenson, & Brotto, 2020). Psychotherapy, a more intense form of therapy, is used when the presence of trauma or family dysfunction is identified.

3. Bibliotherapy

Reading books as a self-help strategy or those recommended by a counselor or therapist is a common intervention for those experiencing sexual difficulties. It is relatively cheap, certainly cheaper than therapy, and accessible for those who can afford to purchase books and interested in reading and self-help as a strategy.

A systematic review of 15 randomized controlled trials concluded that the limitations in the studies of this intervention prevent robust evidence of efficacy (van Lankveld et al., 2021.). However, compared to no treatment, women who read books that they found themselves (unassisted bibliotherapy) showed remission of their sexual problems and both men and women reported greater sexual satisfaction. For women who read books suggested by a counselor or therapist (assisted bibliotherapy), significant improvement in their sexual functioning was reported. Men did not report any improvement in sexual functioning from bibliotherapy.

Physical interventions

For women who may not want to use pharmaceutical products or more invasive therapies, the role of physical interventions may offer benefits. These include partnered sensual massage (sensate focus exercises) and physical therapy, and also vibrators or dilators if vaginal stenosis is the cause of pain with penetration.

1. Sensate focus exercises

Sensate focus exercises were developed by Masters and Johnson (1970) to help couples who were experiencing sexual problems. This graduated home-based program focuses on non-demand, sensation focused, mindful touching. Masters and Johnson (1970) suggest that there are two levels of sensual touching; the first level is to give pleasure to the partner and the second level is to experience pleasure oneself. Many therapists who prescribe this intervention give incorrect instructions that focus the couple on the response of the partner rather than on the individual doing the touching (level two of the Masters and Johnson instruction). This results in counter-therapeutic, partner pleasing practice that may reflect the couple's sexual script where the attention is on the partner's pleasure, resulting in decreased arousal and/or orgasm.

Weiner and Avery-Clark (2017) have written a manual that describes in careful detail how couples should perform these exercises, with specific instructions for diverse populations with specific sexual problems. Box 14.1 presents the guiding principles of sensate focus exercises, but a full description is found in Weiner and Avery-Clark's manual. Prescribing sensate focus exercises should be used in counseling/therapy only by professionals who have been trained and are experienced in the intervention.

Box 14.1 Instructions for sensate focus exercises

The purpose of doing these exercises is to connect you with your own body and its sensations.

- This is a mindful practice; pay attention to the sensations **you** experience without judgment or expectation
- Focus on touch, temperature, pressure, and texture
- **Touch for yourself** rather than for your partner
- If your mind wanders, bring your focus back to what you are feeling through touching your partner
- Ignore thoughts about what your partner is feeling; **this is about YOU**
- Schedule 3 sessions every week
- Do not do the exercises at bedtime

---

2. Physical therapy

The muscles of the pelvic floor are involved in two main areas of sexual function: arousal and orgasm. A hypotonic pelvic floor may result in loss of genital sensation during arousal as well as weak or absent orgasm. A hypertonic pelvic floor is a significant contributor to pelvic pain in both men and women (Rosenbaum, 2007).

Disorders of the pelvic floor are common in women after childbirth and contribute to sexual dysfunction (Verbeek & Hayward, 2019). Pelvic floor physiotherapy uses manual therapy on soft tissue to help alleviate the symptoms of pelvic floor disorders, including pelvic and sexual pain (Ghaderi, Bastani, Hajebrahimi, Jafarabadi, & Berghmans, 2019; Stein, 2019). Pelvic floor exercises, known as Kegel exercises, have been shown to improve arousal, orgasm, and sexual satisfaction in women (Nazarpour, Simbar, Ramezani Tehrani, & Alavi Majd, 2017). Many physiotherapy techniques, including biofeedback, electrical stimulation, and soft tissue manipulation have been shown to be effective in decreasing dyspareunia for women with provoked vestibulodynia (Morin, Carroll, & Bergeron, 2017).

3. Dilators

Plastic or silicone dilators, often sold in a set of graduated sizes, may be used to decrease pain with penetration. Consistent use, multiple times a week, is needed to stretch the vagina (Liu, Juravic, Mazza, & Krychman, 2020). Some women are reluctant to use them, citing discomfort with using a 'sex toy,' even though this is inaccurate (Cullen et al., 2012). Non-adherence to use is significant with women stating that they do not have the time to dedicate to this or lack of privacy as reasons for discontinuing their use (Bakker et al., 2014). Long-term use is needed before any changes are seen (Falk & Bober, 2016).

4. Vibrators

Vibrator use is fairly common among women in the United States with 52.5% of women in a large (3,800 women aged 18–60 years) study reporting that they used the device (Debra Herbenick et al., 2009). Women who used a vibrator were more likely to participate in health promotion such as having a women's health appointment in the previous year and importantly, reported good sexual functioning across all domains of desire, arousal, lubrication, and orgasm). Improvement in genital sensation, sexual function, sexual satisfaction, and reduced distress have been seen in women who use a vibrator (Guess et al., 2017).

However, some women may be resistant to the use of a vibrator for masturbation and may be concerned about their partner's reaction (Marcus, 2011). It is important for health care providers and therapists who suggest using vibrator to consider what the concerns of the woman and her partner may be and to address those along with instructions on how to use the vibrator. The question of whether providers/therapists should sell these and other products to their patients/clients is controversial (Jannini, Limoncin, Ciocca, Buehler, & Krychman, 2012). On the one hand, the provider/therapist should not profit from the sale of any sex aids and should consider the ethics of encouraging something that they sell. However, perhaps any embarrassment or confusion on the part of the patient/client may be avoided if they are able to purchase something directly from their provider/therapist.

5. Laser treatments

The use of laser treatments for so-called 'vulvovaginal rejuvenation' is not approved by the FDA (Romero-Otero et al., 2020) despite widespread use (Enemchukwu, 2017) including in female cancer survivors where interest in non-hormonal interventions is high (Mothes, Runnebaum, & Runnebaum, 2018; Pagano et al., 2017; Pagano et al., 2017). The American College of Obstetricians and Gynecologists also does not approve of this intervention, citing safety concerns (Santen et al., 2017). Studies have small sample sizes (Samuels & Garcia, 2019) and are mostly observational with no control groups and only short-term outcomes are presented (Jha, Wyld, & Krishnaswamy, 2019); many of the study measures are physician- and not patient-reported (Song et al., 2018) and overall are assessed as being of low or very low quality (Pitsouni, Grigoriadis, Falagas, Salvatore, & Athanasiou, 2017). Studies have also reported increased dyspareunia after treatment with the CO_2 laser (Cruz et al., 2018). There are published reports of damage caused by this modality including fibrosis, agglutination, scarring, and penetration injuries (Gordon et al., 2019) as well as vaginal burns and chronic pain (Kaunitz et al., 2019).

There is variation in how many treatments are required, the time between treatments, and the maintenance requirements (Qureshi, Tenenbaum, & Myckatyn, 2018; Song et al., 2018). Costs are significant with an estimated $2,733.00 cited as the average cost for three treatments over one year (Wallace, St Martin, Lee, & Sokol, 2020); however, costs could depend on the individual provider/clinic and if covered by insurance.

Lifestyle interventions

Lifestyle factors such as diet, exercise, nicotine use, and alcohol intake are suggested to impact on sexual functioning in men and women. A systematic review of studies investigating the role of these factors suggests that making lifestyle changes before initiating more invasive interventions can be beneficial (Allen & Walter, 2018). Physical activity has the greatest impact on sexual functioning and eliminating both alcohol and nicotine intake is also recommended.

Weight loss for obese men and women has been shown to improve sexual functioning through multiple pathways including endocrine function, cardiovascular health, and psychosocial factors such as improved self-esteem and body image (Rowland, McNabney, & Mann, 2017). The Mediterranean diet has been shown to alleviate sexual dysfunction in women (Towe et al., 2020). Exercise also has benefits for energy that is important for improved sexual functioning in women in particular (Stanton, Handy, & Meston, 2018).

Conclusion

Despite the prevailing belief that female sexual dysfunction is hard to treat, this chapter has provided a comprehensive, evidence-based approach that includes pharmaceutical, herbal, physical, and psycho-educational interventions. Women thus have many choices to help mitigate the effects of illness or normal aging. It is important to note that off-label use is quite common, so caution is advised before recommending or prescribing some products.

Resources

Brotto, L. (2018). *Better Sex Through Mindfulness: How Women Can Cultivate Desire.* Greystone Books.

Gunter, J. (2019). *The Vagina Bible: The vulva and the vagina--separating the myth from the medicine.* Random House Canada.

Mintz, L. (2018). *Becoming Cliterate: Why Orgasm Equality Matters--And How to Get It.* Harper One.

Nagoski, E. (2015). *Come as You Are: The Surprising New Science that Will Transform Your Sex Life.* Simon & Schuster.

Nagoski, E. (2019). *The Come as You Are Workbook: A Practical Guide to the Science of Sex.* Simon & Schuster.

Perel, E. (2017). *Mating in Captivity: Unlocking Erotic Intelligence.* Harper Paperbacks.

Weiner, L. Avery-Clark, C. (2017). *Sensate Focus in Sex Therapy: The Illustrated Manual.* Routledge.

References

Adam, F., De Sutter, P., Day, J., & Grimm, E. (2020). A randomized study comparing video-based mindfulness-based cognitive therapy with video-based traditional cognitive behavioral therapy in a sample of women struggling to achieve orgasm. *Journal of Sexual Medicine, 17*(2), 312–324. doi: 10.1016/j.jsxm.2019.10.022

Aftab, A., Chen, C., & McBride, J. (2017). Flibanserin and its discontents. *Archives of Women's Mental Health, 20*(2), 243–247. doi: 10.1007/s00737-016-0693-6

Allen, M.S., & Walter, E.E. (2018). Health-related lifestyle factors and sexual dysfunction: A meta-analysis of population-based research. *Journal of Sexual Medicine, 15*(4), 458–475. doi: 10.1016/j.jsxm.2018.02.008

Anderson, R., & Moffatt, C E. (2018). Ignorance is not bliss: If we don't understand hypoactive sexual desire disorder, how can flibanserin treat it? commentary. *Journal of Sexual Medicine, 15*(3), 273–283. doi: 10.1016/j.jsxm.2018.01.001

Arora, N., & Brotto, L.A. (2017). How does paying attention improve sexual functioning in women? A review of mechanisms. *Sexual Medicine Reviews, 5*(3), 266–274. doi: 10.1016/j.sxmr.2017.01.005

Bakker, R.M., Ter Kuile, M.M., Vermeer, W.M., Nout, R.A., Mens, J.W., van Doorn, L.C., de Kroon, C., Hompus, W., Braat, C., & Creutzberg, C.L. (2014). Sexual rehabilitation after pelvic radiotherapy and vaginal dilator use: Consensus using the Delphi method. *International Journal of Gynecological Cancer, 24*(8), 1499–1506. doi: 10.1097/igc.0000000000000253

Basson, R. (2015). Human sexual response. *Handbook of Clinical Neurology, 130*, 11–18. doi: 10.1016/b978-0-444-63247-0.00002-x

Bouchard, C., Labrie, F., Derogatis, L., Girard, G., Ayotte, N., Gallagher, J., ... Moyneur, E. (2016). Effect of intravaginal dehydroepiandrosterone (DHEA) on the female sexual function in postmenopausal women: ERC-230 open-label study. *Hormone Molecular Biology and Clinical Investigation, 25*(3), 181–190. doi: 10.1515/hmbci-2015-0044

Brotto, L.A., Bergeron, S., Zdaniuk, B., & Basson, R. (2020). Mindfulness and cognitive behavior therapy for provoked vestibulodynia: Mediators of treatment outcome and long-term effects. *Journal of Consulting and Clinical Psychology, 88*(1), 48–64. doi: 10.1037/ccp0000473

Brotto, L.A., Bitzer, J., Laan, E., Leiblum, S., & Luria, M. (2010). Women's sexual desire and arousal disorders. *Journal of Sexual Medicine, 7*(1 Pt 2), 586–614. doi: 10.1111/j.1743-6109.2009.01630.x

Brotto, L.A., Chivers, M.L., Millman, R.D., & Albert, A. (2016). Mindfulness-based sex therapy improves genital-subjective arousal concordance in women with sexual desire/arousal difficulties. *Archives of Sexual Behavior, 45*(8), 1907–1921. doi: 10.1007/s10508-015-0689-8

Brotto, L.A., & Goldmeier, D. (2015). Mindfulness interventions for treating sexual dysfunctions: The gentle science of finding focus in a multitask world. *Journal of Sexual Medicine, 12*(8), 1687–1689. doi: 10.1111/jsm.12941

Brotto, L.A., Heiman, J.R., Goff, B., Greer, B., Lentz, G.M., Swisher, E., ... Van Blaricom, A. (2008). A psychoeducational intervention for sexual dysfunction in women with gynecologic cancer. *Archives of Sexual Behavior, 37*(2), 317–329. doi: 10.1007/s10508-007-9196-x

Chubak, B., & Doctor, A. (2018). Traditional Chinese medicine for sexual dysfunction: Review of the evidence. *Sexual Medicine Reviews, 6*(3), 410–418. doi: 10.1016/j.sxmr.2017.11.007

Constantine, G., Graham, S., Portman, D.J., Rosen, R.C., & Kingsberg, S.A. (2015). Female sexual function improved with ospemifene in postmenopausal women with vulvar and vaginal atrophy: Results of a randomized, placebo-controlled trial. *Climacteric, 18*(2), 226–232. doi: 10.3109/13697137.2014.954996

Cruz, V.L., Steiner, M.L., Pompei, L.M., Strufaldi, R., Fonseca, F.L.A., Santiago, L.H.S., ... Fernandes, C.E. (2018). Randomized, double-blind, placebo-controlled clinical trial for evaluating the efficacy of fractional CO_2 laser compared with topical estriol in the treatment of vaginal atrophy in postmenopausal women. *Menopause, 25*(1), 21–28. doi: 10.1097/gme.0000000000000955

Cullen, K., Fergus, K., Dasgupta, T., Fitch, M., Doyle, C., & Adams, L. (2012). From "sex toy" to intrusive imposition: A qualitative examination of women's experiences with vaginal dilator use following treatment for gynecological cancer. *Journal of Sexual Medicine, 9*(4), 1162–1173. doi: 10.1111/j.1743-6109.2011.02639.x

Davis, S.R., Baber, R., Panay, N., Bitzer, J., Perez, S.C., Islam, R.M., ... Wierman, M.E. (2019). Global consensus position statement on the use of testosterone therapy for women. *Journal of Sexual Medicine, 16*(9), 1331–1337. doi: 10.1016/j.jsxm.2019.07.012

Davis, S.R., Robinson, P.J., Jane, F., White, S., White, M., & Bell, R.J. (2018). Intravaginal testosterone improves sexual satisfaction and vaginal symptoms associated with aromatase inhibitors. *Journal of Clinical Endocrinology and Metabolism, 103*(11), 4146–4154. doi: 10.1210/jc.2018-01345

Di Donato, V., Schiavi, M.C., Iacobelli, V., D'oria, O., Kontopantelis, E., Simoncini, T., ... Benedetti Panici, P. (2019). Ospemifene for the treatment of vulvar and vaginal atrophy: A meta-analysis of randomized trials. Part I: Evaluation of efficacy. *Maturitas, 121*, 86–92. doi: 10.1016/j.maturitas.2018.11.016

Dooley, E.M., Miller, M.K., & Clayton, A.H. (2017). Flibanserin: From bench to bedside. *Sexual Medicine Reviews, 5*(4), 461–469. doi: 10.1016/j.sxmr.2017.06.003

dos Santos, C.C.M., Uggioni, M.L.R., Colonetti, T., Colonetti, L., Grande, A.J., & Da Rosa, M.I. (2021). Hyaluronic acid in postmenopause vaginal atrophy: A systematic review. *Journal of Sexual Medicine, 18*(1), 156–166. doi: 10.1016/j.jsxm.2020.10.016

Edwards, D., & Panay, N. (2016). Treating vulvovaginal atrophy/genitourinary syndrome of menopause: How important is vaginal lubricant and moisturizer composition? *Climacteric*, *19*(2), 151–161. doi: 10.3109/13697137.2015.1124259

Enemchukwu, E.A. (2017). CO_2 laser treatment is effective for symptoms of vaginal atrophy: No. *Journal of Urology*, *198*(6), 1228–1229. doi: 10.1016/j.juro.2017.09.004

Falk, S.J., & Bober, S. (2016). Vaginal health during breast cancer treatment. *Current Oncology Reports*, *18*(5), 32. doi: 10.1007/s11912-016-0517-x

Franco, O.H., Chowdhury, R., Troup, J., Voortman, T., Kunutsor, S., Kavousi, M., ... Muka, T. (2016). Use of plant-based therapies and menopausal symptoms: A systematic review and meta-analysis. *JAMA*, *315*(23), 2554–2563. doi: 10.1001/jama.2016.8012

Ghaderi, F., Bastani, P., Hajebrahimi, S., Jafarabadi, M.A., & Berghmans, B. (2019). Pelvic floor rehabilitation in the treatment of women with dyspareunia: A randomized controlled clinical trial. *International Urogynecology Journal*, *30*(11), 1849–1855. doi: 10.1007/s00192-019-04019-3

Goetsch, M.F., Lim, J.Y., & Caughey, A.B. (2015). A practical solution for dyspareunia in breast cnacer survivors: A randomized controlled trial. *Journal of Clinical Oncology*, *33*(30), 3394–3400. doi: 10.1200/JCO.2014.60.7366

Gordon, C., Gonzales, S., & Krychman, M.L. (2019). Rethinking the techno vagina: A case series of patient complications following vaginal laser treatment for atrophy. *Menopause*, *26*(4), 423–427. doi: 10.1097/GME.0000000000001293

Guess, M.K., Connell, K.A., Chudnoff, S., Adekoya, O., Richmond, C., Nixon, K.E., ... Melman, A. (2017). The effects of a genital vibratory stimulation device on sexual function and genital sensation. *Female Pelvic Medicine and Reconstructive Surgery*, *23*(4), 256–262. doi: 10.1097/spv.0000000000000357

Gunst, A., Ventus, D., Arver, S., Dhejne, C., Görts-Öberg, K., Zamore-Söderström, E., & Jern, P. (2019). A randomized, waiting-list-controlled study shows that brief, mindfulness-based psychological interventions are effective for treatment of women's low sexual desire. *Journal of Sex Research*, *56*(7), 913–929. doi: 10.1080/00224499.2018.1539463

Heo, Y.-A. (2019). Prasterone: A review in vulvovaginal atrophy. *Drugs and Aging*, *36*(8), 781–788. doi: 10.1007/s40266-019-00693-6

Herbenick, D., Reece, M., Hensel, D., Sanders, S., Jozkowski, K., & Fortenberry, J.D. (2011). Association of lubricant use with women's sexual pleasure, sexual satisfaction, and genital symptoms: A prospective daily diary study. *Journal of Sexual Medicine*, *8*(1), 202–212. doi: 10.1111/j.1743-6109.2010.02067.x

Herbenick, D., Reece, M., Sanders, S., Dodge, B., Ghassemi, A., & Fortenberry, J.D. (2009). Prevalence and characteristics of vibrator use by women in the United States: Results from a nationally representative study. *Journal of Sexual Medicine*, *6*(7), 1857–1866. doi: 10.1111/j.1743-6109.2009.01318.x

Herbenick, D., Reece, M., Schick, V., Sanders, S.A., & Fortenberry, J.D. (2014). Women's use and perceptions of commercial lubricants: Prevalence and characteristics in a nationally representative sample of American adults. *Journal of Sexual Medicine*, *11*(3), 642–652. doi: 10.1111/jsm.12427

Hickey, M., Marino, J.L., Braat, S., & Wong, S. (2016). A randomized, double-blind, crossover trial comparing a silicone- versus water-based lubricant for sexual discomfort after breast cancer. *Breast Cancer Research and Treatment*, *158*(1), 79–90. doi: 10.1007/s10549-016-3865-1

Hung, K.J., Hudson, P.L., Bergerat, A., Hesham, H., Choksi, N., & Mitchell, C. (2020). Effect of commercial vaginal products on the growth of uropathogenic and commensal vaginal bacteria. *Scientific Reports*, *10*(1), 7625. doi: 10.1038/s41598-020-63652-x

Jaderek, I., & Lew-Starowicz, M. (2019). A systematic review on mindfulness meditation–Based interventions for sexual dysfunctions. *Journal of Sexual Medicine*, *16*(10), 1581–1596. doi: 10.1016/j.jsxm.2019.07.019

Jannini, E.A., Limoncin, E., Ciocca, G., Buehler, S., & Krychman, M. (2012). Ethical aspects of sexual medicine. Internet, vibrators, and other sex Aids: Toys or therapeutic instruments? *Journal of Sexual Medicine*, *9*(12), 2994–3001. doi: 10.1111/jsm.12018

Jaspers, L., Feys, F., Bramer, W.M., Franco, O.H., Leusink, P., & Laan, E.T.M. (2016). Efficacy and safety of flibanserin for the treatment of hypoactive sexual desire disorder in women: A systematic review and meta-analysis. *JAMA Internal Medicine*, *176*(4), 453–462. doi: 10.1001/jamainternmed.2015.8565

Jha, S., Wyld, L., & Krishnaswamy, P.H. (2019). The impact of vaginal laser treatment for genitourinary syndrome of menopause in breast cancer survivors: A systematic review and meta-analysis. *Clinical Breast Cancer*, *19*(4), e556–e562. doi: 10.1016/j.clbc.2019.04.007

Kagan, R., Kellogg-Spadt, S., & Parish, S.J. (2019). Practical treatment considerations in the management of genitourinary syndrome of menopause. *Drugs and Aging*, *36*(10), 897–908. doi: 10.1007/s40266-019-00700-w

Kaunitz, A.M., Pinkerton, J.V., & Manson, J.E. (2019). Women harmed by vaginal laser for treatment of GSM-the latest casualties of fear and confusion surrounding hormone therapy. *Menopause*, *26*(4), 338–340. doi: 10.1097/GME.0000000000001313

Kingsberg, S.A., Althof, S., Simon, J.A., Bradford, A., Bitzer, J., Carvalho, J., … Shifrin, J.L. (2017). Female sexual dysfunction-medical and psychological treatments, Committee 14. *Journal of Sexual Medicine*, *14*(12), 1463–1491. doi: 10.1016/j.jsxm.2017.05.018

Kingsberg, S.A., Clayton, A.H., Portman, D., Krop, J., Jordan, R., Lucas, J., & Simon, J.A. (2021). Failure of a meta-analysis: A commentary on Glen Spielmans's "Re-analyzing Phase III Bremelanotide trials for 'hypoactive sexual desire disorder in women'". *The Journal of Sex Research*, 1–2. doi: 10.1080/00224499.2021.1902926

Kingsberg, S.A., & Krychman, M.L. (2013). Resistance and barriers to local estrogen therapy in women with atrophic vaginitis. *Journal of Sexual Medicine*, *10*(6), 1567–1574. doi: 10.1111/jsm.12120

Kingsberg, S.A., McElroy, S.L., & Clayton, A.H. (2019). Evaluation of flibanserin safety: Comparison with other serotonergic medications. *Sexual Medicine Reviews*, *7*(3), 380–392. doi: 10.1016/j.sxmr.2018.12.003

Kohn, G.E., Rodriguez, K.M., Hotaling, J., & Pastuszak, A.W. (2019). The history of estrogen therapy. *Sexual Medicine Reviews*, *7*(3), 416–421. doi: 10.1016/j.sxmr.2019.03.006

Labrie, F., Archer, D.F., Koltun, W., Vachon, A., Young, D., Frenette, L., … Moyneur, É. (2018). Efficacy of intravaginal dehydroepiandrosterone (DHEA) on moderate to severe dyspareunia and vaginal dryness, symptoms of vulvovaginal atrophy, and of the genitourinary syndrome of menopause. *Menopause*, *25*(11), 1339–1353. doi: 10.1097/gme.0000000000001238

Leavitt, C.E., Lefkowitz, E.S., & Waterman, E.A. (2019). The role of sexual mindfulness in sexual wellbeing, Relational wellbeing, and self-esteem. *Journal of Sex and Marital Therapy*, *45*(6), 497–509. doi: 10.1080/0092623X.2019.1572680

Lethaby, A., Ayeleke, R.O., & Roberts, H. (2016). Local oestrogen for vaginal atrophy in postmenopausal women. *Cochrane Database of Systematic Reviews*, *8*(8), Cd001500. doi: 10.1002/14651858.CD001500.pub3

Liu, M., Juravic, M., Mazza, G., & Krychman, M.L. (2020). Vaginal dilators: Issues and answers. *Sexual Medicine Reviews*. doi: 10.1016/j.sxmr.2019.11.005

Marcus, B.S. (2011). Changes in a Woman's sexual experience and expectations following the introduction of electric vibrator assistance. *Journal of Sexual Medicine*, *8*(12), 3398–3406. doi: 10.1111/j.1743-6109.2010.02132.x

Maseroli, E., & Vignozzi, L. (2020). Testosterone and vaginal function. *Sexual Medicine Reviews*, *8*(3), 379–392. doi: 10.1016/j.sxmr.2020.03.003

Masters, W.H., & Johnson, V.E. (1970). Therapy format. *Human sexual inadequacy*. (pp. 68). New York: Bantam Press Books.

Mayer, D., & Lynch, S.E. (2020). Bremelanotide: New drug approved for treating hypoactive sexual desire disorder. *Annals of Pharmacotherapy*, *54*(7), 684–690. doi: 10.1177/1060028019899152

Morin, M., Carroll, M.-S., & Bergeron, S. (2017). Systematic review of the effectiveness of physical therapy modalities in women with provoked vestibulodynia. *Sexual Medicine Reviews*, *5*(3), 295–322. doi: 10.1016/j.sxmr.2017.02.003

Mothes, A.R., Runnebaum, M., & Runnebaum, I.B. (2018). Ablative dual-phase erbium: YAG laser treatment of atrophy-related vaginal symptoms in post-menopausal breast cancer survivors omitting hormonal treatment. *Journal of Cancer Research and Clinical Oncology*. doi: 10.1007/s00432-018-2614-8

Nazarpour, S., Simbar, M., Ramezani Tehrani, F., & Alavi Majd, H. (2017). Effects of sex education and Kegel exercises on the sexual function of postmenopausal women: A randomized clinical trial. *Journal of Sexual Medicine*, *14*(7), 959–967. doi: 10.1016/j.jsxm.2017.05.006

Pagano, I., Gieri, S., Nocera, F., Scibilia, G., Fraggetta, F., Galia, A., ... Scollo, P. (2017). Evaluation of the CO_2 laser therapy on vulvo-vaginal atrophy (VVA) in oncological patients: Preliminary results. *Journal of Cancer Therapy*, *8*(5), 452–463. doi: 10.4236/jct.2017.85039

Pagano, T., De Rosa, P., Vallone, R., Schettini, F., Arpino, G., Giuliano, M., ... De Placido, G. (2017). Fractional microablative CO_2 laser in breast cancer survivors affected by iatrogenic vulvovaginal atrophy after failure of nonestrogenic local treatments: A retrospective study. *Menopause*. doi: 10.1097/gme.0000000000001053

Palacios, S., & Cancelo, M.J. (2016). Clinical update on the use of ospemifene in the treatment of severe symptomatic vulvar and vaginal atrophy. *International Journal of Women's Health*, *8*, 617–626. doi: 10.2147/IJWH.S110035

Paterson, L.Q.P., Handy, A.B., & Brotto, L.A. (2017). A pilot study of eight-session mindfulness-based cognitive therapy adapted for women's sexual interest/arousal disorder. *Journal of Sex Research*, *54*(7), 850–861. doi: 10.1080/00224499.2016.1208800

Peixoto, C., Carrilho, C.G., Barros, J.A., Ribeiro, T.T., Silva, L.M., Nardi, A.E., ... Veras, A.B. (2017). The effects of dehydroepiandrosterone on sexual function: A systematic review. *Climacteric*, *20*(2), 129–137. doi: 10.1080/13697137.2017.1279141

Pitsouni, E., Grigoriadis, T., Falagas, M.E., Salvatore, S., & Athanasiou, S. (2017). Laser therapy for the genitourinary syndrome of menopause. A systematic review and meta-analysis. *Maturitas*, *103*, 78–88. doi: 10.1016/j.maturitas.2017.06.029

Portman, D.J., Bachmann, G.A., Simon, J.A., & Ospemifene Study Group (2013). Ospemifene, a novel selective estrogen receptor modulator for treating dyspareunia associated with postmenopausal vulvar and vaginal atrophy. *Menopause*, *20*(6), 623–630. doi: 10.1097/gme.0b013e318279ba64

Portman, D.J., Brown, L., Yuan, J., Kissling, R., & Kingsberg, S.A. (2017). Flibanserin in postmenopausal women with hypoactive sexual desire disorder: Results of the PLUMERIA study. *Journal of Sexual Medicine*, *14*(6), 834–842. doi: 10.1016/j.jsxm.2017.03.258

Portman, D.J., Goldstein, S.R., & Kagan, R. (2019). Treatment of moderate to severe dyspareunia with intravaginal prasterone therapy: A review. *Climacteric*, *22*(1), 65–72. doi: 10.1080/13697137.2018.1535583

Pup, L.D., & Sánchez-Borrego, R. (2020). Ospemifene efficacy and safety data in women with vulvovaginal atrophy. *Gynecological Endocrinology*, *36*(7), 569–577. doi: 10.1080/09513590.2020.1757058

Qureshi, A.A., Tenenbaum, M.M., & Myckatyn, T.M. (2018). Nonsurgical vulvovaginal rejuvenation with radiofrequency and laser devices: A literature review and comprehensive update for aesthetic surgeons. *Aesthetic Surgery Journal*, *38*(3), 302–311. doi: 10.1093/asj/sjx138

Romero-Otero, J., Lauterbach, R., Aversa, A., Serefoglu, E.C., García-Gómez, B., Parnhan, A., ... Lowenstein, L. (2020). Radiofrequency-based devices for female genito-urinary indications: Position statements from the European Society of Sexual Medicine. *Journal of Sexual Medicine*, *17*(3), 393–399. doi: 10.1016/j.jsxm.2019.12.015

Rosenbaum, T.Y. (2007). REVIEWS: Pelvic floor involvement in male and female sexual dysfunction and the role of pelvic floor rehabilitation in treatment: A literature review. *Journal of Sexual Medicine*, *4*(1), 4–13. doi: 10.1111/j.1743-6109.2006.00393.x

Rowland, D.L., McNabney, S.M., & Mann, A.R. (2017). Sexual function, obesity, and weight loss in men and women. *Sexual Medicine Reviews*, *5*(3), 323–338. doi: 10.1016/j.sxmr.2017.03.006

Samuels, J.B., & Garcia, M.A. (2019). Treatment to external labia and vaginal canal with CO_2 laser for symptoms of vulvovaginal atrophy in postmenopausal women. *Aesthetic Surgery Journal*, *39*(1), 83–93. doi: 10.1093/asj/sjy087

Santen, R.J., Stuenkel, C.A., Davis, S.R., Pinkerton, J.V., Gompel, A., & Lumsden, M.A. (2017). Managing menopausal symptoms and associated clinical issues in breast cancer survivors. *Journal of Clinical Endocrinology and Metabolism*, *102*(10), 3647–3661. doi: 10.1210/jc.2017-01138

Sauer, U., Talaulikar, V., & Davies, M.C. (2018). Efficacy of intravaginal dehydroepiandrosterone (DHEA) for symptomatic women in the peri- or postmenopausal phase. *Maturitas, 116*, 79–82. doi: 10.1016/j.maturitas.2018.07.016

Segal, J.Z. (2018). Sex, drugs, and rhetoric: The case of flibanserin for 'female sexual dysfunction'. *Social Studies of Science, 48*(4), 459–482. doi: 10.1177/0306312718778802

Shapiro, D., Stevens, D., & Stahl, S.M. (2017). Flibanserin—The female Viagra? *International Journal of Psychiatry in Clinical Practice, 21*(4), 259–265. doi: 10.1080/13651501.2017.1315138

Simon, J.A., Altomare, C., Cort, S., Jiang, W., & Pinkerton, J.V. (2018). Overall safety of ospemifene in postmenopausal women from placebo-controlled Phase 2 and 3 trials. *Journal of Women's Health, 27*(1), 14–23. doi: 10.1089/jwh.2017.6385

Simon, J.A., & Kapner, M.D. (2020). The saga of testosterone for menopausal women at the Food and Drug Administration (FDA). *Journal of Sexual Medicine, 17*(4), 826–829. doi: 10.1016/j.jsxm.2020.01.009

Simon, J.A., & Maamari, R.V. (2013). Ultra-low-dose vaginal estrogen tablets for the treatment of postmenopausal vaginal atrophy. *Climacteric, 16*(Suppl.1), 37–43. doi: 10.3109/13697137.2013.807606

Song, S., Budden, A., Short, A., Nesbitt-Hawes, E., Deans, R., & Abbott, J. (2018). The evidence for laser treatments to the vulvo-vagina: Making sure we do not repeat past mistakes. *Australian and New Zealand Journal of Obstetrics and Gynaecology, 58*(2), 148–162. doi: 10.1111/ajo.12735

Spielmans, G.I. (2021). Irrelevancies and inaccuracies miss the target: A response to Kingsberg et al. *The Journal of Sex Research*, 1–4. doi: 10.1080/00224499.2021.1906399

Stanton, A.M., Handy, A.B., & Meston, C.M. (2018). The effects of exercise on sexual function in women. *Sexual Medicine Reviews, 6*(4), 548–557. doi: 10.1016/j.sxmr.2018.02.004

Stein, A., Sauder, S.K., & Reale, J. (2019). The role of physical therapy in sexual health in men and women: Evaluation and treatment. *Sexual Medicine Reviews, 7*(1), 46–56. doi: 10.1016/j.sxmr.2018.09.003

Stephenson, K.R., & Kerth, J. (2017). Effects of mindfulness-based therapies for female sexual dysfunction: A meta-analytic review. *Journal of Sex Research, 54*(7), 832–849. doi: 10.1080/00224499.2017.1331199

Thompson, J.J., Ritenbaugh, C., & Nichter, M. (2017). Why women choose compounded bioidentical hormone therapy: Lessons from a qualitative study of menopausal decision-making. *BMC Women's Health, 17*(1), 97. doi: 10.1186/s12905-017-0449-0

Towe, M., La, J., El-Khatib, F., Roberts, N., Yafi, F.A., & Rubin, R. (2020). Diet and female sexual health. *Sexual Medicine Reviews, 8*(2), 256–264. doi: 10.1016/j.sxmr.2019.08.004

Vale, F., Rezende, C., Raciclan, A., Bretas, T., & Geber, S. (2019). Efficacy and safety of a non-hormonal intravaginal moisturizer for the treatment of vaginal dryness in postmenopausal women with sexual dysfunction. *European Journal of Obstetrics and Gynecology and Reproductive Biology, 234*, 92–95. doi: 10.1016/j.ejogrb.2018.12.040

van Lankveld, J., van de Wetering, F.T., Wylie, K., & Scholten, R.J.P.M. (2021). Bibliotherapy for sexual dysfunctions: A systematic review and meta-analysis. *Journal of Sexual Medicine, 18*, 582–614. doi: 10.1016/j.jsxm.2020.12.009

Vegunta, S., Kling, J., & Kapoor, E. (2020). Androgen therapy in women. *Journal of Women's Health, 29*(1), 57–64. doi: 10.1089/jwh.2018.7494

Velten, J., Margraf, J., Chivers, M.L., & Brotto, L.A. (2018). Effects of a mindfulness task on women's sexual response. *Journal of Sex Research, 55*(6), 747–757. doi: 10.1080/00224499.2017.1408768

Verbeek, M., & Hayward, L. (2019). Pelvic floor dysfunction and its effect on quality of sexual life. *Sexual Medicine Reviews, 7*(4), 559–564. doi: 10.1016/j.sxmr.2019.05.007

Villena, A., Gimeno, E., Blazquez, M., Zavala, L., García, E., Ilarraza, F., & Chiclana, C. (2018). 643 Mindfulness in sex therapy: A comprehensive review. *Journal of Sexual Medicine, 15*(7), S371–S372. doi: 10.1016/j.jsxm.2018.04.550

Wallace, S.L., St Martin, B., Lee, K., & Sokol, E.R. (2020). A cost-effectiveness analysis of vaginal carbon dioxide laser therapy compared with standard medical therapies for genitourinary syndrome of menopause-associated dyspareunia. *American Journal of Obstetrics and Gynecology, 223*(6), 890.e891–890.e812. doi: 10.1016/j.ajog.2020.06.032

Weiner, L., & Avery-Clark, C. (2017). *Sensate focus in sex therapy.* Oxon, UK: Routledge.

Wheeler, L.J., & Guntupalli, S.R. (2020). Female sexual dysfunction: Pharmacologic and therapeutic interventions. *Obstetrics and Gynecology, 136*(1), 174–186. doi: 10.1097/aog.0000000000003941

Wilkinson, E.M., Łaniewski, P., Herbst-Kralovetz, M.M., & Brotman, R.M. (2019). Personal and clinical vaginal lubricants: Impact on local vaginal microenvironment and implications for epithelial cell host response and barrier function. *Journal of Infectious Diseases, 220*(12), 2009–2018. doi: 10.1093/infdis/jiz412

Zarski, A.C., Berking, M., Fackiner, C., Rosenau, C., & Ebert, D.D. (2017). Internet-based guided self-help for vaginal penetration difficulties: Results of a randomized controlled pilot trial. *Journal of Sexual Medicine, 14*(2), 238–254. doi: 10.1016/j.jsxm.2016.12.232

Zippan, N., Stephenson, K.R., & Brotto, L.A. (2020). Feasibility of a brief online psychoeducational intervention for women with sexual interest/arousal disorder. *Journal of Sexual Medicine, 17*(11), 2208–2219. doi: 10.1016/j.jsxm.2020.07.086

Index

Printed in the United States
by Baker & Taylor Publisher Services